Principles and Practice
of Child Neurology in Infancy
2nd Edition

Principles and Practice of Child Neurology in Infancy
2nd Edition

Edited by

Colin Kennedy
Professor in Neurology and Paediatrics, University of Southampton;
Honorary Consultant in Paediatric Neurology,
University Hospital Southampton NHS Foundation Trust, Southampton, UK

Assistant Editors

Gian Paolo Chiaffoni
Head, Department of Pediatrics,
Conegliano and Vittorio Veneto Hospital, Conegliano, Italy

Leena Haataja
Professor in Pediatric Neurology, University of Helsinki;
Consultant in Pediatric Neurology, Helsinki University Hospital,
Children's Hospital, and Pediatric Research Center, Helsinki, Finland

Richard W Newton
Honorary Consultant Paediatric Neurologist,
Royal Manchester Children's Hospital, Manchester, UK

Thomas Sejersen
Professor, Pediatric Neurologist, Department of Neuropediatrics,
Astrid Lindgren Children's Hospital, Stockholm, Sweden

Jane Williams
Consultant Paediatrician, Neurodisability and Child Health,
Nottingham Children's Hospital,
Nottingham University Hospital NHS Trust, Nottingham, UK

2020
Mac Keith Press

© 2020 Mac Keith Press

Managing Director: Ann-Marie Halligan
Senior Publishing Manager: Sally Wilkinson
Publishing Co-ordinator: Lucy White

The views and opinions expressed herein are those of the authors and do not necessarily represent those of the publisher.

First edition 2012
Second edition 2020

2nd Floor, Rankin Building, 139–143 Bermondsey Street, London, SE1 3UW, UK

British Library Cataloguing-in-Publication data
A catalogue record for this book is available from the British Library

Cover designer: Marten Sealby

ISBN: 978-1-911612-00-1

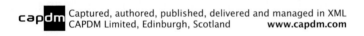 Captured, authored, published, delivered and managed in XML
CAPDM Limited, Edinburgh, Scotland   **www.capdm.com**

Printed by Hobbs the Printers Ltd, Totton, Hampshire, UK

Contents

Author Appointments

Ilona Autti-Rämö
Adjunct Professor, Division of Child Neurology, University of Helsinki Children's Hospital, Helsinki, Finland

Peter Baxter
Paediatric Neurologist, Sheffield Childrens Hospital, Sheffield, UK

Vittorio Belmonti
Child Neuropsychiatrist, IRCCS Fondazione Stella Maris, Pisa, Italy

Gian Paolo Chiaffoni
Head, Department of Pediatrics, Conegliano and Vittorio Veneto Hospital, Conegliano, Italy

Richard FM Chin
Professor in Paediatric Neurosciences and Honorary Consultant Paediatric Neurologist, The University of Edinburgh and Royal Hospital for Sick Children, Edinburgh, UK

Imti Choonara
Emeritus Professor in Child Health, University of Nottingham, Derby, UK

Giovanni Cioni
University Professor and Head, Department of Developmental Neuroscience, Stella Maris Scientific Institute and University of Pisa, Pisa, Italy

J Helen Cross
The Prince of Wales's Chair of Childhood Epilepsy, UCL Great Ormond Street Institute of Child Health; Honorary Consultant Paediatric Neurologist, Great Ormond Street Hospital for Children NHS Trust, London, UK

Leena Haataja
Professor in Pediatric Neurology, University of Helsinki; Consultant in Pediatric Neurology, Helsinki University Hospital, Children's Hospital, and Pediatric Research Center, Helsinki, Finland

Hans Hartmann
Consultant Paediatric Neurologist, Hannover Medical School, Clinic for Paediatric Kidney-, Liver- and Metabolic Diseases, and Child Neurology, Hannover, Germany

Florian Heinen
Professor of Paediatrics and Head of Department, Paediatric Neurology and Developmental Medicine, University of Munich, Hauner Children's Hospital, Center for International Health (CIH), LMU, Munich, Germany

Helgi Hjartarson
Pediatric Neurologist, MD, Department of Neuropediatrics, Astrid Lindgren Children's Hospital, Stockholm, Sweden

Varsine Jaladyan
Doctor, Child Neurology, 'Arabkir' Medical Centre & Institute of Child and Adolescent Health, Yerevan, Armenia

Harriet Joy
Consultant Neuroradiologist, Wessex Neurological Centre, University Hospital Southampton, Southampton, UK

Colin Kennedy
Professor in Neurology and Paediatrics, University of Southampton; Honorary Consultant in Paediatric Neurology, University Hospital Southampton NHS Foundation Trust, Southampton, UK

Fenella Kirkham
Professor of Paediatric Neurology, Developmental Neurosciences Department, UCL Great Ormond Street Institute of Child Health, London, UK

Rachel Kneen
Consultant Paediatric Neurologist, Alder Hey Children's NHS Foundation Trust, Liverpool, UK

Rael Laugesaar
Faculty of Medicine, University of Tartu, Tartu, Estonia

Andrew L Lux
Consultant Paediatric Neurologist, Bristol Royal Hospital for Children; Honorary Senior Clinical Lecturer in Clinical Sciences, Bristol Medical School, University of Bristol, Bristol, UK

Vlatka Mejaški-Bošnjak
Pediatric Neurologist, Children's Hospital Medical School, University of Zagreb, Zagreb, Croatia

Tuuli Metsvaht
Professor, Faculty of Medicine, University of Tartu, Tartu, Estonia

Mary Morgan
Consultant Paediatric Haematologist — retired 2016, University Hospital, Southampton, UK

Alla Nechay
Doctor, Neurology Department, Kyiv City Paediatric Hospital, Kyiv, Ukraine

Charles Newton
Professor, Centre for Geographic Medicine Research (Coast), Kenya Medical Research Institute, Kilifi Kenya; Department of Psychiatry, Oxford University, Oxford, UK

Richard W Newton
Honorary Consultant Paediatric Neurologist, Royal Manchester Children's Hospital, Manchester, UK

Catarina Olimpio
Speciality Registrar in Clinical Genetics, Addenbrookes Hospital, Cambridge, UK

E Juulia Paavonen
Deputy Chief Physician, Child Psychiatry, Helsinki University Hospital, Helsinki Uusimaa Hospital District; Research Manager, Finnish Institute for Health and Welfare, Helsinki, Finland

Alasdair PJ Parker
Consultant Paediatric Neurologist, Addenbrooke's Hospital; Associate Lecturer, University of Cambridge, Cambridge, UK

Barbara Plecko
University Professor; Doctor; Head of the Clinical Department of General Paediatrics, University Clinic for Paediatrics and Adolescent Medicine, Graz, Austria

Audrone Prasauskiene
Child Neurologist, Director at the Children's Rehabilitation Hospital affiliated to the University Hospital; Professor at the Lithuanian University of Health Sciences, Kaunas, Lithuania

Kaija Puura
Professor of Child Psychiatry Tampere University; Chief Child Psychiatrist, Tampere University Hospital, Tampere, Finland

Outi Saarenpää-Heikkilä
Deputy Chief of the Unit of Pediatric Neurology, Department of Pediatrics, Tampere University Hospital, Tampere, Finland

Bernhard Schmitt
Professor of Paediatric Neurology (retired), University Children's Hospital, Zurich, Switzerland

Maryze Schoneveld van der Linde
Owner, Patient Centered Solutions, Varsseveld, the Netherlands

Thomas Sejersen
Professor, Pediatric Neurologist, Department of Neuropediatrics, Astrid Lindgren Children's Hospital, Stockholm, Sweden

John BP Stephenson
Honorary Professor of Paediatric Neurology, University of Glasgow and Retired Consultant Paediatric Neurologist, Fraser of Allander Neurosciences Unit, Royal Hospital for Sick Children, Glasgow, Scotland, UK

Inga Talvik
Head of the Department of Neurology and Neurorehabilitation, Tallinn Children's Hospital, Tallinn, Estonia

Tiina Talvik
Professor Emeritus, Faculty of Medicine, University of Tartu, Tartu, Estonia

Meral Topcu
Professor of Pediatrics and Pediatric Neurologist, Division of Paediatric Neurology, Department of Paediatrics, Faculty of Medicine, Hacettepe University, Ankara, Turkey

Daniele Trevisanuto
Associate Professor of Pediatrics, University of Padova, Padova, Italy

Brigitte Vollmer
Associate Professor of Neonatal and Paediatric Neurology, Clinical Neurosciences, Clinical and Experimental Science, Faculty of Medicine, University of Southampton; Honorary Consultant Paediatric Neurologist, Southampton Children's Hospital, Southampton, UK

Valerie Walker
Honorary Consultant Chemical Pathologist, University Hospital, Southampton, UK

Jane Williams
Consultant Paediatrician, Neurodisability and Child Health, Nottingham Children's Hospital, Nottingham University Hospital NHS Trust, Nottingham, UK

Geoffrey Woods
Professor of Medical Genetics, The Clinical Medical School, University of Cambridge, UK Honorary Consultant in Clinical Genetics, Addenbrookes Hospital, Cambridge, UK

Dilek Yalnizoglu
Professor of Paediatrics, Division of Paediatric Neurology, Department of Paediatrics, Faculty of Medicine, Hacettepe University, Ankara, Turkey

Foreword

This is the second edition of *Principles and Practice of Child Neurology in Infancy*, edited by Professor Colin Kennedy, whose first edition appeared in 2012. The primary objective of this book is to provide a symptom-based guide to the diagnosis and management of neurological disorders in infancy. Each chapter is preceded by a concise summary, updated according to the present best practice and subdivided into 'key messages', 'common errors', and 'when to worry'. In this way the reader has a bird's eye view of the content, points of interest, the most important clinical signs and symptoms, and the pitfalls to avoid.

As can be expected in a second edition, the chapters and references covering the different neurological symptoms have been thoroughly updated to reflect the progress that has been made in recent years in the fields of genomic analysis, neuroimaging pattern recognition, and neurophysiology as well as a concise description of the more recently discovered diseases. Contributions from the book come from widely recognized experts in the field of paediatric and developmental neurology. Many members of the original international working group are again authors in the second edition. However, some updates and a few new topics have been added and covered by the best experts in the field.

The first half of the book now contains 13 chapters and is dedicated to subjects not to be found in ordinary paediatric neurology textbooks such as the principles of working with families, clinical assessments, use of investigations, treatments, and evidence-based medicine. In addition, attention is paid to typical development and its variants. Chapter 4 on 'Promoting child development' has been thoroughly expanded: the topic has been put in a broader context and mentions not only the important role of families in infant development and other positive factors, but now also the common negative social factors for development such as psychoactive drugs, poverty, and stress, especially important when present together. An important new section on neurological aspects of vaccination has been added alongside the updated sections on prevention and screening. Two important new chapters are added that were sorely missed in the first edition:

first, a very helpful and practical chapter on 'Neurological examination beyond the neonatal period' and, second, a chapter, also much needed, on 'Genetic testing'. This last chapter offers a concise introduction to inheritance patterns, common types of genetic mutations, and an overview of currently available types of genetic testing, what to expect from them and their strengths and limitations. Many examples of everyday clinical situations where genetic testing can be of use are discussed.

The second half of the book addresses the major disorders that may present in neonates and infants in a symptom-based manner. Topics include neonatal encephalopathy, neonatal seizures, acute febrile and nonfebrile encephalopathies (now including malaria), epileptic and nonepileptic paroxysmal disorders, macrocephaly (now including brain tumours), cerebral palsy and movement disorders other than cerebral palsy, as well as progressive loss of skills. The chapters on microcephaly (with extended consideration of genetic aspects and inclusion of Zika virus) and the floppy infant have been largely revised for this edition. Also new for this edition are authoritative but concise chapters on stroke and on inherited neurometabolic diseases — with valuable information on the clinical manifestations, the approach in the diagnosis and therapy of both well-known and newly identified disorders. Another new and very useful chapter has been added covering normal and abnormal patterns of infant sleep and behaviour. This is an important topic because sleep disturbances are common and may be quite disruptive to family life. The Appendix provides WHO growth charts for skull circumference, length, and weight and a colour-coded chart for use in conjunction with Gross Motor Function Classification System.

The authors have filled the chapters not only with their knowledge but also with the wisdom of many years of clinical practice. They emphasize the importance of clinical assessment, adequate history taking, and skillful neurological examination as key diagnostic tools. Mastering these delicate skills is a prerequisite to successfully solving a neurological problem while involving parents and caretakers, investigating selectively, and avoiding over-treatment. This approach limits the burden on and increases the benefits to the child and parents. The book thus provides the reader with important tools to improve both technical and ethical aspects of acute and long-term care of the child.

The first edition of this book was an immediate and great success. This updated and extended second edition was, like the first edition, written to provide strong guidance for paediatric neurologists, whether in practice or still in training, in both resource-poor and resource-rich countries. The book will also provide a quick general update for more senior paediatric neurologists who mainly work in a highly specialized field — such as for example epileptology, sleep disorders, or neuromuscular diseases — and may serve as a reference guide for those who are teaching paediatric neurology in medical schools. Because of its strong clinical approach, the book is also very accessible and helpful for all physicians, either in training or practice, who need guidance in the care of infants with neurological problems, be they paediatricians, neurologists, developmental specialists, or rehabilitation specialists.

The content of the first edition of the book was the basis of a series of very successful and much appreciated teaching courses in Eastern Europe (Tbilisi 2015, Astana 2012, 2017, Tashkent 2019) and of the European Paediatric Neurology Society (EPNS) teaching courses in western Europe. Thus, the chapter authors, and especially the book's editor Professor Colin Kennedy, have contributed to the training of a generation of young paediatric neurologists from all countries of Europe and beyond, not only by providing practical knowledge on neurological diseases in neonates and infants but also by stimulating a critical attitude to the diagnostic process based on clinical epidemiological data and evidence-based medicine.

The second edition will be no less influential given the fact that two very informative online courses based on the chapters of this book have been created by Mac Keith Press.

Coriene Catsman-Berrevoets MD, PhD
Assistant Professor of Paediatric Neurology
Board member and Chair of the Education and Training Committee of EPNS
Chair of the European Committee of National Advisors to EPNS
Erasmus Medical Centre, Sophia Children's Hospital, Erasmus University
Rotterdam, the Netherlands

Preface

The favourable response to the first edition of *Principles and Practice of Child Neurology in Infancy* created the challenge of updating the book to remain portable but also to include methods and diagnoses of increasing importance in 2020. Additions to the first edition include four chapters (*Neurological examination beyond the neonatal period, Genetic testing, Inherited metabolic encephalopathies of infancy,* and *Infant sleep and behaviour*) and five completely new sections within chapters (*Vaccination, Immune-mediated encephalitis, Malaria, Zika virus infection,* and *Intracranial space-occupying lesions*). All chapters have been updated and there have been major redrafts and a change or addition to the authorship of three other chapters (*Promoting child development, Microcephaly, including congenital infections,* and *The floppy infant*). The number of hyperlinks to online resources has been substantially increased.

Taken together, these improvements provide a major revision of the first edition. They will also provide the basis for two online courses related to the book which have been developed in partnership with Mac Keith Press and the European Paediatric Neurology Society (EPNS).

I am grateful to all the authors for updating chapters and providing new ones, and to Sally Wilkinson at Mac Keith Press for her inexhaustible patience.

Colin Kennedy, Southampton, UK
December 2019

CHAPTER 1

Terms, definitions, and concepts

Colin Kennedy

Key messages

- The precautionary principle, 'first do no harm', was established 2500 years ago. Justification for the use of a treatment remains the responsibility of the treating physician.
- For many centuries 'ecologies of care' rather than definition of illness was the predominant paradigm of medical practice and this continues to be relevant to the young because the relationships between a child, the family, and the wider environment remain important determinants of health outcomes, especially in infancy.
- Discussion of the management of disease is greatly facilitated by internationally agreed definitions of disease and these are available as the International Classification of Diseases, 11th Revision (www.who.int/classifications/icd/en/).
- Evidence-based medicine provides an objective method for the systematic evaluation of the evidence of the benefit and harm of medical interventions.

Common errors

- Use of imprecise terms for which international agreement is lacking, for example, the syndrome of raised intracranial pressure, hydrocephalus syndrome, myotonic syndrome, hyperexcitability syndrome.
- Imprecise or incorrect use of terms for which precise definitions exist, for example, perinatal encephalopathy, epilepsy.
- Generalization of uncommon conditions to common clinical situations, for example, attributing trembling of the chin, feeding problems, excessive crying, or febrile seizures to neurological disorders.

> ## When to worry
>
> - Separation of infants from their families (one should facilitate bonding between an infant and his/her main carer).
> - Use of poorly evaluated, potentially harmful interventions in many infants to treat rare neurological problems (one should use common sense and look at international recommendations of good practice).
> - Resistance to evaluation of the benefits and harms of current treatments (one should consider both the potential benefits and potential risks of all interventions).

THE BASIS OF MEDICAL PRACTICE

This book offers knowledge, only some of which is truly evidence-based, and a framework for incorporating evidence into the clinical care of infants in whom there is concern about neurological function or developmental progress.

Historically, the starting point was myth and wise myths will continue to have their place in medical practice. According to the ancient Greeks, Apollo was the god of healing and Asclepius, his son, was rescued by Apollo from the womb of his dying human mother, Coronis. Asclepius' daughters were Hygeia, the goddess of health, and Panacea, the goddess of cures. Asclepius also had sons and Hippocrates, according to myth, was a descendant of one of those sons. Hippocrates was a practising physician nearly 2500 years ago and author of the Hippocratic Oath (www.pbs.org/wgbh/nova/body/hippocratic-oath-today.html), the most famous text in Western medicine. The most widely quoted section of that oath states: 'I will use treatments for the benefit of the ill in accordance with my ability and my judgement, but from what is to their harm and injustice, I will keep them'. In addition to this statement of the precautionary principle (i.e. 'first do no harm'), other sections of the oath bind the practitioner to resist all temptations that their privileged position as physicians offer, to acknowledge the limits of their competence and refer to specialist practitioners when necessary, to leave surgery to the surgeons, to respect patient confidentiality, to treat one's professional teachers as one's parents, and to pass on the art of medicine to the next generation. Thus, many of the issues of key importance to clinical practitioners and the health systems within which they work are identified within the oath.

THE PRECAUTIONARY PRINCIPLE IN THE CONTEXT OF NEUROLOGICAL PROBLEMS IN INFANCY

The precautionary principle is especially relevant in the assessment and management of neurological and neurodevelopmental problems in infancy, when medical intervention may unwittingly hinder the role of the parents in the child's development, whether typical or impaired; hospitalization or other institutionalization should be avoided whenever possible (Chapters 2 and 4). Any system of medical activity that involves surveillance of typically developing children should be based on explicit principles of screening (Chapter 7), including evidence that the benefit of early intervention, whether special investigation (Chapters 8, 9, 10 and 11) or treatment (Chapters 12 and 13), outweighs the potential for harm. The range of 'normal', better termed 'typical', neurological development in infancy is broad. In cases of doubt, continuing clinical surveillance and support for normal parenting is needed. This has less potential for harm than either enthusiastic separation into medical categories in the border zones of normality or the use of treatments for which benefit is not established or is outweighed by risk of harm. Any system of practice that categorizes more than a few per cent of infants as neurologically atypical must itself be suspect. Such a system is incompatible with the epidemiology of neurological disorders in childhood and will, by definition, expose many typical children to the risk of being wrongly categorized as impaired. This is a particular example of the need for any form of screening to fulfil several criteria additional to those that apply to the treatment of the illness (Chapter 7).

Neurological and developmental assessment and neurological examination of an infant (Chapters 5 and 6) is a practical skill of central importance that requires hands-on experience as well as knowledge. The importance of the physiological state of the infant (hungry or fed, wakeful or drowsy, contented or distressed), the need to rely on best performance (as opposed to poorer performance on a single occasion), and the extent to which clinical features are consistent over time are more important to bear in mind at this age than any other factor. Almost any finding with respect to deep tendon reflexes, other than complete absence of them, for example, is within the typical (i.e. normal) range in some physiological states or at some age within the first year.

ECOLOGIES OF CARE AND CATEGORIES OF ILLNESS

On the foundations expressed by Hippocrates, the art of clinical practice in Western countries evolved in the pre-scientific era using a system of knowledge based on the eminence and experience of senior practitioners. For many centuries before the more modern description of categories of illness as the basis of medical practice, ecologies of care for maintenance of health and for the treatment of illness acknowledged the importance of the relationship between the patient and the wider environment and provided the predominant paradigm of care. In the case of the child-patient, family relationships are of primary importance and are fundamental to the Head Start (USA) and Sure Start (UK) programmes for the improvement of the health and well-being of young children (Blair and DeBell, 2011). These issues are discussed in Chapters 2, 4, and 7.

THE INTERNATIONAL CLASSIFICATION OF DISEASES

The World Health Organization (WHO) was founded by international treaty in 1948 as a specialized agency of the United Nations with unique authority to establish global health standards and to secure international agreement on defining disease. The 193 member states of the WHO have agreed to use the International Classification of Diseases (ICD), the most recent version of which, the 11th Revision (ICD-11), was released on 18 June 2018 (www.who.int/classifications/icd/en/) and endorsed at the World Health Assembly in May 2019 for use from January 2022. Classification of mental disorders, which include neurological disorders, is complex and controversial, both because underlying pathophysiology cannot be observed directly and because many symptoms are contiguous with normal phenomena. Nowhere are these issues more relevant than in the neurology and neurodevelopment of infants. The ICD classification is predominantly driven by the clinical utility and public health outcomes of the disease entities and, despite these controversies, is, therefore, an appropriate framework for clinical practice (Reed et al. 2011).

The ICD provides the basis of the discussion for classifying the phenomena observed in the clinical contexts that are discussed in Chapters 14 to 29. A number of entities (e.g. brain tumours of infancy) are included in the differential diagnosis but not covered in detail in this volume for lack of space. Other entities do not appear because they are based on classifications of disease other than the ICD. Such diagnostic classifications, including some listed in the paragraphs below, may claim to identify disease entities requiring active management in a substantial percentage of neonates or infants. In some cases, the criteria for making such diagnoses are vague, their relationships with disorders of later childhood unknown, and the rationale for intervention is obscure (Mustafayev et al. 2020).

International clinical guidelines depend upon this shared nosology and classification of illnesses and disease: the foundation for rational management requires knowledge of what treatments are of benefit and what are harmful, which in turn requires specific disease definitions that are shared by all those involved in providing care.

RELEVANT TERMS AND DEFINITIONS

The brief discussion of terms below is intended to help the reader to navigate through later chapters of the book but is not intended to be exhaustive.

Encephalopathy is defined as 'a disease in which the functioning of the brain is affected by some agent or condition' (*New Oxford Dictionary*). Because this definition is so inclusive, it is of little practical value in clinical medicine. While 'acute' means 'of short duration' or 'experienced to an intense or severe degree' (*New Oxford Dictionary*), the medical definition of *acute encephalopathy* includes alteration in conscious level as an essential criterion (Chapter 17) and to that extent, is a more clinically useful term for the formation of a plan of investigation and management.

The term *perinatal encephalopathy* does not indicate whether the observed effect on the functioning of the brain is of short duration or whether it involves an alteration of conscious level. Furthermore the term 'perinatal' includes the period before birth when the infant's level of consciousness is usually not known to the clinician. However, the general term 'encephalopathy' is no more useful in the perinatal period than it is generally, especially since there is often disagreement as to whether or not commonly observed neonatal or post-neonatal behaviour (e.g. tremor of the chin) indicates abnormal brain functioning. This carries a significant potential for harm in exposing many infants, the vast majority of whom will have no known subsequent medical disorder, to the risks associated with medical diagnoses of doubtful validity (Mustafayev et al. 2020). In practice therefore, the definition of neonatal (not perinatal) encephalopathy (NE) includes alteration of the level of consciousness (Chapter 14). It is, in effect, the special case of 'acute encephalopathy' in a newborn baby. Other more inclusive uses of the term *perinatal encephalopathy* are to be avoided and will not be further discussed here.

Hydrocephalus is used to mean an excess of cerebrospinal fluid within the head but excluding those situations where that condition has arisen purely from atrophy or failure of the brain substance to develop (sometimes called hydrocephalus *ex vacuo*). The presence of hydrocephalus cannot be confirmed or excluded based on the dimensions of the third cerebral ventricle alone (see Chapter 23 for further discussion).

Hydrocephalus and *raised intracranial pressure* frequently co-exist and specific clinical signs, often including disturbed consciousness, can be combined with cranial imaging to provide evidence for the presence of both entities (see especially Chapters 17 and 23). By contrast, 'the syndrome of intracranial hypertension' and 'hydrocephalus-intracranial-hypertension syndrome' are not internationally recognized as diagnostic entities (Mustafayev et al. 2020) and should not be confused with the rare condition of older children and adults known as pseudotumor cerebri syndrome (and also as idiopathic intracranial hypertension) (Matthews et al. 2017).

A *seizure* may be epileptic (Chapter 20) or nonepileptic (Chapter 21). Epilepsy is defined as recurrent unprovoked epileptic seizures. Febrile seizures are provoked by a rising fever and are not conventionally regarded as falling within the above definition of an epilepsy. These chapters also provide further discussion of these definitions and of the syndromes that constitute disease entities within them.

Myotonia is defined as the inability of muscle fibres to relax after muscle contraction and can be demonstrated by myotonic discharges on electromyography. This is a very rare phenomenon in infancy and even in an infant with congenital myotonic dystrophy (Chapter 24), myotonia is usually only demonstrable in an affected parent.

The term *myotonic syndrome*, in which abnormality of muscle tone is the dominant feature, is not an internationally recognized diagnostic entity in infants.

Hyperexcitability syndrome is not a generally accepted diagnostic disease entity term in infancy and internationally accepted criteria for its definition are lacking. Problems with one or more of sleeping, feeding, or excessive crying in infancy are reported in up to 30% of all infants and are usually transient. Most cases may, therefore, be regarded as falling within the spectrum of typical development and need not be conceptualized as indicating an underlying neurological disorder. Associations do, however, exist between multiple problems with these functions (often referred to as early regulatory problems) and long-term behavioural outcomes in childhood, including attention-deficit/hyperactivity disorder. These problems are attributable partly to biological predisposition in the infant, partly to parenting behaviours, and partly to interactions between the two. Interventions that alter parenting behaviours may help (see Chapter 25). Support to parents to help prevent or reduce early regulatory problems is typically given in the context of general paediatric nursing or medical assessment of the infant and advice to families rather than as treatment of a disease entity.

EVIDENCE-BASED MEDICINE

The accumulated wisdom of previous generations of medical practitioners has, since the 19th century, been progressively supplanted by the concept of 'evidence', of greater or lesser quality, to support the use of treatments. Myth has been progressively replaced by evidence, although the process has sometimes been hindered by political interference (McKee, 2007). Hopefully the value of certain myths, starting with Hygeia and Panacea, will continue to be recognized. Evidence-based medicine has only emerged within the second half of the 20th century and has been an increasing influence on medical practice in the 21st century. It is, as described in Chapter 3, the systematic construction of a body of knowledge about interventions for medical illnesses with explicit, objective criteria for rating the quality of the evidence upon which that knowledge is based. The great strength of evidence-based medicine lies in its capacity for constant improvement as new information comes to light and without *ad personam* arguments about the authority of the individuals advocating any particular treatment, which had dominated previous medical thought since Hippocrates, sometimes referred to as 'eminence-based medicine'.

Unfortunately, the quality of much of the evidence upon which we must currently rely for guidance in the treatment of neurological disorders in infancy is poor. Furthermore, the traditional measures of quality of evidence are sometimes difficult to apply when studying rehabilitation, including physiotherapeutic interventions (Rosenbaum, 2010; Autti-Ramo, 2011). The methodology of evidence-based medicine can also help us to identify those situations where evidence is lacking and serve to remind us that justification is always required for medical intervention, especially in an infant, and the responsibility for this rests with the physician.

REFERENCES

Autti-Ramo I (2011) Physiotherapy in high-risk infants — a motor learning facilitator or not?*Dev Med Child Neurol* 53: 200—201.

Blair M, DeBell D (2011) Reconceptualising health services for school age children in the 21st century. *Arch Dis Child* 96: 616—618.

McKee M (2007) Cochrane on Communism: the influence of ideology on the search for evidence. *Int J Epidemiol* 36: 269—273.

Matthews YY, Dean F, Lim MJ, et al. (2017) Pseudotumor cerebri syndrome in childhood: incidence, clinical profile and risk factors in a national prospective population-based cohort study. *Arch Dis Child* 102: 715—721.

Mustafayev R, Seyid-Mammadova T, Kennedy C, et al (2020) Perinatal encephalopathy, the syndrome of intracranial hypertension and associated diagnostic labels in the Commonwealth of Independent States: a systematic review. *Arch Dis Child* 105: 921-926.

Reed GM, Dua T, Saxena S (2011) World Health Organization responds to Fiona Godlee and Ray Moynihan. *BMJ* 342: 1380.

Rosenbaum P (2010) The randomized controlled trial: an excellent design, but can it answer the big question in neurodisability?*Dev Med Child Neurol* 52: 111.

Resources

Edelstein L. The Hippocratic Oath. Text, translation and interpretation by L. Edelstein, 1943, p. 56. https://www.pbs.org/wgbh/nova/body/hippocratic-oath-today.html

ICD-11 codes in advance release. https://www.who.int/classifications/icd/en/

CHAPTER 2

Interprofessional working: user and carer involvement

Audrone Prasauskiene and Maryze Schoneveld van der Linde

Key messages

- Be aware of the social and cultural environment of the child, such as nationality, language dependence, religion, family situation, etc.
- Use all possible means to avoid separating the child and parents.
- Inform and talk to parents about their child's health problems.
- Inform the child about their health condition in an age-appropriate manner.
- Listen to parents' feelings regarding their child's condition.
- Include parents in the treatment plan for their child, so that they have some control over their child's problem.
- Encourage parents to develop a good, strong emotional bond with their child.
- Provide parents and children with a window of hope without denying the seriousness of the child's health situation.
- Good quality of life with a disability is certainly possible but needs creativity and flexibility of approach. If parents are having difficulty finding the way forward, try to assist them to find perspectives on life with their child from which they could derive pleasure and satisfaction.
- Discuss with the professional healthcare team their ideas, solutions, and feelings regarding the health of the patient.

Common errors

- Being too focused on the medical aspects of treatment and forgetting the psychological and emotional well-being of the affected child, the parents, and, sometimes, the healthcare professionals confronted by very difficult situations.
- Forgetting that the patient is not only a sick body, but also a human being with social, emotional, and psychological needs.
- Failing to include the parents in the treatment plan of their child. The parents are the main carers of the child in all situations.

When to worry

- Signs of depression in the parents and/or the child.
- Parental interest in institutions that take care of disabled children. This can indicate that a family plans to leave their disabled child there.
- Denial by parents that the child has a health problem.
- Parents avoiding their child. This can be a sign of psychological difficulty in coming to terms with the child's health problems.

THE HOLISTIC APPROACH TO CHILDHOOD DEVELOPMENT

Holism is a concept derived from the meaning of its Greek root *holos*, which means 'all' or 'total'. The term 'holistic' means looking at something as a whole rather than in separate parts. This approach is often linked to health, where the patient may be treated holistically, in the sense that mental, physical, emotional, and spiritual well-being are all considered.

Holistic care is based upon valuing the whole child and understanding the young child as an individual in the context of family, community, and culture. It is impossible to separate the normal physical and emotional development of the child from their place in their family. From the first hours of life of the newborn infant it is very important to ensure that, despite the need to use all available technologies, infants have close contact with their parents/primary caregivers.

A holistic approach to the child's development and education has to involve physical, emotional, and psychological domains of general well-being. As highlighted above, the holistic approach leads to better understanding of a child's individual needs and multiple factors which are likely to affect growth and development. So, care of a child that is typically developing or has a developmental disorder must be based on four main principles:

- *Client-centered*, with the child's and family's needs prioritized.

- *Strength-focused*, based on the strengths of the child and family rather than on their weaknesses.

- *Solution-oriented*, based on eliciting a child's strengths and abilities rather than focusing on the roots of his/her deficits.

- In partnership with the family, irrespective of the child's diagnosis, family social status, and cultural background.

USER AND CARER INVOLVEMENT

Care of the newborn infant

The 'kangaroo care' technique was developed for newborn infants. *Kangaroo care* is the term used for maintaining skin-to-skin contact between the infant and mother/father for several hours each day over a period of days or weeks after birth. Typically, the infant, wearing only a nappy, is held against the mother's/father's bare chest, with the mother's/father's shirt or hospital gown wrapped under and around the infant's bottom for support. Maternal and paternal contact appears to have a calming effect on the newborn infant in addition to enhancing bonding. For infants born preterm the benefits can be even greater, with the mother's and father's body directly responding to the infant's and helping to regulate temperature, for example, more naturally and smoothly than an incubator. Kangaroo care has also been shown to help stabilize heartbeat and breathing of an infant born preterm. Physicians have found that kangaroo care can help to wean an infant off a ventilator sooner than might otherwise be possible.

Another worldwide initiative supported by the World Health Organization (WHO) and United Nations International Children's Emergency Fund (UNICEF) is the development of infant-friendly hospitals. In these hospitals close contact between mother and infant is maintained and breastfeeding is supported by all means possible.

Care of infants and children more generally

A child, especially in the early years and particularly when developmental problems are suspected, should not be separated from his/her parents or carers, even if the child is sick and has to be hospitalized. There is scientific evidence that long-term continuity of parental care is very beneficial to all children except, of course, in cases where parents neglect or abuse their children. Long-term hospitalization with isolation from parents during the first year of life may have the same consequences for psychological and emotional development as institutionalization and can cause:

- *Social and behavioural abnormalities* (aggressive behavioural problems, inattention/hyperactivity, delays in social/emotional development, syndromes mimicking autism).

- *Poor growth:* institutionalized children cared for without involvement of the family lose 1 month of growth every 3 months; decreased emotional reactivity: children living outside of family care demonstrate deficient understanding of and response to facial emotion and other impairments in sensory perception.

Disability, developmental disorder, and developmental delay

The concept of *disability* refers to limitations resulting from physical and/or cognitive dysfunction. Disability is not something that happens to only a minority of humanity. About 15% of the world's population lives with some form of disability, of whom 2% to 4% experience significant difficulties in functioning (WHO and World Bank, 2011). It is also important to appreciate that there are different views and opinions on the concept of disability. To clarify and specify the concept and the impact of disability on health and health-related domains, the WHO created the International Classification of Functioning, Disability and Health (ICF) in 2001 (WHO, 2001). The ICF acknowledges that *every* human being can experience a decrement in health and, thereby, experience some degree of disability.

The ICF defines disability as an umbrella term for impairments, activity limitations and participation restrictions. It denotes the negative aspects of the interaction between an individual (with a health condition) and that individual's contextual factors (environmental and personal factors (WHO, 2001). The ICF, thus, brings disability into the mainstream of experience and recognizes it as a universal human experience. The ICF takes into account the social aspects of disability and does not see disability only as a medical or biological dysfunction. By including contextual and environmental factors, the ICF allows recording of the impact of the environment on a person's functioning.

The rapid growth and changes occurring in the first 20 years of life were not well captured in the ICF, and so in 2007 the ICF for Children and Youth (ICF-CY; WHO, 2007) was developed and subsequently merged with the ICF between 2012 and 2015 (https://www.who.int/classifications/icf/en/). It addresses this important developmental period in greater detail and enables disability to be seen as part of life and the care of disabled people a social responsibility of every society. The ICF-CY can assist clinicians, educators, researchers, and parents to document and measure health and disability in populations of children and young people (WHO, 2007).

In Western cultures, disability is conceptualized as dependence on others and loss of autonomy but, on closer examination, dependency and autonomy are universal in social relationships. Reliance upon another person may be encompassed by love and a feeling of mutuality, and the value of family and community membership may, in some cultures, outweigh that of individual ability. Dependency also varies according to the characteristics of those with whom a person with a disability lives and the ability of the person with a disability to develop as an individual (Ingstad and Reynolds Whyte, 1995). The meaning and consequences of dependency, therefore, vary.

The concept of *impairment*, by contrast, is more restricted and describes a lack or loss of structure or function within an individual. It does not address the effects on function or social participation of the individual caused by their personality and ability to take responsibility, or by their family setting, or by their legal and sociopolitical context, or by the meaning of being different in their society. Autonomy, dependency, capacity, identity, and the meaning of loss, which are central to the effect of disability, are thus not captured by describing disability in terms of the individual's impairment. To describe disability simply in terms of the underlying impairment, therefore, raises metaphysical and ethical difficulties.

Cerebral palsy, intellectual disability, epilepsy, autism, and spina bifida are examples of developmental disorders, and there are many others. They often, but not always, lead to developmental disability, i.e. limitations in functioning resulting from disorders of the developing nervous system. Developmental delay refers to delays in reaching developmental milestones, indicating lack of function in one or multiple domains (cognition, motor, speech, vision, hearing, behaviour).

The term *developmental disability* refers to lifelong disabilities primarily attributable to mental and/or physical impairments manifested before 18 years of age. But parents need to understand that a child with developmental disability has different life opportunities. The occurrence of developmental disability can be a single event in a family or can have a genetic basis. Having a disability, whether mild or severe, does not mean that a child has no future. A family and community can create an environment at home and at school where the child can be safe and grow and thrive physically and emotionally. Many children with a mental and/or physical impairment can work, albeit at a very low level in some cases. When the child gets the necessary support, their full developmental potential can be realized and they can have a good life among the people who care about and love them.

THE NEEDS OF THE CHILD

Early intervention for developmental disorders

Guralnick (1997), Heckman and Masterov (2007), Kolb and Gibb (2011), Hensch and Bilimoria (2012), and other researchers have presented reliable evidence in support of theories that early childhood offers the best opportunity to promote development and to prevent or minimize consequences of biological and environmental risk factors to a child's development. Furthermore, politicians, professionals, and parents in most countries agree that it is the responsibility of a mature society to provide early inter-vention programmes for children with established disabilities or who are at risk of compromised development.

Children who have a developmental disorder or any other health problem early in life need all the support they can get to guarantee the highest possible quality of life; to feel safe, be able to play and enjoy life, and to receive unconditional love, respect, care, attention, and explanation about what they may be experiencing. So first a child has to be pain-free, properly fed, and all his/her individual needs should be professionally assessed with the corresponding tool and/or method for his/her age, health problem, and culture.

The family at the heart of developmental interventions

Therapy methods must be acceptable for the child and their family, goal-oriented, and evidence-based. The reasons for their selection have to be adequately explained to the parents and the child (if possible). Explaining to the child what is happening or going to happen shows the child that he/she is being taken seriously and that his/her feelings, questions, fear, anxiety, and pain are being acknowledged. It also involves the child in the rehabilitation/habilitation treatment which, like the involvement of the parents and other caregivers, is crucial to success.

A child functions within the family. His/her quality of life, access to the health and social care, and education facilities, therefore, depend on family characteristics. Single parenting, young parents, poor parenting skills, and poverty might aggravate a devel-opmental disorder and its outcomes. Children learn best when they are motivated and inspired. Mahoney and MacDonald (2007) estimated that caregiver−child purposeful interactions at home or in a related child-friendly environment that occur for just 1 hour a day, 7 days a week would provide 220 000 learning opportunities each year, while a 30-minute therapy session once a week for a whole year would provide only 7500 such opportunities.

FAMILY NEEDS AND THE NEEDS OF THE CHILD

Evaluating a family's situation

No family ever dreams of having a child with disability. So being told that their child has been born with neurodevelopmental disorder that will lead to disability might be as traumatizing for the parents as learning about their child's death, and they may exper-ience emotional shock, fear, disbelief, rejection, and frustration. Their dreams about the child's future and achievements are left in tatters. Later they might feel grief 'for the loss of the perfect child'. A model of grief, expounded by Kübler-Ross (1969, 2005) identifies five stages: denial, anger, bargaining, depression, and acceptance, which may be 'used as a tool to help frame and identify what we may be feeling'. Every person's response to loss is different, depending on personality and coping abilities. Some families finally accept their child with a disability and love him/her for who he/she is and generate new dreams related to the child's and family's life. Others 'get stuck' in their sadness: they never experience a full acceptance and live a life of unending sorrow. This may lead to loss of self-esteem, depression, and constant feelings of guilt, disruption of family life and marriage, and neglect of the other children and the extended family.

Siblings and family relationships

Childhood disability affects not only the parents but also the brothers and sisters of the affected child. Typically developing siblings may be potentially forgotten, disregarded, and neglected. Typically developing siblings of children with cancer may 'experience similar stress to that of the ill child' (Murray, 2000). A review by Knecht, Hellmers, and Metzing (2015) identified and discussed several themes in the experiences of typically developing siblings of a disabled child:

- *Emotional deprivation:* experiences of loss associated with the lack of parental availability, separation anxiety caused by frequent hospitalization, loneliness, unimportance, feelings of being ignored, displaced, neglected, or rejected.

- *Somatic complaints:* eating problems, sleep disturbances, headaches, etc.

- *Developmental experiences:* restriction of personal growth, independence, and maturity in healthy siblings.

- *Experience of family:* difficulties with sibling–sibling bonds, the parent–child relationship, and the functioning of the family as a whole.

- *Experiences of everyday life: social isolation and withdrawal.* The siblings may on the other hand, develop better communicative and collaborative skills, empathy, compassion, and patience.

Grandparents, other extended family members, and family friends form a group that can have positive and negative effects on the family's coping with the disability. Their support is very important for the family.

The pattern of relationships within a family is the most important factor influencing a child's development. Personal characteristics of parents (empathy, resilience, devotion), social support, marital relationship, economic well-being, and the child's temperament are critical factors unrelated to the child's disability that have a great impact on the functioning of the family. Other factors that influence the impact of the child's disability on the well-being of the family are information needs, interpersonal and family distress, resource needs and loss of confidence. Family involvement in early intervention programmes strengthens the confidence and competence of family members

(Dunst et al. 2007; Morgan et al. 2014, 2015, 2016) and affects the child's developmental outcomes (Guralnick, 1997).

THE CONTRIBUTION OF HEALTHCARE PROFESSIONALS

Accurate assessment of the family's situation and needs is, therefore, crucial not only in order to organize the necessary help and stimulate coping processes, but also to involve family members in the programme of habilitation. So far, there are no specific tools to assess the needs of a family with a young, developmentally disabled child. The family situation can be evaluated by using tests to assess family stress (Parental Stress Index) and stigma (Family Interview Stigma Scale). Providers of the child's healthcare need to discuss these aspects with parents and other caregivers in order to evaluate their emotional, social, informational, practical, spiritual, and physical needs.

Family needs might change over time. Therefore, regular monitoring of those needs should be included in clinical practice and can help in setting individual rehabilitation priorities and treatment plans.

Healthcare professionals cannot cure developmental disabilities, solve all family problems, and make everyone happy and safe. But they can and must make a positive difference to the lives of families with a child with a developmental disorder. Early and correct clinical and developmental diagnosis is usually just the beginning of the long path that the family and the child have to travel. Therefore, a well-informed team of healthcare professionals must build a team around the child and his/her family. This includes giving parents time and attention or a shoulder to cry on and can have a positive impact on building up family's strength and self-confidence. Parents are empowered by being provided with understandable, up-to-date, culturally adapted verbal and written information about the causes, prognosis, and treatments (methods and effectiveness) of the child's disorder. This is one of the most important factors in building trust and future collaboration with the family and the foundation for developing and implementing individual intervention plans.

It is important for healthcare professionals always to be honest, not to promise anything, and not to offer a negative prognosis too quickly, especially when uncertainty remains. Healthcare professionals should help the family to identify their expectations and values related to the child and his/her future. They should give hope by drawing attention to positive experiences the child and the parents can both look forward to enjoying in the future. Without hope it will be difficult for parents to find energy to continue to support their child as best as they can. Providing a window of hope for whatever kind of future the child has is essential. Tell parents that there will be reasons that their child will be glad to be alive, even if he/she is severely disabled and can be expected to do little except to share in family life. It can be helpful to seek connection with them via their spiritual faith. Although providing information, respect, support, and explaining the medical cause of the child's disability is very important, compassion is essential. It is good to show parents that as well as being a healthcare professional, you empathize with them in their situation.

TEAMWORK IN CARING FOR CHILDREN WITH DEVELOPMENTAL DISABILITIES

Katzenbach and Smith (1993) defined a team as 'a small group of people with complementary skills who are committed to a common purpose, performance goals, and approach for which they are mutually accountable'. The team working with children who have developmental disorders require skills, including joint working with other professionals in multiple medical, social, and psychological disciplines. This is especially important when the diagnosis of the developmental disorder of the child has just been established and is new to the family. According to Patel, Pratt, and Patel (2008), a multidisciplinary approach in healthcare delivery produces the following benefits:

- Improves quality of care;

- Reduces errors in healthcare delivery;

- Reduces duplication of services;

- Provides cost-effective care;

- Enhances efficiency of healthcare delivery;

- Addresses medical and psychosocial aspects of care;

- Is more convenient for the patient and family or caregiver;

- Increases patient and family or caregiver satisfaction;

- Promotes development of innovative approaches and solutions to complex problems;

- Meets the mandates of applicable laws;

- Increases collaboration and networking among professionals; and

- Enhances individual professional development.

There is, however, still not enough evidence that multidisciplinary approaches are cost-effective, improve quality of care, or reduce errors in delivery of healthcare. More research-based evidence in the context of provision of care to children with developmental disabilities is required, to supplant decisions made on intuition and experience.

The effectiveness of a team largely depends on the culture of the organization and the professional competencies and communication skills of the team members. A team coordinator who is responsible for communication with the family and for the organization of teamwork is essential. Therefore, the parents and, if applicable, the child must be equal members of the team and their needs have to be prioritized in setting goals for rehabilitation/habilitation.

The team may experience a wide range of emotions and its members need a means to vent their feelings, for example at team meetings. This requires good collaboration and mutual trust within the team. Good team working will help team members support the parents, the child, and each other, address problems, communicate with each other regarding the treatment of the child, and focus on the child's future with parents and family, even when the child is severely disabled.

The development of a child is a complicated and diverse process, influenced by multiple factors. To provide professional and effective healthcare or habilitation/rehabilitation services for the child and family, several professionals should be involved. It is very important that these professionals work as a team.

There are three types of cross-professional working (Thylefors, Persson, and Hellström, 2005), as detailed below.

- *Multiprofessional:* each team member is focused on their own tasks and not on collective working. Contributions are made either in parallel or sequentially to each other with minimal communication. Each contribution stands alone and can be performed without input from others. Independent contributions have to be coordinated. Traditionally, the physician takes the lead. This type of cross-professional work is often the method used in Eastern European countries. In this type of team, the members rely on their own individual assessments to deduce the needs of the family, while the parents stay outside the team.

- *Interprofessional (the product is more than a simple sum of its parts):* this model implies a high level of communication, mutual planning, collective decisions, and shared responsibilities; outcome requires interactive effort and contribution of the professionals involved. Everyone involved in the process must take everyone else's contribution into consideration. This type of teamwork involves all the staff members working with the child and parents. This team is more likely to concentrate on the needs and goals of the child and the family than on purely medical goals.

- *Transprofessional:* the opposite end of the continuum from multiprofessional working. The team uses integrative work processes so that disciplinary boundaries become partly dissolved. Professionals, by close interpersonal and interprofessional communication, become more sensitive to the needs of the child and the family; they can build treatment strategies that help to achieve functional goals. Communication also helps to share knowledge, solve conflicts, and to generally improve services.

There are no strict rules or guidelines about the composition of the team around the child with a developmental disorder. This will vary with the organizational level of the services (local, regional, national), financial capability of the country, and needs of the child and his/her family. But the main principle to be adhered to is that professionals should have specialized education, training, and professional experience in providing services for this very vulnerable and very specific group of patients. Professionals that may be involved in the care of a child with developmental disability are listed below.

- *Paediatrician:* a medical specialist focused on children. They diagnose and treat infants and children with a diversity of diseases, sometimes including metabolic diseases, and give advice on feeding, respiratory problems, catheterization, bowel evacuation, etc. In some countries there are developmental, neurodevelopmental, or developmental-behavioural pediatricians who specialize in taking care of children with developmental disorders.

- *Paediatric neurologist:* a medical specialist focused on the diagnosis and treatment of neuromuscular diseases, epilepsy, developmental disorders (including delayed speech, motor milestones, and coordination issues), cerebral palsy, myelomeningocele, intellectual disability, traumatic brain injuries, metabolic and progressive disorders, and childhood variants of neurological diseases that also affect adults.

- *Orthopaedic surgeon:* a surgeon who treats scoliosis, club foot, hip dysplasia, contractures, and other joint or bone problems related to muscle weakness or imbalance.

- *Speech and language therapist or logoped:* helps to diagnose and treat a variety of speech, voice, and language disorders, and feeding and swallowing difficulties.

- *Ear, nose, and throat (ENT) specialist:* treats ear, nose, and throat impairments. Both ENT specialists, audiological physicians, and audiologists diagnose and treat hearing loss. Every child with a developmental disability should be examined for hearing disorders.

- *Ophthalmologist:* treats diseases of the eye and visual impairments. Every child with developmental disability should be examined for vision disorders.

- *Dietician:* creates nutrition plans to manage weight loss, malnutrition, and swallowing problems.

- *Social worker:* helps parents to cope with practical concerns such as educational and financial issues.

- *Psychologist:* helps parents with their fears and worries and tries to assist them to find a way to deal with the new situation of having a child with a developmental disorder. Evaluates the child's cognitive and other abilities to identify the profile of cognitive strengths and weaknesses.

- *Occupational therapist or ergotherapist:* helps parents to learn new ways to do everyday tasks, adjust their home for the needs of the child, and deals with fine motor problems. Advises on aids and equipment, including wheelchairs.

- *Physiotherapist or kinesiotherapist:* helps the child to do physical exercises, strengthen weak muscles, prevent contractures, improve stamina, improve motor abilities, and reach specific functional goals.

- *Special needs teaching assistant or special pedagogue:* helps to evaluate and develop the child's educational and developmental skills to ensure the maximum is done to support the child to be as independent as possible.

- *Genetic counsellor:* discusses issues related to family risk and family planning and arranges for prenatal diagnoses when applicable and requested by the family.

- *Clinical geneticist:* recognizes patterns of malformation and recurrence risk. Advises on diagnostic genetic testing, including prenatal testing in cases where future children are at risk of a genetic condition.

THE LIFE TRAJECTORY OF THE CHILD WITH A DEVELOPMENTAL DISORDER

When a child with a developmental disability grows up, the needs of both the child and the parents may change. Every stage in a child's life will involve change for the child and the parents. This means that it is important that child and parents are followed-up appropriately by the healthcare team. The team can identify what additional support or services a child and their parents need. For parents it is usually good to be closely involved in the treatment plan for their child. For them, knowing what is done, why it is done, and what healthcare professionals hope to achieve is usually important. Taking care of a child with a developmental disability is a lifelong commitment, but the commitment of parents, healthcare professionals, society, and, of course, the child him/herself can enable a child to live life to the fullest, within their own capabilities.

REFERENCES

Dunst CJ, Trivette CM, Hamby DW (2007) Meta-analysis of family-centered help-giving practices research. *Ment Retard Dev Disabil Res Rev* 13: 370—8.

Guralnick MJ, editor (1997) *The Effectiveness of Early Intervention*. Baltimore: Brookes.

Heckman JJ, Masterov DV (2007) The productivity argument for investing in young children. *Review of Agricultural Economics* 29: 446–493.

Hensch TK, Bilimoria PM (2012) Re-opening windows: manipulating critical periods for brain development. *Cerebrum*: 11.

Ingstad B, Reynolds Whyte S (1995) *Disability and Culture*. Los Angeles: University of California Press, pp. 3–11.

Katzenbach JR, Smith DK (1993) *The Wisdom of Teams: Creating the High-Performance Organiza- tion*. Boston, Massachusetts: Harvard Business School Press.

Knecht C, Hellmers C, Metzing S (2015) The perspective of siblings of children with chronic illness a literature review. *J Pediatr Nurs* 30: 102–116.

Kolb B, Gibb R (2011) Brain plasticity and behaviour in the developing brain. *J Can Acad Child Adolesc Psychiatry* 2: 265–276.

Kübler-Ross E (1969) *On Death and Dying*. New York: Routledge.

Kübler-Ross E (2005) *On Grief and Grieving: Finding the Meaning of Grief Through the Five Stages of Loss*. New York: Simon & Schuster Ltd.

Mahoney G, MacDonald J (2007) *Autism and Developmental Delays in Young Children: The Respons- ive Teaching Curriculum for Parents and Professionals*. Austin, TX: PRO-ED.

Morgan C, Novak I, Dale RC, Badawi N (2015) Optimising motor learning in infants at high risk of cerebral palsy: a pilot study. *BMC Pediatr* 15: 30.

Morgan C, Novak I, Dale RC, Guzzetta A, Badawi N (2014) GAME (Goals – Activity – Motor Enrichment): protocol of a single blind randomised controlled trial of motor training, par- ent education and environmental enrichment for infants at high risk of cerebral palsy. *BMC Neurol* 14: 203.

Morgan C, Novak I, Dale RC, Guzzetta A, Badawi N (2016) Single blind randomised controlled trial of GAME (Goals – Activity – Motor Enrichment) in infants at high risk of cerebral palsy. *Res Dev Disabil* 55: 256–267.

Murray JS (2000) Attachment theory and adjustment difficulties in siblings of children with cancer. *Issues Ment Health Nurs* 21: 149–169.

Patel DR, Pratt HD, Patel ND (2008) Team processes and team care for children with develop- mental disabilities. *Pediatr Clin North Am* 55: 1375–1390.

Thylefors I, Persson O, Hellström D (2005) Team types, perceived efficiency and team climate in Swedish cross-professional teamwork. *J Interprof Care* 19: 102–114.

World Health Organization (2001) *International Classification of Functioning, Disability and Health (ICF)* resolution WHA 54.21 (https://apps.who.int/classifications/icfbrowser/)

World Health Organization (2007) *International Classification of Functioning, Disability and Health – Children and Youth Version (ICF-CY)*. Geneva: World Health Organization.

World Health Organization, The World Bank (2011) *World Report on Disability*. (https://www.who. int/disabilities/world_report/2011/report.pdf?ua=1)

CHAPTER 3

Clinical epidemiology and evidence-based medicine

Andrew L Lux

Key messages

- A good understanding of evidence-based medicine and clinical epidemiology is essential for the effective practice of all clinicians.
- Although there are good sources of aggregated data and clinical practice guidelines, effective clinical practice often requires decisions based upon small studies or series of descriptive data and the ability to interpret those studies reliably.
- You can adopt your own 'ABC' for the evaluation and interpretation of reported clinical studies by considering Assumptions, Bias, Confounding, and Chance.

Common errors

- We are all prone to recognizing causal patterns from associations where effects are due to chance or other factors such as bias and confounding.
- Many reported studies force the reader to 'lose touch' with the data by reporting modelled and adjusted estimates of effect without first reporting the crude or unadjusted effect estimates.
- Published reports tend to have a 'positive' finding and similar studies that fail to detect an important or significant difference are less likely to get submitted and published. This might lead to publication bias.

> ## When to worry
>
> - When published evidence contrasts with your personal experience. The definitions and ideas in this chapter should help you determine why your experience is so different and to assess the validity of the reported findings.
> - When published evidence is based on *p*-values and hypothesis testing alone rather than on reported estimates of effect and confidence intervals. This latter approach allows the clinician to better assess the magnitude and importance of any reported effect.
> - When effect estimates, confidence intervals, or *p*-values are reported without clear reference to the statistical tests from which they are calculated.

INTRODUCTION

Epidemiology is the study of the incidence, distribution, determinants, and possible control of disease and other factors relating to health in populations. In *clinical epidemiology* the principles and techniques of epidemiology are applied to clinical settings. It is concerned with activities such as defining cases and exposure to risk-modifying factors, assessing measures of risk, and assessing the impact and effects of treatment interventions. It was first described as 'a marriage between quantitative concepts used by epidemiologists to study disease in populations and decision-making in the individual case, which is the daily fare of clinical medicine' (Paul, 1938). In other words, its key function is to provide tools allowing the clinician to make good decisions.

Evidence-based medicine (EBM) is a movement that provides a context for clinical epidemiology and espouses 'the conscientious, explicit and judicious use of current best evidence in making decisions about the care of individual patients' (Sackett et al. 1996). It attempts to take into account the patient's physical and clinical circumstances and the beliefs and values of the patient and their family. This chapter provides an overview of some key elements of clinical epidemiology and EBM, but it is by no means a comprehensive or systematic review.

SOME BASIC CONCEPTS IN CLINICAL EPIDEMIOLOGY

Case definitions and severity   In clinical studies and in rigorous clinical practice, it is necessary to define the features of a disease or condition that make it reasonable to state that the patient is genuinely affected by that condition. These features may be considered necessary, sufficient, or merely consistent with the diagnosis. In defining cases, it is often necessary to also define exclusion criteria, in other words, features that would make one consider that this is a different health condition. It is worth noting that a condition can exist with variable degrees of severity, and so it may be necessary to categorize cases further in order to make true comparisons between groups.

Syndrome   A syndrome is a confluence of features. For example, onset of focal motor seizures in middle childhood with sleep-activated epileptiform discharges in the central-midtemporal area would be consistent with the epilepsy syndrome of 'benign childhood epilepsy with central-midtemporal spikes'. However, if the patient has a focal neurological deficit and a temporal lobe tumour, then it would be inappropriate to use this syndromic label since we would have identified clear exclusion criteria (see 'Case definitions and severity' above). Precise inclusion and exclusion criteria for the definition of a syndrome are crucially important for communication between health-care providers and are, in effect, the basis of the international classification of disease.

Bias   A bias is a factor or process that makes results, analyses, or their interpretation (the 'inference') deviate from the truth. Systematic bias is a bias that affects validity. There are many potential forms of bias. For example, Sackett (1979) identified 35 forms of bias relating solely to sampling and measurement. (In spoken presentations, the term 'bias' is often confused with 'skewness', which is a measure of asymmetry of a probability distribution).

Publication bias   This refers to the distorting effect of studies being more likely to be accepted for publication when there are positive findings and less likely to be published when no association or causal relationship has been identified. This will particularly affect the conclusions derived from aggregated data (such as systematic reviews) since the review is biased towards positive results by identifying only the papers that have been accepted for publication. There are techniques for analysing data aggregated from multiple studies, such as funnel plot analyses (Sterne and Egger, 2001), that can identify the presence of publication bias.

Regression to mean effect   This is another form of bias. The degree or severity of a condition will tend, over time, to a certain average value. An apparent beneficial effect might be falsely attributed to a treatment intervention — for example, the addition of a new antiepileptic drug added at a time when seizures are particularly frequent or severe — where there is no true effect, since what is observed is the condition tending back to its baseline (mean effect) with respect to the outcome being measured, such as frequency or severity. One way of adjusting for this bias is to perform a randomized controlled trial (RCT) in which some patients receive a placebo medication.

Confounding   This is a form of bias that confuses the effects of the exposure of interest with other effects that might be operating to influence the outcomes. The defining characteristic of a confounding factor is that it is associated both with the exposure being studied and the outcome of that exposure. For example, the severity of hearing impairment would be expected to be associated with age at diagnosis of the impairment (with more severe impairments being diagnosed earlier) and with subsequent language abilities (with more severe impairments being associated with poorer language development). In this example, the association between early diagnosis and subsequently poorer language skills is said to be confounded by the severity of the hearing impairment.

Association and causality   Statistical tests can identify associations between random variables (study factors) but clinicians and researchers need to exercise reason and judgement to decide whether such relationships are likely to be causal, rather than being due to chance, bias, or confounding.

Hill's criteria Hill's criteria (Hill, 1965) are useful for investigating possible causal relationships (see Table 3.1). It is also important to consider the possibility of reverse causality. For example, in a study showing that the attendance of a paediatrician at the resuscitation of a newborn infant is associated with a higher statistical risk of the infant having a subsequent neurological problem. The explanation is far more likely to be that paediatrician attendances are in response to an increased risk of injury rather than directly increasing those risks!

Table 3.1   Sir Austin Bradford Hill's causal criteria

Criterion	Features
Strength	Strong associations are more likely to be causal, but weaker associations are more likely to be due to unidentified biases.
Consistency	The same association is found in different populations and in different circumstances.
Specificity	The cause leads to a single effect rather than multiple effects.
Temporality	The cause necessarily occurs before the effect.
Biological gradient	The presence of a dose-response effect, either linear (monotonic) or with threshold effects.
Plausibility	The causal relationship makes sense in terms of current knowledge of biological and social systems (although this is not an absolute requirement: the explanatory mechanism may follow the epidemiological finding).
Coherence	The causal interpretation aligns with what is known about the biological or social system.
Experimental evidence	It might be better to regard this as a means of testing a causal hypothesis.
Analogy	A criterion that seems to lend support to plausibility.

(Hill, 1965)

Validity   Validity is the extent to which a tool measures what it purports to measure.

Precision   Precision is the extent to which measurements are reliable and repeatable, in other words, the extent of freedom from random error.

Statistical tests and parameters   A parameter is a measurable feature of a population, such as the mean (which, like the median and the mode, is a measure of the location of a value) or a standard deviation (which, like the range and interquartile range, is a measure of dispersion of values). Statistical tests are often designed to calculate the degree to which we can be confident that measures like these (referred to as *estimates*) of parameters of a sample of participants included within a study are reliable and precise. Sometimes the statistical tests involve assessing the 'goodness of fit' between the study sample data and a theoretical probability distribution, such as the normal (Gaussian) distribution.

Type I error rate (alpha)   This is a 'false positive' study conclusion in which the null hypothesis of a test is rejected where in fact no true association exists; it equals the significance level of the statistical test. In other words, if the significance level of a set of study observations is $p=0.05$, the possibility of those observations arising by chance is 5%.

Type II error rate (beta)   This is a 'false negative' study conclusion in which the null hypothesis of a test is accepted where in fact a true association exists. For a given strength of association between study factors, a larger study will have a smaller beta value. Power calculations (see below) are based on achieving an acceptably low chance of failing to detect a true association and so they are related to the beta value.

Statistical power   This is a measure of the study's sensitivity to detect a genuine association or causal relationship and is equal to one minus the Type II error. A power of 90% means a 10% chance (beta=0.1) of failing to detect a true association. Such calculations should be undertaken *before* embarking on a study.

Significance versus importance   In general, it is prudent to reserve the term 'significant' to refer to statistical and analytical elements of a study and to discuss the clinical 'importance' of the findings independently. A large study, for example, might find a statistically significant difference in mean blood pressure outcomes of 2mmHg between two groups, but the clinical importance of this finding would be questionable. Another study might find a 15-point (1 standard deviation) difference in mean developmental quotients between two groups that could be clinically important but is not statistically significant because the study is underpowered or did not enrol sufficient participants before study completion.

Confidence interval (CI)   In classical (frequentist) statistics, a 95% CI is calculated from the sample observations and forms the range of values that would be expected to contain the true parameter value (such as the mean, for example) 95% of the time if repeated on samples from the same population. In other words, the CI provides a measure of the precision of the best estimate of the value of the parameter. This conveys more information about the potential range of size of an association than does a *p*-value. For example, a study of the benefit of universal newborn hearing screening (UNHS) for permanent childhood hearing loss (PCHL) switched the UNHS programme back and forth between pairs of hospitals every few months during the study. It then measured the association between birth at a hospital during a period of UNHS and receptive language skills at a mean follow-up interval of 7.9 years (Kennedy et al. 2006). The adjusted group mean difference (95% CI) between the group mean receptive language z-score of children with PCHL born in periods with UNHS and those born in periods without UNHS was 0.82 (0.31–1.33), *p*=0.004. The 95% CI indicates that the true benefit to receptive language group mean z-score has a 95% chance of falling within the range 0.31 to 1.33. This conveys more information about the potential size of the association range than the *p*-value, which tells you only that the observed benefit had a 0.4% chance of occurring by chance.

Measures of disease frequency   *Prevalence* is the amount of a disease or condition present at a given time. This is often expressed as a proportion, i.e. the number of cases per number in the study population. *Incidence* refers to the number of newly identified cases over a given time and is usually expressed as a rate per unit time. Prevalence and incidence have different relative values for different conditions. Thus, a condition that is long-lasting (like cerebral palsy) will have a higher prevalence relative to its incidence than a condition that is brief and self-limiting. In Table 3.2, *prevalence* is represented by the ratio $(a + c)/(a + b + c + d)$. The prevalence proportion can be used as a *prior probability* for a disease or condition, representing the clinician's belief, informed by baseline data, about the probability that the condition is present before any clinical tests are performed on a patient.

Table 3.2   Contingency table showing relationships between clinical investigation results and the presence or absence of a disease or condition

		Disease or condition		
		Present	Absent	
Test result	Positive	a True positive	b False positive	$a + b$
	Negative	c False negative	d True negative	$c + d$
		$a + c$	$b + d$	$a + b + c + d$

(Reproduced from Nongena et al. 2010 with permission from BMJ Publishing Group Ltd)

Sensitivity   The true positive rate, $a/(a+c)$; the probability that the test result is positive when the disease is present.

Specificity   The true negative rate, $d/(b+d)$; the probability that the test result is negative when the disease is absent.

Positive predictive value   The probability that the disease is present if the test is positive, $a/(a+b)$.

Negative predictive value   The probability that the disease is absent if the test is negative, $d/(c+d)$.

Probabilities   We often think of probabilities in terms of percentages, but they are easier to manipulate mathematically if expressed within the range from 0 to 1, where 0 indicates an event that can never occur and 1 indicates that an event is certain to occur.

Odds and odds ratios   Odds are the ratio of one probability to its complement. The complement of probability p (where p lies in the range $[0 \leq p \leq 1]$ is $(1-p)$.

Likelihood ratios (LRs)   For a positive test, the *positive likelihood ratio* (LR+) is given by (sensitivity)/(1 − specificity); and for a negative test, the *negative likelihood ratio* (LR-) is given by (1 − sensitivity)/(specificity). An example of the application of LRs to indicate the predictive value of particular clinical or imaging features after intraventricular haemorrhage in infancy is given in Table 3.3.

Statistical models   These are mathematical equations that generally describe possible relationships between an outcome (dependent) variable and predictor (explanatory) variables. For example, a *linear regression model* describes a mathematical relationship between an outcome variable (often represented as Y) and the combination of a constant parameter (say a) and one or more predictor variables (X_1, X_2, etc.) that are multiplied by parameters (b_1, b_2, etc.) that are referred to as *regression coefficients*. For example,

$$Y = a + b_1 x_1 + b_2 x_2$$

An example of a relationship that might be simplified (and probably oversimplified) into such a form would be postnatal height in cm (on the y-axis) against age in months (on the x-axis) so that height in cm equals a constant, a (equal to height in cm at birth) plus a coefficient, b, multiplied by x, x in this example being the age in months.

The linear regression method models continuous data that follow a *normal distribution* but there are other statistical regression models for data modelled by other probability distributions. For binary (yes/no) outcome data, for example, we can use a logistic regression model, where the regression coefficients represent estimated values for the logarithm of the odds ratio adjusted for the effects of other predictor variables in that model; in other words, adjusted odds ratios. Similarly, Poisson regression models permit analyses for data describing the rate of events over time. And Cox (proportional hazards) regression models permit analysis of data describing survival times, that is intervals of time to a specific event, such as death or recurrence of an epileptic seizure.

Table 3.3   Prediction of abnormal neuromotor function by cranial ultrasound. An example of an analysis using prior and posterior probabilities

| Ultrasound test result | Pre-test probability | Cerebral palsy | | |
		Likelihood ratios (95% CI)	Post-test probability (95% CI)	Heterogeneity among studies (I^2)
Normal scan	9%	0.5 (0.4—0.7)	5% (4—6%)	90%
Grade 1 or 2 IVH	9%	1 (0.4—3)	9% (4—22%)	88%
Grade 3 IVH	9%	4 (2—8)	26% (13—45%)	82%
Grade 4 haemorrhage (any)	9%	11 (4—31)	53% (29—76%)	84%
Cystic PVL	9%	29 (7—116)	74% (42—92%)	90%
Ventricular dilatation	9%	3 (2—4)	22% (17—28%)	0%
Hydrocephalus	9%	4 (1—13)	27% (10—56%)	97%

(Reproduced from Nongena et al. 2010 with permission)

Normal scan refers to absence of haemorrhage within the brain parenchyma or ventricles, cysts, or ventricular dilation. The grade of intraventricular haemorrhage (IVH) is given according to the Papile classification. Ventricular dilation indicates moderate to severe ventricular dilation not meeting the criterion for hydrocephalus. Hydrocephalus indicates massive ventricular dilation >4mm above the 97th centile. Pre-test probability refers to the prevalence of cerebral palsy based on the EPIPAGE study (Larroque et al. 2008). The likelihood ratio is the probability that a patient with cerebral palsy has a positive test (abnormal ultrasound result). Post-test probability is the probability that a patient with a specific abnormality on cranial ultrasound will have abnormal neuromotor function. Heterogeneity is a measure of similarity between studies and the validity of statistical pooling. PVL, periventricular leukomalacia.

STUDY DESIGN

Observational study   The participants' lifestyle or care pathway is not altered by being part of the study (e.g. the investigator does not determine whether participants receive or do not receive a particular treatment). For an observational study, the investigator observes the outcome of participants after their exposure (or nonexposure) to a particular intervention or lifestyle, such as a surgical procedure, a lifestyle factor (e.g. breastfeeding), or screening for a health condition. The study may be done prospectively or retrospectively. Classic types of observational studies are cohort studies and case–control studies. In observational studies, the intervention is usually being given as part of the standard care pathway and in this respect, the clinical element of the study protocols tends to be simpler.

Interventional study   The participants' exposure to a particular intervention (e.g. care pathway or lifestyle) are influenced by participating in the study. For example, the research protocol determines whether a participant receives a particular intervention, such as a drug, a screening test for a health condition, a surgical procedure, or an alteration of lifestyle (e.g. exercise). These studies are prospective. Clinical trials are the most common type of interventional study. 'Before-and-after studies' are another type of interventional study as they assess participants before and after introducing a particular intervention.

Cohort study   A form of longitudinal study in which a sample group of participants, the cohort of interest, is studied systematically over time with collection of data at more than one point in time. The cohort shares important and relevant common characteristics or a common experience, such as exposure to a suspected risk factor.

Case—control study   A form of study that is usually retrospective but can be prospective and in which participants with a disease or condition are compared with control cases without the disease. Data from such studies can be used to estimate relative risks for exposures or risk factors of interest, but they need to be combined with cohort or population data in order to estimate absolute risks.

Randomization and cluster randomization   Randomization is a process for assigning a treatment intervention to study participants in a predictable and equal way. This is usually an equal chance of receiving an active treatment or a placebo. Cluster randomization is a process in which participants are sampled or given treatments in groups rather than as individuals.

Blinding and masking   These terms are generally used synonymously and refer to the state of knowledge of the study participants, healthcare providers, and investigators assessing outcomes for a randomized intervention. Although terms such as single-blind, double-blind, and triple-blind have been used traditionally, the CONSORT statement (Schulz et al. 2010) recommends instead giving a description of which study members were unaware of treatment assignment.

Systematic reviews and meta-analysis   A systematic review is a method for identifying, collecting, appraising, selecting, and synthesizing published evidence relating to a specific clinical or research question. Where relevant unpublished evidence can be identified, this might also be included in order to reduce the effects of publication bias. Meta-analysis is the body of statistical methods used to combine and summarize the results of relevant studies. It produces summary statistics that, because they contain more data than the original individual studies, usually have greater precision.

Statistical heterogeneity Studies included within a meta-analysis should ideally have been performed using similar definitions and techniques, which would lead them to have statistical estimates that vary solely because of chance variation. In real life, however, it is common for a meta-analysis to show greater variation in the statistical estimates between studies than would have occurred merely by chance, and this phenomenon is referred to as *statistical heterogeneity* or, more simply, as *heterogeneity*.

SOME MYTHS

'Only researchers need to be interested in statistics.'

Most medical research leads to innovations in practice by clinicians other than those undertaking the research. Therefore, all clinicians should have a working knowledge of statistical reasoning.

'P-values are best used to accept or reject a treatment choice.'

In practice, deciding upon a treatment relies on knowledge of estimates of effect size and clinical judgement about the impact and clinical importance of such an effect. CIs convey information about the precision of a study finding that p-values do not.

'There is only one way to approach a clinical study and all factors need to be closely controlled.'

Clinical studies can be performed with an emphasis on one of two paradigms: *efficacy* or *effectiveness*. The former study design attempts to control factors closely, but with the latter design, sometimes referred to as a *pragmatic study*, the emphasis is on real-world effects that might include factors such as diagnostic misclassification and non-adherence to treatment in some study participants.

APPROACHES TO EBM

You can add EBM activities to your clinical practice, especially if you meet with your colleagues to incorporate small-group learning that is directly relevant to your clinical context (Al Achkar and Davies, 2016).

In the final chapter of their book on practising and teaching EBM, Straus et al. (2019) suggest methods that fall into one of three teaching modes: (1) role modelling evidence-based practice; (2) weaving evidence into teaching clinical medicine; and (3) targeting specific EBM skills. Alongside those teaching modes they suggest the 10 situations that are most likely to lead to success in teaching EBM:

1. When it centres on real clinical decisions and action.

2. When it focuses on learners' actual learning needs.

3. When it balances passive ('diastolic') with active ('systolic') learning.

4. When it connects 'new' knowledge to 'old' knowledge (what learners already know).

5. When it involves everyone on the team.

6. When it attends to all four domains of learning: affective, cognitive, conative (i.e. involving the will to perform an act), and psychomotor.

7. When it matches and takes advantage of the clinical setting, available time, and other circumstances.

8. When it balances preparedness with opportunism.

9. When it makes explicit how to make judgements, whether about the evidence itself or about how to integrate evidence with other knowledge, clinical expertise, and patient preferences and circumstances.

10. When it builds learners' lifelong learning abilities.

They also suggest 10 ways in which to make it fail (but those are not reproduced here) and 10 ways in which to teach EBM in clinical teams and small groups.

With appropriate strategies, EBM and teaching activities can be incorporated into all sorts of rounds (such as admission rounds, morning reports or handover rounds, and specific teaching rounds) and into the various outpatient settings. It is also helpful to incorporate EBM into specific learning environments, such as journal clubs, team case discussions, and morbidity and mortality meetings (Das, Malick, and Khan, 2008). And, of course, whenever we are teaching, we are also learning.

The four steps of EBM

Step 1: Formulating clear clinical questions

A combination of clinical questions will be well structured if it considers both the 'background' and a more specific 'foreground' (Straus et al. 2019). The background question will have a question root (who, what, where, when, how, why) with a verb; and an area of healthcare that is the main focus, such as disorder, test, or specific treatment. An example background question is: 'What is the best treatment of infantile spasms?'

Foreground questions search out specific knowledge and draw upon four essential components, which can be remembered using the PICO acronym (Haroon and Phillips, 2009).

Patient, population, predicament, or problem.
Intervention, exposure, test, or other agent.
Comparison intervention, exposure, or test (or comparator or control).
Outcomes of clinical importance, often considering time factors.

Therefore, the foreground question might become, for example: 'In infants presenting with epileptic spasms (P), does vigabatrin (I), compared with prednisolone or tetracosactide (C) lead to better seizure control and neurodevelopmental outcomes (O)?'.

There are some variations in this model. While PICO is suited to quantitative studies, qualitative research designs might use PICo:

Population, problem, or patient.
Interest (activity, event, experience, or process).
Context (setting or distinct characteristics).

The SPICE and SPIDER models might work well for quantitative or qualitative studies:

SPICE	SPIDER
Setting	Sample
Population or Perspective	Phenomenon of
Intervention	Interest
Comparison	Design
Evaluation	Evaluation
	Research type

The effectiveness of these models upon the quality of search strategies has itself been subject to systematic review (Eriksen and Frandsen, 2018).

Step 2: Finding appropriate evidence

As EBM and, more broadly, evidence-based healthcare and evidence-based practice, have become established, there is now more ready access to relevant evidence that has already been subject to some degree of aggregation and appraisal. A well-established approach has been to grade evidence as having increasing quality in the following order:

- Lowest quality: expert opinion, non-EBM guidelines, and general background information.

- Moderate quality: individual case reports, observational studies, and case series.

- Higher quality: experimental studies, with non-RCTs being inferior to RCTs.

- Best quality: critical appraisal of the literature leading to evidence-based practice guidelines, systematic reviews, and meta-analyses.

However, although systematic reviews, with or without meta-analysis, have tended to be considered the criterion standard in terms of evidence quality, their position in this hierarchy has been challenged (Murad et al. 2016) because:

- the process of a rigorous systematic review can take years to complete and findings can therefore be superseded by more recent evidence;

- the methodological rigor and strength of findings must be appraised by the reader before being applied to patients;

- a large, well-conducted RCT may provide more convincing evidence than a systematic review of smaller RCTs.

Step 3: Synthesizing and evaluating the evidence

As the quality and range of EBM evidence has grown, other pyramids of quality have been developed, with one recent version, the evidence-based healthcare pyramid 5.0, focusing more exclusively on pre-appraised evidence and guidance (Alper and Haynes, 2016). In that pyramid, evidence is graded in the following order of increasing quality and usefulness:

1. Studies (with synopses and filtered views).

2. Systematic reviews (also with synopses and filtered views).

3. Systematically derived recommendations (guidelines with syntheses of information from levels 1 and 2).

4. Synthesized summaries (integrating the content of the three lower levels in order to meet the needs of clinical reference).

5. Systems (in which the evidence and guidance from the four lower levels is integrated within electronic health records and computerized decision support systems).

Within this hierarchy of research evidence, most of the papers available on MEDLINE (PubMed) are excluded (or not yet included) because they have not been subject to the process of pre-appraisal for clinical relevance and quality. Systematic reviews should now conform to the recommendations of the Preferred Reporting Items for Systematic Reviews and Meta-Analyses (PRISMA) statement (Moher et al. 2009), which provides a structured checklist that ensures easier navigation of such reviews. One important source of such reviews is the Cochrane Library.

Although it is the responsibility of the clinician to make a specific decision for a particular patient, evidence has sometimes been organized into a user-friendly guideline. Guidelines are available from institutions in many countries. These include, for example, those at the UK National Institute for Health and Care Excellence (NICE) (e.g. www.nice.org.uk/guidance/ng127/chapter/Recommendations-for-children-aged-under-16), the Scottish Intercollegiate Guidelines Network (SIGN) (e.g. www.sign.ac.uk/sign-145-assessment,-diagnosis-and-interventions-for-autism-spectrum-disorders), and the Policy and Guidelines section of the American Academy of Neurology, which has a section on child neurology (www.aan.com/Guidelines/home/ByTopic?topicId=14). There are a number of resources which, with varying degrees of scope, currency, and quality, provide synthesized summaries at Level 4 of this model. These include BMJ Best Practice, DynaMed Plus, and UpToDate (Alper and Haynes, 2016).

Level 5 of the evidence-based healthcare pyramid 5.0 is being developed as Evidence-Based Medicine electronic Decision Support system (EBMeDS), creating a scenario in which the healthcare practitioner would no longer need to initiate a search because it would have been made by the computerized system. This systems approach has been subject to an RCT in primary healthcare (Kortteisto et al. 2014).

In terms of evaluating the quality of evidence and strength of recommendations, many organizations now use the GRADE system. In the first of five articles on the GRADE system, Guyatt et al. (2008) stated that: 'Not all grading systems separate decisions regarding the quality of evidence from strength of recommendations. Those that fail to do so create confusion. High quality evidence doesn't necessarily imply strong recommendations, and strong recommendations can arise from low quality evidence'. As an example, they cite the case of treating infants and children with chicken pox with either aspirin or paracetamol. Even though there is only weak evidence that aspirin causes harm (Reye syndrome) in this situation, the fact that paracetamol is considered safe and to have a similar treatment effect leads to a strong recommendation that it is used in place of aspirin.

Depending upon the scope and focus of the original clinical question, full evaluation of the evidence usually requires consideration of the synthesized data from the guideline or systematic review as well as some consideration of the data and arguments from some of the original papers. Factors to consider include the following:

- Are the conclusion and message important, credible, and consistent with other research in this area?

- Are there any ethical or design problems with the research?

- Are the study objectives and methods clear?

- Are there any sources of funding that might bias the reporting and conclusions?

- Are there any authorial competing interests that might affect the authenticity and reliability of the research?

Step 4: Applying the evidence to your specific clinical question

Having acquired and appraised appropriate evidence, it is necessary to decide upon the best way of 'integrating EBM with clinical judgment, taking into account clinical circumstances, choices and values' (Malick, Das, and Khan, 2008). At this level, one needs to consider, among other things, the beliefs and values of the patient. In deciding about the applicability of the search findings to a specific patient, the clinician needs to consider the following questions:

1. Is the patient so different from those reported in the studies that the results do not apply?

2. Is the treatment feasible and appropriate to my setting?

3. What are the likely benefits and harms from the intervention?

4. How do the values and beliefs of my patient or the family influence my decision?

EBM in practice

There are many areas of paediatric neurology in which there are few RCTs and where other study designs provide less strong evidence. Therefore, it is often necessary to appraise an individual study or a small number of studies and to extrapolate to the specific case in question. This means that it remains important to continually sharpen the skill of critically appraising a paper (Greenhalgh, 2014).

One useful distinction in EBM is that between *primary studies* and *integrative studies* (Oxman et al. 1993). A **primary study** might have a focus on *therapy, diagnosis,* the *risk of harm* (side effects), or *prognosis*. Before deciding upon the usefulness of such studies, the reader might wish to ask questions assessing the validity and value of such studies with questions such as:

- Was assignment to treatment groups randomized?

- Were all enrolled study participants followed up reliably?

- Was the diagnostic test compared with some form of reference (criterion) standard?

- If there were harms, were exposures assessed similarly in all of the groups being studied?

- Was follow-up sufficiently long and complete?

Integrative studies might be an *overview* or *systematic review, practice guidelines,* a *decision analysis,* or an *economic analysis.* Relevant questions to address to such studies might include:

- Was the review question clearly focused?

- Were the articles undergoing review selected in an appropriate fashion?

- Was there a clear and transparent process behind the choice of outcome measures and how the evidence was combined?

- Did the decision analysis address a clinically important question in a fashion that reflects that actual process of clinical decision-making?

- Were any estimates of probabilities and utilities (positive value to the patient or the healthcare system) based upon valid and reliable evidence?

- Did the economic analysis compare clearly described alternatives?

Useful examples of EBM in practice are regularly published in the paediatric literature. For example, McGovern et al. (2019) present the scenario of a 3-week-old infant with a corrected gestational age of 27 weeks in whom a blood culture grows a coagulase-negative staphylococcus (CONS). One of the doctors on the ward round asks about the possible neurodevelopmental consequences of this finding, which leads to the following structured question: 'Do preterm neonates (patient) requiring treatment for CONS sepsis (intervention) have poorer neurodevelopmental outcomes (outcome) compared with neonates without sepsis (comparison)?' The article describes details of the specific search terms used on databases within the Cochrane Library and on PubMed and how this identifies seven relevant studies (one systematic review and meta-analysis, four prospective cohort studies, one retrospective cohort study, and one case—control study). The key features of these studies' design and results are tabulated and a commentary provides a context for all the findings. On the basis of their search and appraisal, the authors conclude that there is grade B evidence linking CONS sepsis with later developmental impairment.

There are many online tools that help the practitioner to practice EBM. For example, the Centre for Evidence-Based Medicine in Oxford provides critical appraisal tools and the Critical Appraisal Skills Programme (CASP) has a collection of editable appraisal checklists for reviews, RCTs, cohort studies, case—control studies, economic evaluations, diagnostic studies, qualitative studies, and clinical prediction rules. These are included in the Resources section below.

SUMMARY AND CONCLUSION

Clinical epidemiology and EBM underpin all good clinical practice. In all clinical practice, quality and improvement are dependent upon appropriate research and innovation. Clinical epidemiology and EBM provide the basic tools for organizing our thinking and for designing, performing, and interpreting such research. Interpreting clinical studies and other clinical information is as important as producing the original studies, and there are now many sources of synthesized evidence and guidelines and online tools that assist with the process of critical appraisal.

ACKNOWLEDGEMENTS

I thank Clare Thornally and Tom Osborne at the Department of Library and Knowledge Services, University Hospitals Bristol NHS Foundation Trust for their useful suggestions on new developments in evidence-based practice.

REFERENCES

Al Achkar M, Davies MK (2016) A small group learning model for evidence-based medicine. *Adv Med Educ Pract* 7: 611—615.

Alper BS, Haynes RB (2016) EBHC pyramid 5.0 for accessing preappraised evidence and guidance. *Evid Based Med* 21: 123—125.

Das K, Malick S, Khan KS (2008) Tips for teaching evidence-based medicine in a clinical setting: lessons from adult learning theory. Part one. *J Soc Med* 101: 493—500.

Eriksen MB, Frandsen TF (2018) The impact of patient, intervention, comparison, outcome (PICO) as a search strategy tool on literature search quality: a systematic review. *J Med Libr Assoc* 106: 420—431.

Greenhalgh T (2014) *How to Read a Paper: the Basics of Evidence-based Medicine* (5th edition). Oxford: John Wiley and Sons.

Guyatt GH, Oxman AD, Vist GE, et al. (2008) GRADE: an emerging consensus on rating quality of evidence and strength of recommendations. *BMJ* 336: 924—926.

Haroon M, Phillips R (2009) 'There is nothing like looking if you want to find something' — asking questions and searching for answers — the evidence-based approach. *Arch Dis Child Educ Pract Ed* 95: 34—39.

Hill AB (1965) The environment and disease: association or causation?*Proc R Soc Med* 258: 295—300.

Kennedy CR, McCann DC, Campbell MJ, et al. (2006) Language ability after early detection of permanent childhood hearing impairment. *N Engl J Med* 354: 2131—2141.

Kortteisto T, Raitanen J, Komulainen J, et al. (2014) Patient-specific computer-based decision support in primary healthcare — a randomized trial. *Implementation Sci* 9: 15.

Larroque B, Ancel PY, Marret S, et al. (2008). EPIPAGE Study group. Neurodevelopmental disabilities and special care of 5-year-old children born before 33 weeks of gestation (the EPIPAGE study): a longitudinal cohort study. *Lancet* 371: 813—820.

Malick S, Das K, Khan KS (2008) Tips for teaching evidence-based medicine in a clinical setting: lessons from adult learning theory. Part two. *J R Soc Med* 101: 536—543.

McGovern M, Flynn L, Coyne S, Molloy EJ (2019) Question 2: Does coagulase negative staphylococcal sepsis cause neurodevelopmental delay in preterm infants. *Arch Dis Child* 104: 97—100.

Moher D, Liberati A, Tetzlaff J, Altman DG, and the PRISMA Group (2009) Preferred reporting items for systematic reviews and meta-analyses: the PRISMA statement. *J Clin Epidemiol* 62: 1006—1012.

Murad MH, Asi N, Alsawas M, Alahdab F (2016) New evidence pyramid. *Evid Based Med* 21: 125—127.

Nongena P, Ederies A, Azzopardi DV, Edwards AD (2010) Confidence in the prediction of neuro developmental outcome by cranial ultrasound and MRI in term infants. *Arch Dis Child Fetal Neonatal Ed* 95: F388—F390.

Oxman AD, Sackett DL, Guyatt GH for the Evidence-Based Medicine Working Group (1993) Users' guides to the medical literature: I. How to get started. *J Am Med Assoc* 270: 2093—2095.

Paul JR (1938) Clinical epidemiology. *J Clin Invest* 17: 539—541.

Sackett DL (1979) Bias in analytic research. *J Chronic Dis* 32:51—63.

Sackett DL, Rosenberg WM, Gray JA, et al. (1996). Evidence-based medicine: what it is and what it isn't. *BMJ* 312: 71—72.

Schulz KF, Altman DG, Moher D, CONSORT Group (2010) CONSORT 2010 statement: updated guidelines for reporting parallel group randomised trials. *BMJ* 340: 698—702.

Sterne JAC, Egger M (2001) Funnel plots for detecting bias in meta-analysis: guidelines on choice of axis. *J Clin Epidemiol* 54: 1046—1055.

Straus SE, Glasziou P, Richardson WS, Haynes R (2019) *Evidence-Based Medicine: How to Practice and Teach EBM* (5th edition). Amsterdam: Elsevier Health Sciences.

Resources

BMJ Best Practice: https://www.bestpractice.bmj.com/info/

Critical Appraisal Skills Programme (CASP): https://www.casp-uk.net/casp-tools-checklists/

Centre for Evidence-Based Medicine Critical Appraisal tools: http://www.cebm.net/2014/06/critical-appraisal/

Cochrane Library: www.cochranelibrary.com/

DynaMed Plus: https://www.dynamed.com/

Garrido MV, Kristensen K, Nielsen CP, Busse R (2008) *Health Technology Assessment and Health Policy-making in Europe.* Copenhagen: WHO.

Greenhalgh T (2019) *How to read a paper: the basics of evidence-based medicine* (6th edition). Oxford, John Wiley and Sons, 2019. (This book provides a concise and insightful overview of EBM).

Hunink M, Glasziou P (2001) *Decision Making in Health and Medicine: Integrating Evidence and Values*. Cambridge: Cambridge University Press.

Medical Calculator (MDCalc): https://www.mdcalc.com/ebm-guide#glossaryand links to other useful resources https://www.mdcalc.com/ebm-guide#evidence(accessed January 2019). (An EBM Guide is available on the app MDCalc, with a glossary of terms).

UpToDate: https://www.uptodate.com/home

CHAPTER 4

Promoting child development

Audrone Prasauskiene

Key messages

- Care for the development of the child should start long before conception.
- The infant in isolation does not exist — look at the family.
- The main obstacle to reaching goals is not lack of money; it is almost always a lack of imagination and knowledge.

Common errors

- Not listening to the parents' and carers' concerns.
- Seeing the development of the child as a purely medical problem.
- Blaming parents.

When to worry

- When the child starts losing his/her skills at any age.
- When parents deny developmental problems of their child.
- When parents avoid developmental screenings, vaccinations, or feeding recommendations.
- When parents are too engaged in 'treating' (requesting medications, hospitalizations, complicated assessments, etc.) an early developmental impairment/disorder.

There are several definitions of child development. Depending on their background, researchers, professionals, educators, and lay people describe it as:

- the sequence of physical, language, thought, and emotional changes that occur in a child from birth to the beginning of adulthood (Nikolova and Georgiev, 2017);

- the patterns of growth, change, and stability that occur from conception through adolescence that are amenable to scientific study (Punjabi, 2015);

- a product of the continuous dynamic interactions of the child and the experience provided by his or her social settings (Sameroff, 2009);

- the process that ends when the child invites his/her parents for dinner at a restaurant and pays the bill (author unknown).

Opinions vary as to whether development starts at conception or at birth and when it ends, but we have to agree that it is a dynamic process of change, extending throughout childhood and far beyond. Developmental changes follow an orderly pattern that enhances survival and becomes more complex.

Childhood may be divided into five age-related stages:

- *Prenatal:* from conception to birth;

- *Infancy and toddlerhood:* birth to 2 years;

- *Early childhood:* 2 to 6 years;

- *Middle childhood:* 6 to 12 years;

- *Adolescence:* 12 to 19 years.

Development is divided into several domains of function: gross motor, fine motor, social, emotional, language, and cognition. Within each of these domains, there are developmental sequences of age-related functional changes leading to particular milestones. For example, in language development the child starts cooing during the first 3 months, coos and babbles at age 4 to 6 months, and starts to use gestures and say one or two words at age 7 to 12 months.

An understanding of child development permits the paediatric professional to detect delay or the emergence of unusual behaviours in early development and to discuss their observations and concerns with the parents. The development of the child has intrigued philosophers and researchers for centuries. In the medieval period (6th–15th centuries), children were seen and treated as undersized adults: they were dressed like an adult, could be married, and had to work. In the 16th century attitudes to children and childhood started to change: puritan religion proclaimed that children were born evil and must be civilized, so children were raised based on that belief. In the 17th century, the idea evolved that children develop in response to nurturing. In the 18th century, Jean-Jacques Rousseau developed the notion of stages of development. In the 19th century, Charles Darwin developed his theories of natural selection and survival of the fittest. He also made parallels between human and animal prenatal growth. In the 20th century, psychoanalytical, behavioural and social learning, biological, cognitive, and developmental systems theories about children's development expanded around the world. Childhood received special attention, and international and national laws protecting children came into existence. Based on these and other theories, biopsychosocial models of development were created that recognize the importance of internal (biological) and external (environmental) factors for child development.

The internal and external factors related to child development cannot be analysed separately; they interact and change over time. Mackay et al. (2016) linked nationwide records of education (annual pupil census) and maternity (Scottish Morbidity Record 02) databases for 801 592 singleton children attending Scottish schools in 2006 to 2011. They found cyclicity in the rates of children with special educational needs: the highest (8.9%) among the children conceived in the first quarter of the year (January–March) and lowest (7.6%) among those conceived in the third quarter (July–September). Seasonal variations were specific to autism spectrum disorder (ASD), intellectual disabilities, and learning difficulties (e.g. dyslexia) and were absent for sensory or motor/physical impairments and mental, physical, or communication problems (Mackay et al. 2016).

BRAIN DEVELOPMENT

Brain development encompasses several stages (see Box 4.1) that can be divided into two phases (Kolb et al. 2011) as follows:

1. The genetically determined sequence of events in utero that can be modulated by the maternal environment.

2. Pre- and postnatal periods when the connectivity of the brain is very sensitive to the environment and to the patterns of brain activity produced by experiences.

Stage of neurogenesis

The nervous system begins to form about 3 weeks after fertilization. The neural tube contains cells that will later form the central nervous system. At about 6 weeks' gestation, neural stem cells become elongated to form radial glial cells in the area called the subventricular zone, adjacent to the central fluid-filled cavity of the neural tube, and divide to produce intermediate neuronal precursors and neurons. These migrate radially over long distances to form the cortical plate, which will become the central cortex. At about 14 weeks, the brain has its outline shape, but as yet does not have

---

Box 4.1 Stages of brain development

1. Cell birth (neurogenesis, gliogenesis)
2. Cell migration
3. Cell differentiation
4. Cell maturation (dendrite and axon growth)
5. Synaptogenesis (formation of synapses)
6. Cell death and synaptic pruning
7. Myelogenesis (formation of myelin)

(Adapted from Kolb et al. 2011 with permission from the Canadian Academy of Child and Adolescent Psychiatry)

---

sulci or gyri. The process of neurogenesis is very intense: at its peak, about 250 000 neurons are produced per minute and it is largely complete by 5 months' gestation. Neuroscientists used to believe that the central nervous system was incapable of neurogenesis and unable to regenerate. However, stem cells were discovered in parts of the adult brain in the 1990s and adult neurogenesis is now accepted to be a normal process that occurs in the healthy brain.

Stages of migration and differentiation

In the stage of migration, neurons start to migrate from the subventricular zone to the cortex, following pathways formed by the fibres of radial glial cells. The subventricular region appears to have a map of the cortex that predisposes the cells formed in a specific area of the subventricular zone to move to a particular cortical area. Those cells are stem cells, and they can develop into neural or glial progenitor cells that can migrate into cerebral white or grey matter, even in adulthood. As they reach their destination point, the interaction of genes, maturation, and environmental influences determine their differentiation into a particular cell type. At the same time, the *maturation stage* starts: cells begin to mature by growing dendrites and extending the axons necessary for synapse formation. Dendrite formation begins prenatally and continues after birth.

During the *stage of synaptogenesis*, more than 100 000 trillion (10^{14}) synapses are formed. The peak of synapse formation is at the age of 1 to 2 years. Dendrites and spines demonstrate high plasticity in response to experience and can form synapses hours and minutes after the experiences (Greenough and Chang, 1989). In the next stage of cell death and synaptic pruning, overproduced cells and synapses that were not involved in the forming of cerebral circuitry are eliminated. In some areas, this process lasts until age 20 years and correlates with behavioural development.

The final step of brain development is the stage of *myelogenesis*. Although axons can function before myelination, normal function can be attained only after myelination is complete. This continues until the age of 18 years in some brain regions.

The developing brain is very plastic and susceptible to the effects of environmental factors. There is enough scientific evidence now to show that epigenetic changes, which can be defined as changes in developmental outcomes, including regulation of gene expression by mechanisms other than change in the DNA itself (Blumberg, Freeman, and Robinson, 2010), affect developmental outcome. Importantly, some of those mechanisms react to environmental changes only in a specific time window. These periods are called critical or 'sensitive'. The evolution of sensitive periods, according to the age and neurodevelopmental stage of the individual (Thompson and Nelson, 2001), is illustrated in an often cited diagram of the developmental course of human brain development (Figure 4.1). The busiest time for human brain development is the first 1000 days of life when all stages of the development start and most of them end. This provides the foundation for the development of language, vision, hearing, cognition, and movement. For example, for the successful development of language, the child has to be exposed to verbal communication with other human beings (not with television, computers, or tablets). If the child is born deaf and his/her hearing loss is not corrected before the age of 2.5 to 3 years, he/she will probably never develop fluent language. Likewise, if a child born with a visual problem that prevents him/her from seeing (e.g. cataracts) is not diagnosed and treated early enough, the child will develop amblyopia ('lazy eye') as a result of the lack of visual stimulus in the specific period of development of visual circuits.

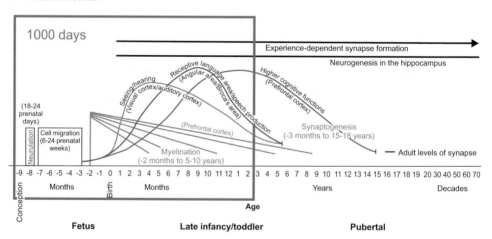

Figure 4.1 The course of human brain development. (Adapted from Thompson and Nelson, 2001 with permission from the American Psychological Association.) A colour version of this figure can be seen in the colour plate section.

FACTORS THAT AFFECT THE DEVELOPMENT OF THE CHILD AND HIS/HER BRAIN

Sensory and motor experiences

Multiple studies on animals show that raising them in severely deprived environments has a deleterious effect on their development, including poor mental and physical health and atypical social functioning, and that enriched environments have the reverse effect. Studies on children that were raised in institutions show similar developmental outcomes. Researchers from the Bucharest Early Intervention Project studied the effects of foster and institutional care on the development of 136 children aged 7 to 33 months. The study showed that the developmental quotient of children who had never been institutionalized was around 100. Children placed in foster care had a higher developmental quotient than those who were institutionalized. Children taken from the institution and placed into foster care before age 24 months had a higher developmental quotient (see Box 4.2) at 54 months than those placed after 24 months (Nelson et al. 2014, McLaughlin et al. 2015). Institutionalization early in life was associated with decreased executive function performance, increased deficits in working memory, and response inhibition typical of attention-deficit/hyperactivity disorder (ADHD) (Tibu et al. 2016) and alterations in white matter microstructure throughout the brain, specifically involving the body of the corpus callosum, cingulum, fornix, anterior and superior corona radiata, external capsule, retrolenticular internal capsule, and medial lemniscus. The foster care group did not significantly differ from the never-institutionalized group in measurements of these tracts, except for the body of the corpus callosum and superior corona radiata (Bick et al. 2015).

Box 4.2   Calculating the developmental quotient

Developmental quotient (%) = (Developmental age/Biological age) × 100

For example: an infant born at term whose developmental age is 6 months (child sits independently) and postnatal age is 12 months has a motor developmental quotient of 50%.

Institutionalization currently remains a powerful influence on child development throughout Europe. According to the World Health Organization (WHO) (Figure 4.2), there are still children aged 0 to 2 years living in institutions (WHO, 2018). The report also reveals information about hospitalization, which can equally lead to neglect, overuse of medications, and unnecessary medical procedures, etc. Hospitalization rates vary widely within the region and by age group. The lowest hospitalization rate for children under 5 years was 25 per 10 000 in Portugal and the highest, 570 per 10 000, in the Republic of Moldova, with a subregional average of 252 per 10 000. In the 5 to 9 years

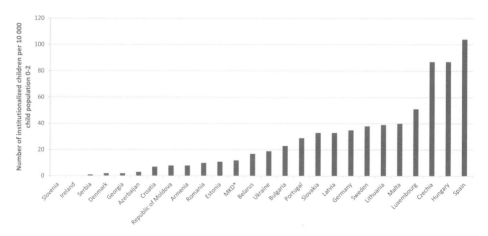

Figure 4.2 Rates of 0–2-year-old children in institutional care, per 10 000. *MKD: the former Yugoslav Republic of Macedonia (MKD is an abbreviation of the ISO). (Reprinted from WHO, 2018. Licence: CC BY-NC-SA 3.0 IGO.)

group, the lowest rate was 15 per 10 000 in Norway and the highest 188 per 10 000 in Lithuania, with a subregional average of 83 per 10 000 (WHO, 2018).

Multiple studies by Greenough and Chang (1989), Kolb (1995), and others, on the effect of enriched environments on animal development have revealed that visual or tactile stimuli or environments providing opportunities for complex play and movement increase brain size, cortical thickness, neuron size, dendritic branching, spine density, synapses per neuron, number and complexity of glia, and vascular arborization. These changes in brain organization were related to enhancement of skilled motor performance and spatial learning.

Parent–child relationships

Infants can survive physically and psychologically only in the context of their social relationships. So, during their development, infants have to learn to identify, remember, and prefer their caregivers.

Therefore, parent–child relationships are critical and play a key role in brain development. Differences in the nature of early mother and infant relations and interactions shape long-term developmental outcomes that persist into adulthood (Myers et al. 1989). The effect of maternal-newborn infant skin-to-skin contact using kangaroo care was examined in 73 infants born preterm. The findings demonstrated reduced maternal anxiety, increased maternal attachment, and long-term impact on the children's physiological organization and behavioural control at age 10 years (Feldman, Rosenthal, and Eidelman, 2014).

The first year of life is critical for the baby to acquire gross motor skills, such as gaining head control, ability to roll, crawl, sit, stand and walk, to explore an environment efficiently. There are numerous infant carriers for parents to place infants safely into, such as slings and backpacks, nursing pillows or cushions, floor seats, car seats and high chairs, jumpers or walkers, and infant swings. All these items can be seen as 'containers'. Extended time spent in this equipment may cause developmental and other health issues currently dubbed 'container baby syndrome'.

Time spent at a screen (television, tablet, or phone) is another example of potentially extended time spent 'in' and 'with' new technical devices with a consequent reduction in communication and play. Data from a study on 2441 children revealed that higher levels of screen time at 24 months and 36 months were significantly associated with lower, not higher, performance on developmental screening tests at 36 months (Madigan et al. 2019). The American Academy of Paediatrics in 2016 and WHO in 2019 released guidelines regarding safe maximum time for a child to spend at a screen to avoid deprivation of social interaction and to increase quality time for the child and his parents. The American Academy of Paediatrics guidelines recommend that children aged less than 18 months should avoid screens, other than video chats, and that children aged less than 2 years should only be exposed to 'high-quality programming' with educational value that can be watched with a parent to help the child understand what they are seeing (Council on Communications and Media, 2016). WHO guidelines recommend that children under 1 year should not be exposed to screens at all, that children under 5 years of age should not spend more than one hour per day watching screens and that less is better (WHO, 2019).

Psychoactive substances

Prenatal exposure of the fetus to alcohol has a damaging effect on brain development. The child born to a mother drinking any kind of alcohol at any time during pregnancy is at increased risk of learning difficulties, ADHD, behavioural problems, and multiple defects in other systems. Those children also have a specific phenotype (see Chapter 26). Studies in rats have shown that psychostimulants, such as amphetamine or methylphenidate, alter the development of the prefrontal cortex and are related to behavioural abnormalities later in life (Kolb et al. 2011). Children may also be exposed to antipsychotics, antidepressants, and anxiolytics in the prenatal period. These medications have a damaging effect on cortical development (Kolb et al. 2011). The recent systematic review by Yeoh et al. (2019) revealed that prenatal opioid use had a negative impact on cognitive and motor development discernible as early as 6 months after birth and persisting into adulthood.

Poverty and stunting

The number of children younger than 5 years living in low- and middle-income countries at risk of not attaining their developmental potential because of extreme poverty

---

Box 4.3 WHO guidelines on physical activity, sedentary behaviour, and sleep for children under 5 years of age

Infants (less than 1 year) should:

☑ **Be physically active several times a day in a variety of ways**, particularly through interactive floor-based play; more is better. For those not yet mobile, this includes **at least 30 minutes in prone position** (tummy time) spread throughout the day while awake.

☑ **Not be restrained for more than 1 hour at a time** (e.g. prams/strollers, high chairs, or strapped on a caregiver's back). Screen time is not recommended. When sedentary, engaging in reading and storytelling with a caregiver is encouraged.

☑ Have 14—17 hours (0—3 months of age) or 12—16 hours (4—11 months of age) of good quality sleep, including naps.

Children 1—2 years of age should:

☑ **Spend at least 180 minutes in a variety of types of physical activities at any intensity**, including moderate-to-vigorous-intensity physical activity, spread throughout the day; more is better.

☑ **Not be restrained for more than 1 hour at a time** (e.g. prams/strollers, high chairs, or strapped on a caregiver's back) or sit for extended periods of time. **For 1-year-olds, sedentary screen time (such as watching television or videos, playing computer games) is not recommended. For those aged 2 years, sedentary screen time should be no more than 1 hour per day; less is better.** When sedentary, engaging in reading and storytelling with a caregiver is encouraged.

☑ **Have 11—14 hours of good quality sleep**, including naps, with regular sleep and wake-up times.

Children 3—4 years of age should:

☑ **Spend at least 180 minutes per day in a variety of types of physical activities** at any intensity, of which at least 60 minutes is of moderate to vigorous intensity physical activity, spread throughout the day; more is better.

☑ **Not be restrained for more than 1 hour at a time** (e.g. prams/strollers) or sit for extended periods of time. **Sedentary screen time should be no more than 1 hour per day; less is better.** When sedentary, engaging in reading and storytelling with a caregiver is encouraged.

☑ **Have 10—13 hours of good quality sleep**, which may include a nap, with regular sleep and wake-up times.

(Reproduced from WHO, 2019. Licence: CC BY-NC-SA 3.0 IGO)

---

and growth disorder remains as high as 43% (Black et al. 2017). Poverty is related to lower language and cognitive functioning at 1 year and has even greater deleterious effects at 3 years and 5 years (Rubio-Codina et al. 2015). Poverty was mainly related to socioeconomic status (SES) (parents' education, home environment) and postnatal growth during the first 2 years of life. Later stunting was found to be less related to cognitive function, but positive changes in the home environment had a beneficial effect on neurodevelopmental progress by 63 months of age (Hamadani et al. 2014). Changes in the poverty level after age 36 months still affect cognitive development and executive function (Hackman et al. 2015). A study in the 1960s by Hart and Risley (2003) provides a striking example of how the SES of a family may affect child development. They followed 42 families for 2.5 years and found that 86% to 98% of the words used by each child by the age of 3 years was derived from their parents' vocabularies. The children also used nearly identical words and that the number of words and the speech patterns were similar to those of their caregivers. They also found that children from lower SES families (families on welfare) heard about 616 words per hour, children from middle/lower SES families heard 1251 words per hour, and those from higher SES (professional) families heard 2153 words per hour. Higher SES families provided their children with far more words of praise (ratio of six encouragements for every discouragement) compared to children from low-income families (two encouragements to one discouragement). In that study, the developmental level of a child at age 3 years was highly predictive of functioning at the ages of 9 years and 10 years on various vocabulary, language development, and reading comprehension measures.

Their study thus showed that a child from a high SES family would experience 30 million more words within the first 4 years of life than a child from a low SES family, more words of encouragement (560 000 vs 125 000 words) and fewer words of discouragement. These differences increase over time as does the resulting benefit to the vocabulary of the child (Figure 4.3 and Figure 4.4) (Hart and Risley, 2003).

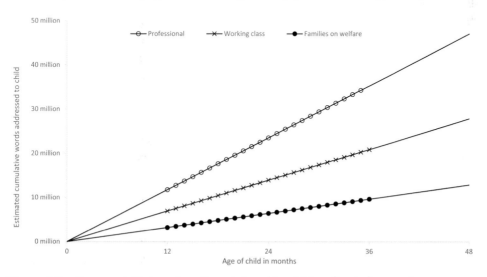

Figure 4.3 The cumulative number of words heard by children (by age) across income groups. (Reprinted from Hart and Risley, 2003.)

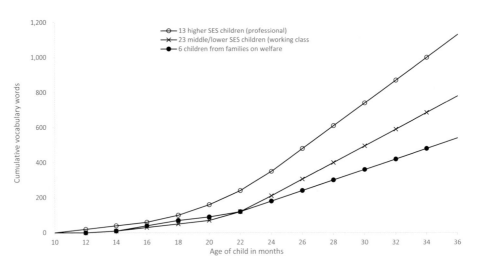

Figure 4.4 The cumulative number of words used by a child (vocabulary) by age across the income groups. SES, socioeconomic status. (Reprinted from Hart and Risley, 2003.)

Stress

The term 'stress' was coined by Hans Selye in 1936 and refers to 'the nonspecific response of the body to any demand. A stressor is an agent that produces stress at any time' (Selye 1976). A typically developing brain, developing in a child-friendly environment, learns to handle stressful experiences. Stress can be positive (infrequent, short, and mild, eliciting normal response, necessary for a child's development), tolerable (more severe, frequent, or sustained, all systems recover if adversity is buffered by carers), or toxic (intense, persistent and/or prolonged adversity, such as physical or emotional abuse, chronic neglect, caregiver substance abuse or mental illness, exposure to violence, and/or the accumulated burdens of family economic hardship, without adequate adult support).

Prolonged, or caused by multiple adversities, toxic stress might cause cumulative damage to the individual's physical and mental health all his/her life. The more adverse experiences the child has during his/her life, the higher the risk he/she has for developmental delays and later health problems.

The more adverse experiences in childhood, the higher the likelihood of developmental delays, immune dysregulation followed by increased risk and frequency of infections in childhood and later health problems, including alcoholism, chronic obstructive pulmonary disease, depression, cancer, obesity, increase in suicide attempts, and ischemic heart disease. Research indicates that awareness of early childhood adversity risk and resultant downstream effects of toxic stress is critical. Prevention must begin early with the targeting of at-risk populations. Protection of children from toxic stress requires a multifaceted approach, including interventions that will target the child, the caregiver, and the environment. Strengthening the stability of the family, as well as the community, affords environmental protection against the effects of toxic stress in childhood (Franke, 2014).

Effect of multiple negative factors

In many cases, several negative factors coexist in a child's life and, therefore, their adverse impact on the child's development is much more evident. In 2008, a group of researchers on behalf of the US Department of Health and Human Services released a report 'Developmental Status and Early Intervention Service Needs of Maltreated Children' (Barth et al. 2007). The authors analysed the data from their own study as well. They found that 55% of maltreated children aged 0 to 3 years had at least five risk factors associated with developmental problems. Specific risk factors that were examined (with the percentage of children that experienced that risk factor) included child maltreatment (100%), caregiver mental health problem (30%), minority status (58%), low caregiver education (29%), single caregiver (48%), biomedical risk condition (22%), poverty (46%), adolescent caregiver (19%), domestic violence (40%), four or more children in home (14%), and caregiver substance abuse (39%). They also found that only about 5% of children that were exposed to a single risk factor in addition to maltreatment had a developmental delay, but 76% to 99% of children who experienced between five and seven risk factors had developmental delay (Figure 4.5) (Barth et al. 2007).

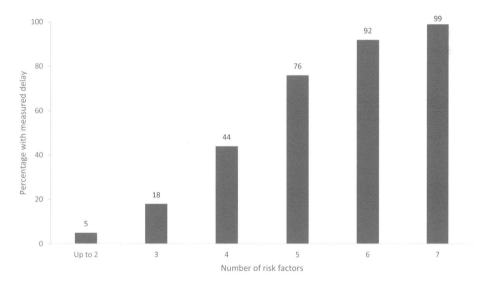

Figure 4.5 Percentage of infants and toddlers with a developmental delay by the number of risk factors. (Adapted from Barth et al. 2007.)

Assessment of development and biodiversity

In this chapter, we have mainly discussed factors that affect the development of the child. Here, we will explain briefly what is 'normal' and what is not, and when to worry that something is not right. First of all, for purpose of assessment or intervention in the development of an infant, it is crucial to bear in mind that he/she does not exist in isolation. This means that the child has not only to be examined in the presence of his caregivers, but the results and possible intervention plan should be considered in the context of the family situation.

Developmental milestones vary with genetic and cultural factors, and so must be inter-preted with caution. The study by Karasik et al. (2015) showed that at the age of 5 months Italian children do not sit, but 17% to 25% in the USA, South Korea, and Argentina, 67% of Kenyan, and 92% of Cameroonian children sit independently at 5 months. In 2016, a systematic review which concluded that standardized motor devel-opment assessments of children aged 0 to 2 years have limited validity in cultures other than the one in which the normative sample was obtained and, thus, their use can result in under- or over-referral to medical services (Mendonça et al. 2016). So this develop-mental diversity could be called a cultural variation of 'normality' or an example of biodiversity.

Neurodiversity is a term referring to another aspect of biodiversity. It originated as a movement among individuals labelled with ASDs who wanted to be seen as different, not disabled, and was first used by Judy Singer in her 1999 PhD thesis (Singer, 1999) and the same ideas were also developed by Harvey Blume at around the same time. The term refers to variation in the human brain regarding sociability, learning, attention, mood, and other mental functions (Armstrong, 2011). The concept of neurodiversity is usually used to explore the origin of mental conditions like autism, ADHD, dyslexia, anxiety, and also of left-handedness and sexual orientation. In this context, these con-ditions may best be described on the one hand as a 'disease', or, on the other as a 'disa-bility', 'disorder', or 'difference'. For example, the autism spectrum encompasses vast diversity, from individuals that are nonverbal and have intellectual disability, to high-functioning individuals with average and above average IQ and typical language devel-opment. But all individuals with ASDs have (according to DSM-5) 'persistent deficits in social communication and social interaction across multiple contexts' and 'restricted, repetitive patterns of behavior, interests, or activities'. Autism is sometimes also associ-ated with cognitive strengths, notably in domains such as attention to detail, memory for detail, and a drive to detect patterns (or 'systematizing') (Baron-Cohen, 2006).

Baron-Cohen (2017) offers less medicalized definitions for the terms used in medical practice. 'Disorder' should be used when there is nothing positive about the condi-tion, or when despite trying different environmental modifications, the person is still unable to function. 'Disease' should be used when the biomedical mechanistic cause of a disorder becomes known, perhaps through medical testing or through scientific research. 'Disability' should be used when the person falls below an average level of functioning in one or more psychological or physical functions and where the individual needs support or intervention. 'Difference' should be used when the person is merely atypical, for biological reasons, relative to a population norm, but where this difference does not necessarily affect functioning or well-being. Using these definitions, we should remain open-minded that some forms of autism are correctly thought of as a disorder, and others not, given the heterogeneity that exists within this diagnostic category (Baron-Cohen, 2017).

So use of the term 'neurodiversity' is not a sentimental ploy to help people with mental illness and their caregivers 'feel good' about their disorders. Rather, it is a powerful concept, backed by substantial neuroscience, evolutionary psychology, anthropology, and other fields, that can help revolutionize the way we look at mental illness (Armstrong, 2011).

Box 4.4   Points to remember about the concept of neurodiversity

1. There is no single way for a brain to be normal, as there are many different ways for the connectivity of the brain to develop on the developmental pathway that continues into adulthood.

2. We need more ethical, non-stigmatizing language and concepts for thinking about people who are different and/or who have disabilities.

3. We need a framework that does not pathologize and focus disproportionately on what the person struggles with, and instead takes a more balanced view, to give equal attention to what the person can do.

4. Genetic or other kinds of biological variation are intrinsic to the person's identity, their sense of self, and personhood, which seen through a human rights lens, should be given equal respect alongside any other form of diversity, such as sex.

(Adapted from Baron-Cohen, 2017)

THE RIGHT TO 'LIVE HAPPILY EVER AFTER'

In the year 2000, the United Nations released Millennium Development Goals, a document that aimed at reducing maternal and child mortality by 75% and 66% respectively. The document was signed by 189 countries. National and international activities (vaccinations, effective healthcare, and other measures) helped to reduce mortality in children younger than 5 years from 10 million deaths in 2000 to 5.4 million in 2017. But children's healthcare situation remains complicated: nearly 15 000 children die before the age of 5 years each day; there is no strategy to integrate planning and healthcare for children into healthcare systems or link them to sectors outside health, such as education, social safety, housing, and environmental health. Inequalities persist and are often associated with poverty, migration, ethnicity, conflict, and environment because there has been insufficient attention to child health and development in global strategies (Bhutta and Black, 2019; GBD, 2017). Therefore, in 2015, the United Nations released a plan for 'people, planet and prosperity' called 'Transforming Our World: the 2030 Agenda for Sustainable Development' (UN General Assembly, 2015). The ultimate commitment of the document is to 'leave no one behind'; 193 member states adopted the plan. The Agenda has 17 sustainable development goals and 169 targets. Promotion of child development, healthy lives, and quality education are prioritized in Goal 3: 'Ensure healthy lives and promote well-being for all at all ages', and Goal 4: 'Ensure inclusive and equitable quality education and promote lifelong learning opportunities for all'. The document has ambitious goals to advocate for a more holistic understanding of health and addresses social determinants of health across diverse sectors.

Box 4.5   Global progress has saved millions of childhoods since the year 2000

Now there are:

- ☑ 4.4 million (49%) fewer child deaths per year
- ☑ 49 million (33%) fewer children with growth disorder
- ☑ 115 million (33%) fewer children out of school
- ☑ 94 million (40%) fewer child labourers
- ☑ 11 million (25%) fewer females married before 18 years
- ☑ 3 million (22%) fewer adolescent births per year
- ☑ 12 000 (17%) fewer child homicides per year

(Adapted from Save the Children, 2019)

Aiming to promote children's health in Europe, the WHO Regional Office for Europe developed a strategy for child and adolescent health for the period of 2015 to 2020, which was adopted by all 53 European member states. The priorities of the strategy are broad and include actions around supporting early childhood development, reducing exposure to violence, and tackling mental health problems in adolescence (Alemán-Díaz et al. 2018).

There cannot be too much attention given to children's health and well-being. The policies mentioned above in this chapter and the results of implementing them show that joint activities can improve our world. In 2018, WHO, UNICEF, and other international organizations launched one further document: 'Nurturing care for early childhood development: a framework for helping children survive and thrive to transform health and human potential' (WHO, 2018). Nurturing care refers to a stable environment created by parents and other caregivers that ensures children's good health and nutrition, protects them from threats, and gives young children opportunities for early learning through interactions that are emotionally supportive and responsive (WHO, 2018). This document contains a resumé of the scientific evidence, giving a holistic view and grounding of child development, and emphasizes the need 'to leave no one behind', indicating that the needs of all children (healthy, poor, disabled, refugees, newborn infants, adolescents, victims of country or family wars, etc.) have to be addressed. If we fail to recognize those needs, it indicates that we are inexperienced or that we are relying on insensitive instruments of measurement. It also includes guiding principles and describes strategic actions for everyone from policymakers to families (see Box 4.6). The community of developmental and child neurology scientists and practitioners has to act in partnership to undertake the task for which we are best prepared, namely to 'promote the health and well-being of all children, and enable all to reach their full potential' (Wertlieb, 2019).

Box 4.6   Recommended ways for the health sector to make nurturing care happen

1.   Ensuring access to good-quality services.

2.   Making services supportive of nurturing care.

3.   Increasing outreach to families and children with the greatest risk of suboptimal development.

4.   Establishing inclusive services for children with developmental difficulties and disabilities.

5.   Collaborating with other sectors to ensure a continuum of nurturing care.

(Adapted from WHO, 2018. Licence: CC BY-NC-SA 3.0 IGO)

REFERENCES

Alemán-Díaz AY, Backhaus S, Siebers LL, et al. (2018) Child and adolescent health in Europe: monitoring implementation of policies and provision of services. *Lancet Child Adolesc Health* 2: 891—904.

American Psychiatric Association: Diagnostic and Statistical Manual of Mental Disorders: Diagnostic and Statistical Manual of Mental Disorders, Fifth Edition. Arlington, VA: American Psychiatric Association, 2013.

Armstrong T (2011) *The Power of Neurodiversity: Unleashing the Advantages of your Differently-wired Brain.* Cambridge, MA: Da Capo Lifelong.

Baron-Cohen S (2006) Two new theories of autism: hyper-systemising and assortative mating. *Arch Dis Child* 91: 2—5.

Baron-Cohen S (2017) Editorial Perspective: Neurodiversity — a revolutionary concept for autism and psychiatry. *J Child Psychol Psychiatry* 58: 744—747.

Barth RP, Scarborough A, Lloyd EC, Losby J, Casanueva C, Mann T (2007) *Developmental Status and Early Intervention Service Needs of Maltreated Children*. Washington, DC: U.S. Department of Health and Human Services, Office of the Assistant Secretary for Planning and Evaluation.

Bhutta ZA, Black RE (2019) Current and future challenges for children across the world. *JAMA* 321: 1251—1252.

Bick J, Zhu T, Stamoulis C, Fox NA, Zeanah C, Nelson CA (2015) Effect of early institutionalization and foster care on long-term white matter development: a randomized clinical trial. *JAMA Pediatr* 169: 211—219.

Black M, Walker S, Fernald L, et al. (2017) Early childhood development coming of age: science through the life course. *Lancet* 389: 77—90.

Blumberg MS, Freeman JH, Robinson SR (2010) A new frontier for developmental behavioral neuroscience. In: Blumberg MS, Freeman JH, Robinson SR, editors, *Oxford Handbook of Developmental Behavioral Neuroscience*. New York, NY: Oxford University Press, pp. 1—6.

Council on Communications and Media (2016) Media and young minds*Pediatrics* 138: e20162591.

GBD (2017) Diseases, Injuries, and Risk Factors in Child and Adolescent Health, 1990 to 2017: Findings From the Global Burden of Diseases, Injuries, and Risk Factors 2017 Study. *JAMA Pediatr* 173: e190337.

Greenough WT, Chang FF (1989) Plasticity of synapse structure and pattern in the cerebral cortex. In: Peters A, Jones EG, editors, *Cerebral Cortex*, Vol 7 New York NY: Plenum Press, pp 391—440.

Feldman R, Rosenthal Z, Eidelman AI (2014) Maternal-preterm skin-to-skin contact enhances child physiologic organization and cognitive control across the first 10 years of life. *Biol Psychiatry* 75: 56—64.

Franke HA (2014) Toxic Stress: Effects, Prevention and Treatment. *Children (Basel)* 1: 390—402.

Hackman DA, Gallop R, Evans GW, Farah MJ (2015) Socioeconomic status and executive function: developmental trajectories and mediation. *Dev Sci* 18: 686—702.

Hamadani JD, Tofail F, Huda SN, et al. (2014) Cognitive deficit and poverty in the first 5 years of childhood in Bangladesh. *Pediatrics* 134: e1001—08.

Hart B, Risley TR (2003) The Early Catastrophe: The 30 Million Word Gap by Age 3 *American Educator*. Available at https://www.aft.org//sites/default/files/periodicals/TheEarlyCatastrophe.pdf

Karasik LB, Tamis-LeMonda CS, Adolph K, Bornstein MH (2015) Places and postures: A cross cultural comparison of sitting in 5-month-olds. *J Cross Cult Psychol* 46: 1023—1038.

Kliegman R, Stanton B, St Geme J, Schor N, Behrman R, editors. (2016) *Nelson Textbook of Pediatrics*. Edition 20. Phialdelphia, PA: Elsevier.

Kolb B, Gibb R, Clarke M, Ghali L (2011) Plasticity and behaviour in the developing brain. *J Can Acad Child Adolesc Psychiatry* 20: 265—276.

Kolb B (1995) *Brain Plasticity and Behaviour*. London: Psychology Press.

Mackay DF, Smith G, Cooper S, et al. (2016) Month of conception and learning disabilities. a record-linkage study of 801,592 children. *Am J Epidemiol* 184: 485—493.

Madigan S, Browne D, Racine N, Mori C, Tough S (2019) Association between screen time and child development. *JAMA Pediatr* 173: 244—250.

Myers MM, Brunelli SA, Squire JM, Shindledecker R, Hofer MA (1989) Maternal behavior of SHR rats in its relationship to offspring blood pressure. *Dev Psychobiol* 22: 29—53.

McLaughlin KA, Sheridan MA, Tibu F, Fox NA, Zeanah CH, Nelson CA (2015) Causal effects of the early caregiving environment on development of stress response systems in children. *Proc Natl Acad Sci USA* 112: 5637—42.

Mendonça, B, Sargent B, Fetters L (2016) Cross-cultural validity of standardized motor development screening and assessment tools: a systematic review. *Dev Med Child Neurol* 58: 1213—1222.

Nelson CA, Fox NA, Zeanah CH (2014) *Forgotten Children: What Romania Can Tell Us About Institutional Care*. Available at www.adoptioninstitute.org/news/forgotten-children-what-romania-can-tell-us-about-institutional-care/

Nikolova A, Georgiev V (2017) A Method for Assessing the Development of Children under Six Years of Age. In Proceedings of Seventh International Conference on Digital Presentation and Preservation of Cultural and Scientific Heritage, Veliko Tarnovo, 7-10 September 2017, Bulgaria (pp. 223—227). Veliko Tarnovo: Institute of Mathematics and Informatics — BAS. http://dipp.math.bas.bg/8-archives/17-archives-2017

Punjabi S (2015) *Child Development and Pedagogy for CTET & STET*, 2nd Edition. Delhi, Disha Publications.

Rubio-Codina M, Attanasio O, Meghir C, Varela N, Grantham-McGregor S (2015) The socioeconomic gradient of child development: cross-sectional evidence from children 6—42 panel in Bogota. *J Hum Resour* 50: 464—83.

Save the Children (2019) Changing lives in our lifetime. Global Childhood Report, 2019. https://www.savethechildren.org/content/dam/usa/reports/advocacy/global-childhood-report- 2019-pdf.pdf

Sameroff A, editor, (2009) *The Transactional Model of Development: How Children and Contexts Shape Each Other*. New York: Wiley.

Selye H (1976) Forty years of stress research: principal remaining problems and misconceptions. *Can Med Assoc J* 115: 53—56.

Singer J (1999) 'Why can't you be normal for once in your life?' From a 'problem with no name' to the emergence of a new category of difference. In Corker M, French S (eds.). Disability Discourse. McGraw-Hill Education (UK) pp. 59—67.

Thompson RA, Nelson CA (2001). Developmental science and the media: Early brain development. *Am Psychol* 56: 5—15.

Tibu F, Sheridan MA, McLaughlin KA, Nelson CA, Fox NA, Zeanah CH (2016) Disruptions of working memory and inhibition mediate the association between exposure to institutionalization and symptoms of attention deficit hyperactivity disorder. *Psychol Med* 46: 529—541.

UN General Assembly (2015) *Transforming Our World: the 2030 Agenda for Sustainable Development*. Available at: https://www.refworld.org/docid/57b6e3e44.html

Wertlieb D (2019) Nurturing care framework for inclusive early childhood development: opportunities and challenges. *Dev Med Child Neurol* 61: 1275—1280.

WHO (2018) *Situation of child and adolescent health in Europe. World Health Organization*. Available at: http://www.euro.who.int/en/publications/abstracts/situation-of-child-and-adolescent-
health-in-europe-2018

WHO (2018) *Nurturing care for early childhood development: a framework for helping children survive and thrive to transform health and human potential.* Geneva: World Health Organization, United Nations Children's Fund, World Bank Group. Available at https://apps.who.int/iris/bit-stream/
handle/10665/272603/9789241514064-eng.pdf

WHO (2019) *Guidelines on physical activity, sedentary behaviour and sleep for children under 5 years of age.* World Health Organization. Available at https://apps.who.int/iris/handle/10665/311664

Yeoh SL, Eastwood J, Wright IM, et al. (2019) Cognitive and motor outcomes of children with prenatal opioid exposure: a systematic review and meta-analysis. *JAMA Netw Open* 2: e197025.

CHAPTER 5

The neonatal examination and neurodevelopmental assessment

Leena Haataja, Vittorio Belmonti, and Giovanni Cioni

Key messages

- Distinguish development that is too slow or too different from normal variation.
- Use standardized protocols for neurological and neurodevelopmental assessments.
- Realize that there is no criterion standard: different protocols have different goals.

Common errors

- Misinterpreting a normal variant as abnormal.
- Suspecting neurological disorders without comprehensive examination.
- Failing to adapt the neurological examination derived from adult neurology to the examination of infants.
- Delaying diagnosis and intervention.

When to worry

- Abnormal quantity or quality of movement repertoire.
- Neurological findings that are not seen in typically developing infants.
- Late developmental milestones.

- Loss of developmental skills at any age.
- Concerns about vision or hearing (parental or professional).

MAIN FEATURES OF TYPICAL NEUROLOGICAL DEVELOPMENT

Morphological and functional development

The development of the central nervous system (CNS) is a complex and highly coordinated causal chain of events (Table 5.1). Morphological disorders (i.e. CNS malformations) may arise at any moment from a variety of causative factors, not only genetic but also external ones (e.g. inflammation, maternal substance abuse). The causative mechanisms are still largely unknown, while the timing (phase of onset) of each pattern of malformation (phenotype) is rather consistent. Therefore, all traditional classification schemes of CNS malformations are mainly based on phenotypical and temporal criteria (e.g. disorders of proliferation, migration, organization, etc.). This approach to CNS malformations has increasingly been replaced with an integrated one, including aetiological criteria (especially genotype) whenever possible.

In a clinical context, however, the dependency of the nature of morphological abnormalities, including those resulting from perinatal or postnatal brain injuries, on the age at onset seems to provide easier and more general guidance than aetiology. This, for instance, is one of the bases of most modern classifications of cerebral palsy, which include the timing of the lesion as a fundamental criterion.

Even if neurons in most brain regions do not continue to proliferate after birth, it is evident that maturational processes extend far into postnatal life, even into adult life. Brain plasticity and reorganization after insults are inherent features of the immature brain, which is capable of effective rearrangements of pathways and of regional specialization. For example, language areas may shift from the dominant to the contralateral hemisphere, while the damaged primary motor area may reorganize, either around the lesion or contralaterally, depending on timing and extent of the lesion.

A crucial question is how such a wide variation as that found in typical neurological development could be explained. The major developments in imaging and neurophysiological techniques during the last few decades have allowed us to understand that infant motor activity is a complex process driven by the CNS and involving interaction between afferent information, and spinal and supraspinal controlling networks. The current prevailing neuronal group selection theory (NGST) is based on the synergy between genetic and environmental determinants of activity that influence the maturation of infant development. According to NGST, the abundant variation in the repertoire of motor behaviours is expressed from fetal life onwards and continues through infancy when selection of the functionally most effective motor pattern happens at a particular age that is specific to the motor function.

Table 5.1   The main stages of central nervous system (CNS) development and peak gestational age (GA) for their occurrence and the main disorders which may arise

Gestational age	Stage of CNS development	Disorders that may arise
2 weeks	Formation of the neural plate	Enterogenous cysts and fistulae
3–4 weeks	Dorsal induction/neurulation (the neural tube and crest are formed)	Blastopathies (e.g. anencephaly, encephaloceles, spina bifida, meningoceles)
4–7 weeks	Dorsal induction/caudal neural-tube formation	Diastematomyelia, Dandy-Walker syndrome, cerebellar hypoplasia
5–6 weeks	Ventral induction (forebrain and face emerge; cleavage of the forebrain into two cerebral vesicles, formation of optic and olfactory placodes and of diencephalon)	Disorders of ventral induction (holoprosencephaly, median cleft face syndrome)
8–16 weeks	Neuronal and glial proliferation (cells proliferate in ventricular and subventricular zones; early differentiation of neuroblasts and glioblasts)	Disorders of proliferation (microcephaly, megalencephaly)
12–20 weeks	Migration (mainly radial migration of neurons towards the cortex)	Disorders of migration (e.g. lissencephaly-subcortical band heterotopia-pachygyria spectrum, nodular heterotopias), agenesis of corpus callosum
24 weeks onwards	Organization (alignment, orientation and layering of cortical neurons, synaptogenesis, programmed cell death, glial proliferation and differentiation)	Disorders of organization (e.g. polymicrogyria, focal cortical dysplasias)
24 weeks gestational age to 2 years post-term	Myelination	Dysmyelination, clastic insult (24-36 wks GA: typically deep white matter damage; 36 wks GA-early post-term age: cortical-subcortical damage)

(Adapted from Aicardi, 2018)

TYPICAL DEVELOPMENTAL MILESTONES

There is a wide biological variation in attaining developmental milestones; for example, walking independently in neurologically typical infants may happen at any given time between 8 months and 18 months of age or even beyond the age of 2 years in 'bottom shufflers'. If the infant was born preterm (i.e. >37wks' gestation) reaching developmental milestones is expected according to the corrected age, i.e. the age from the estimated due date for the 2 years after birth.

Another characteristic feature of typical development is the general forward direction of development with the various developmental skills usually appearing in a predictable sequence. Typically, there are periods of rapid progress in attaining a new skill alternating with developmentally stable periods. Even though typical development allows discontinuity, the typically developing infant does not lose learned skills.

It is a common myth that males would attain motor skills and females communication skills faster compared to the opposite sex. Research evidence does not support systematical, clinically significant differences between sex, and accordingly, the norms for developmental milestones are not given separately for males and females.

Typical development is a dynamic and multifaceted process which is a challenge to accurately measure. Nevertheless, the use of formal developmental screening tools and validated neurological examinations improves the early identification of infants with development problems, thus improving the prospects for interventions.

Norms and variability

Child development consists of gross motor, fine motor, language, cognitive, and social-behavioural domains of development. Taking into consideration the wide normal variation in attaining any developmental milestone, it is important to emphasize that the norms for developmental screening are more in the form of reference ranges than clear-cut differences between typical and atypical. Above all, an atypical developmental finding implies the need for close follow-up and, depending on the case, the need for further consultation and intervention to enable all the available developmental potential to be realized (see especially Chapter 13 in this volume). Late developmental milestones or loss of developmental skills act as red flags that suggest atypical development to the assessor. The references for developmental milestones, which should be regarded as for guidance rather than absolutely invariable, are given in the subsections that follow. In particular, it is important not to place too much reliance on a single milestone falling outside the reference ranges provided.

Gross motor milestones

The World Health Organization (WHO) Child Growth Standards (WHO Multicentre Growth Reference Study Group, 2006) collected longitudinal data on the attainment of six gross motor milestones (sitting without support, hands-and-knees crawling, standing with assistance, walking with assistance, standing alone, and walking alone) in a total of 816 children aged 4 to 24 months in Ghana, India, Norway, Oman, and the

United States (these growth charts are reproduced in Appendix 1 of the report and can be downloaded from www.who.int/childgrowth/standards/en/).The normal variation in the ages of mastering any given milestone was described with a concept of 'a window'; that is, a time interval during which typically developing infants learn a specific motor task. It is also of interest that 4.3% of infants never crawled on hands and knees, which is also reported in other studies as the milestone often missed out as a variation of normal. In 90% of infants the milestones were achieved in a fixed order, the most common sequence, seen in 42% of infants, being sit, crawl, stand, assisted walking, then unassisted walking. The upper age limits for attaining the six main motor milestones in typically developing infants are given in Table 5.2 and the range is shown in Figure 5.1. A simplified rule of thumb is that infants should sit independently before 10 months and walk independently no later than at age 18 months.

Table 5.2 The upper age limits for attaining motor milestones during infancy

Milestone	Age (months)
Sitting without support	9
Hands-and-knees crawling	14
Standing with assistance	11
Walking with assistance	14
Standing alone	17
Walking alone	18

Fine motor milestones

Separating fine motor function from gross motor development is somewhat arbitrary during the first year of life since developmental changes happen in interplay, for example attaining posture control and independent sitting position are prerequisites for the most efficient development of hand function. The upper age limits of attaining fine motor milestones in typically developing infants are presented in Table 5.3. A simplified rule of thumb is that the infant should voluntarily grasp an object by 5 months and show a mature pincer grip before 12 months of age.

Language and social milestones

Typically developing infants produce different reflexive sounds associated with internal states (e.g. crying for hunger) from birth onwards. The vowel sounds are increasingly produced between 2 months and 6 months, and canonical babbling (babbling long utterances including consonants) begins between 6 months and 10 months. Laughing aloud is usually present by 6 months of age. The comprehension of spoken language

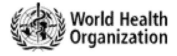

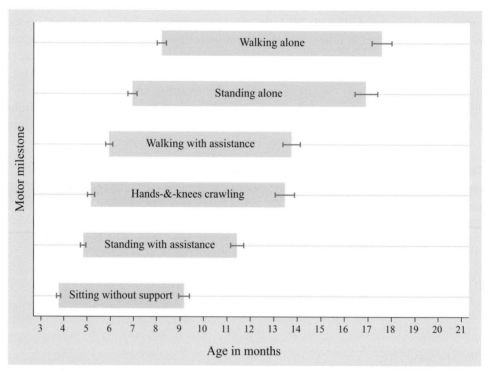

Figure 5.1 Windows of achievement for six gross motor milestones. (Reproduced from WHO Multicentre Growth Reference Study Group, 2006 with permission from Taylor & Francis.)

Table 5.3 The upper age limits for attaining fine motor milestones during infancy

Milestone	Age (months)
Reaches for an object	4
Grasps using whole hand	5
Changes object from one hand to another	7
Pincer grasp	11

precedes expressive language in early development. Infants recognize their own name by 8 months of age and start understanding single words between 8 months and 10 months of age. Infants with typical hearing start the production of true words — that is, verbal utterances used consistently to indicate specific stimuli in the external world — by 10 to 12 months of age.

Generally, by 8 months of age, the infant should produce canonical babbling and show consistent reaction when called by name. By 12 months of age, typically developing infants show understanding of a few words. If there is a suspected delay in sound production and/or receptive language it is always advisable to have the child's hearing checked. If their hearing is normal, this would then raise the question of whether the infant shows signs of a specific language or autism spectrum disorder or a significant general impairment of early development.

Typically developing infants show a smile in response to external sensory stimuli by 2 months of age, and a selective social smile, for example to their caregiver, by 3 months of age. Around 7 months of age infants start distinguishing between familiar persons and strangers, and they start showing anxiety when approached by strangers. By 8 to 10 months of age infants start showing attempts at interactive play. They typically first start to release or cast toys with the expectation of somebody giving the toys back to them. By 12 months of age infants become capable of playing give-and-take games and waving goodbye.

Absence of the smile response is a red flag for the need of visual assessment. The absence of any attempt at interactive play and joint engagement by 12 months requires a thorough investigation of the psychosocial environment of the child in addition to the medical differential diagnostic work-up as outlined above for speech delay.

STRUCTURED NEURODEVELOPMENTAL SCALES

There is a wide selection of neurodevelopmental scales available, and the goal of the assessment should guide the selection of a specific scale (e.g. whether used as a screening tool by a community paediatrician or as a detailed standardized scale for an infant at high risk for developmental problems). Unlike the tools for neurological examination, neurodevelopmental scales are not aimed at a categorical diagnosis (e.g. of cerebral palsy or behavioural disorder), but at an assessment of the infant's functioning on certain dimensions of development. Most scales are multidimensional and provide a developmental profile, but there are also unidimensional ones, specifically for motor function, cognition, or language. All structured scales must be administered by a specifically trained examiner. They are usually relatively time-consuming compared with neurological examinations. They are, however, important for the assessment of high-risk infants: poor functioning in one or more developmental areas, and especially in cognitive, perceptual-motor and visual-spatial abilities, language, and/or behaviour, is much more common than a definite neurological disorder at toddler and school age. Moreover, neurodevelopmental assessment allows the planning and monitoring of intervention protocols, individualized to suit the infant's strengths and weaknesses and prioritized to achieve functional goals.

The standardized scales for assessing development from birth to 2 years are shown in Table 5.4. Among them the Bayley Scales of Infant and Toddler Development, Third

Edition and Griffiths Mental Development Scales are the ones used most frequently in follow-up and other clinical studies. One of the key characteristics of standardized tests is the derivation of standardized scores, based on a previous standardization process involving a large sample of typically developing infants. Importantly, the standardization of a test does not guarantee properties such as validity and reliability, which vary greatly among the tests. The selection of a particular scale may also be determined by considerations other than its psychometric properties, such as availability, proven validity for a specific class of disorders or presence of particular risk factors (e.g. infants born preterm, visual or auditory defects, etc.), or personal experience. A crucial feature that should always be checked, is whether standardized scores for a given population (e.g. non-English-speaking populations) are provided.

MAIN ITEMS OF CLINICAL NEUROLOGICAL ASSESSMENT

Box 5.1   Items included in systematic history taking

- ☑ The course of pregnancy and birth
- ☑ Achieved developmental milestones (e.g. first smile, rolling onto side)
- ☑ Enquiry about any unusual behavior patterns
- ☑ Previous and current health problems
- ☑ Previous and present medications
- ☑ Parental concerns about the child
- ☑ Social situation of the family
- ☑ Family history of neurological disorders

Clinical neurological assessment always comprises three main aspects: history taking, physical examination, and neurological assessment. Systematic history taking should include the items listed in Box 5.1.

Physical examination including growth pattern, especially the increase in head circumference over time plotted on a growth chart with z-scores or centiles for age (see Growth Charts, Appendix 1 at the end of this volume), may give a crucial 'diagnostic handle' in cases of atypical development (see especially Chapters 22, 23, and 29).

The examiner must be sensitive to both the state and clinical condition of the infant, especially those under the age of 1 year. The optimal timing of the neurological examination relative to the infant's state is important and findings in a crying, irritable infant may be misleading. In neonatal examinations it is advisable to assess the newborn infant in the middle third of the time interval between feeds to avoid disturbing the

Table 5.4 Standardized scales for assessing development from birth to 2 years

Name	Age range	Duration	Domains
Bayley Scales of Infant Development, Second Edition	1–42 months	25–60 min	Mental Development, Motor Development, Behaviour Rating Scale
Bayley Scales of Infant and Toddler Development, Third Edition	1–42 months	30–90 min	Cognitive, Language, Motor, Social-Emotional (parent report), Adaptive Behaviour (parent report)
Griffiths Scales of Child Development, Third Edition	Birth to 6 years	35–60 min	Foundations of Learning, Language and Communication, Eye and Hand Coordination, Personal–Social–Emotional, Gross Motor
Mullen Scales of Early Learning	Birth to 5 years 8 months	15–30 min (depends on age)	Gross Motor, Fine Motor, Visual Reception, Receptive Language, Expressive Language
Battelle Developmental Inventory II	Birth to 8 years	1–2 h	Personal-Social, Adaptive, Motor, Communication, Cognitive
Merrill-Palmer Revised	1 month to 6 years 6 months	30–40 min	Cognitive, Fine Motor, Receptive Language, Memory, Visual-Motor, Speed of Processing, Expressive Language, Gross Motor, Social-Emotional, Self-Help/ Adaptive Temperament
Alberta Infant Motor Scale	Birth to 18 months	20–30 min	Gross Motor Skills (assessed in four postures)
Peabody Developmental Motor Scales, 2nd edn.	Birth to 5 years 11 months	45–60 min	Gross and Fine Motor

(Adapted from Cioni and Mercuri, 2007)

infant's sleeping cycle and to make the assessment before the infant becomes hungry for the next feed.

The internationally used Dubowitz examination is an example of a structured neonatal assessment. It includes 34 items, under the main item headings shown in Box 5.2. This method provides reference ranges for typically developing infants born at term tested during the first days after birth and low-risk infants born preterm at term age (see Dubowitz et al. 1999; Ricci et al. 2008). Videos teaching this examination are accessible free of charge (http://hammersmith-neuro-exam.com/videos/#wpforms-21). It is important to note that typically developing infants born preterm show less limb flexor tone and poorer head control at term age than infants born at term. Furthermore, infants born preterm tend to be more hyperexcitable (brisk reflexes, startles, tremors) and have less mature visual behavior compared with infants born at term.

Box 5.2 The main item headings included in the neonatal examination

☑ Orientation and behavior (e.g. visual and auditory orientation, alertness, consolability)

☑ Tone and tone pattern including assessment both prone and supine

☑ Neonatal reflexes and tendon reflexes:

  ○ suck and gag

  ○ palmar/plantar grasp, placing and Moro reflexes, tendon reflexes

☑ Movements: quantity and quality

☑ Abnormal signs: abnormal hand/toe posture, excessive tremor, startle

---

Isolated abnormal clinical findings in the neonatal examination have little diagnostic value, but merely indicate the need for later reassessment. Abnormal findings that require further assessment are listed in Box 5.3.

Box 5.3 Clinical signs suggesting central nervous system involvement

☑ Altered state of consciousness

☑ Convulsions

☑ Abnormal tone patterns (e.g. opistothonus, marked leg extension with strong arm flexion)

☑ Abnormal auditory or visual responses

☑ Sucking/swallowing difficulties

☑ Abnormal posture of hand or toes (e.g. continuous fisting or big toe extension)

The Hammersmith Infant Neurological Examination (HINE) is an example of a structured infant assessment. HINE is based on the same methodological principles as the neonatal Dubowitz examination, and it has been developed for use after the neonatal period up to 24 months of age. This method can be used to make a distinction between typical and atypical development and to predict future outcomes. The examination (which can be viewed in a teaching video at http://hammersmith-neuro-exam.com/videos/#wpforms 21) includes 26 items evaluating posture, active and passive tone, assessment of cranial nerve function, movements, reflexes, and protective reactions (Box 5.4). The examination has been standardized based on findings in a cohort of low-risk infants born at term at 12 months and 18 months, and the norm references are available both for infants born at term and infants born preterm (Romeo et al., 2016).

In addition to the items listed in Box 5.4, it is advisable to assess systematically, especially in infants with suspected neurological problems, hearing, visual function, growth, and physical abnormalities that could be related to neurological diseases, such as axial, proximal and distal muscle bulk, tone and power (i.e. muscle strength) (see also Chapter 24 in this volume).

Box 5.4 Items included in the Hammersmith infant neurological examination

- ☑ Assessment of cranial nerve function:
  facial appearance, eye appearance, auditory response, visual response, sucking/swallowing

- ☑ Posture:
  head and trunk in sitting, arms, hands, legs, feet in supine, sitting and standing

- ☑ Spontaneous movements:
  quantity and quality

- ☑ Tone:
  scarf sign, passive shoulder elevation, pronation/supination, adductors, popliteal angle, ankle dorsiflexion, pull to sit, ventral suspension

- ☑ Reflexes and reactions:
  tendon reflexes; protective upper limb reflexes on falling from sit (lateral propping); arm extension on moving head toward floor (forward parachute)

COMPLEMENTARY APPROACH TO NEUROLOGICAL EVALUATION IN THE FIRST YEAR OF LIFE

General Movement Assessment: methodology and purposes

A method of neonatal assessment, based on the observation and categorization of normal and abnormal spontaneous movement patterns in the fetal period, neonatal period, and in the first months of life was proposed in the 1990s by Heinz Prechtl. Among others, the so-called general movements (GMs), global movements involving all body parts, were identified as particularly suitable for assessment. This gave rise to Prechtl's Method on the Qualitative Assessment of General Movements in Preterm, Term and Young Infants (Einspieler et al. 2005).

GM assessment has proven to be reliable and to have predictive value not only for later cerebral palsy, but also for minor neurological disorders, Rett syndrome, and cognitive and autism spectrum disorders.

Normal GMs involve the whole body in a complex sequence of arm, leg, neck, and trunk movements. They wax and wane in intensity, force, and speed, and have a gradual beginning and end. Rotations along the axis of the limbs and slight changes in the direction of movements make them fluent and elegant and create the impression of complexity and variability. GMs appear as early as 9 to 12 weeks post-menstrual age and continue after birth without substantially changing their form, irrespective of when birth occurs. The typical time course of normal GM patterns is described in Table 5.5.

Table 5.5 Typical time course of the normal patterns of general movements

Pattern	Age (weeks post-menstrual age)	Disorders that may arise
Writhing movements	Range: 9—49 Peak: 40 (term)	Variable amplitude, slow to moderate speed, typically ellipsoid limb trajectories lying close to the sagittal plane with superimposed rotations
Fidgety movements	Range: 46—64 Peak: 52	Smaller than writhing movements, moderate average speed with variable acceleration in all directions, migrating through all body parts as an ongoing flow of movement. Continual in the awake infant, except during fussing, crying and focused attention

GMs of infants with cerebral impairment lack complexity, fluency, and/or variability. Abnormal GM patterns are divided into two groups depending on whether they are observed in the writhing movements (WMs) or in the fidgety movements (FMs) period Table 5.6). In the FM period, various other motor patterns gradually emerge and mingle with GMs, thus building up the so-called associated motor repertoire, whose richness and age-adequacy have been related to the optimality of later motor coordination.

The 'global' visual (Gestalt) perception of movement quality has proven a powerful and reliable instrument, but only if carefully applied after specific training in this form of assessment. A thorough description of the standardized assessment procedure can be found in Einspieler et al. (2005). Notably, the standard GM assessment is based on video recording, but it has also proven reliable (especially in the FM period) when employed by the examiner's observation as a part of the neurological examination.

Table 5.6   Main abnormal patterns of general movements

Pattern	Description
(a) Writhing movements period	
Poor repertoire	Monotonous sequences, few movement components, repetitive and not so complex as in normal writhing movements. Fluency may be reduced too (but usually more spared than complexity and variability).
Cramped-synchronized	No complexity, fluency and variability: all limb and trunk muscles contract and relax almost simultaneously.
Chaotic	Large amplitude, high jerk and chaotic order without any fluency or smoothness. Rare, often evolving into cramped-synchronized.
(b) Fidgety movements (FM) period	
Absent FMs	FMs are never observed in the whole period.
Abnormal FMs (AF)	Fidgety-like movements, but amplitude, average speed and jerkiness are exaggerated.

Diagnostic and prognostic validity of GMs assessment

Although several developmental disorders are related to GM abnormality, the most reliable GM markers concern the prediction of cerebral palsy (Novak et al. 2017). These markers are: (1) a consistent cramped-synchronized (CS) pattern throughout the WM period and (2) the absent FM pattern. Consistent CS movements, though not common, have a 100% specificity for the diagnosis of cerebral palsy, while the absent FM pattern has both a high sensitivity and specificity for cerebral palsy. The other abnormal patterns are less reliable, possibly leading to a normal neurological outcome. In unilateral cerebral palsy, additional assessment of selective distal movements will identify the laterality of the lesion.

PRACTICAL CONCLUSIONS

Modern techniques of exploration of the nervous system, such as genetic tests, electrophysiological measures (electroencephalography, evoked potentials) and neuroimaging, cannot replace the essential contribution of neurological clinical examination to diagnosis and prognosis of neurodevelopmental disorders in the young infant. The examiner should be competent in the assessment of 'normal' or, more precisely, 'typical' development, to be able to distinguish between the normal biological variation and abnormal development. The essential items to be examined and the red flags to be taken into account have been described in this chapter.

The use of comprehensive and standardized protocols is always preferable to limited and personal lists of items. There is no consensus for a unique criterion standard, and the examiner should be aware of the advantages and limitations of the assessment method applied. Spontaneous and elicited gross and fine motor skills, perceptual, social, and attentional functions should be included in a comprehensive assessment. The appropriate use of comprehensive neurological assessment is not a single event, but it has the great advantage of being easily repeatable to obtain developmental trajectories, which are much more informative than a single assessment. They can be used either to reassure doctors and parents by detection of positive changes in development or, on the contrary, to lead to suspicion of static or delayed development or a progressive neurological disorder. In these situations, they may help to identify appropriate investigations or treatments for the underlying cause.

REFERENCES

Arzimanoglou A, editor (2018) *Aicardi's Diseases of the Nervous System in Childhood*, 4th edition. London: Mac Keith Press.

Dubowitz LMS, Dubowitz V, Mercuri E (1999) *The Neurological Assessment of the Preterm and Full-term Newborn Infant*, 2nd edition. Clinics in Developmental Medicine Series. London: Mac Keith Press.

Einspieler C, Prechtl FR, Bos A, Ferrari F, Cioni G (2005) *Prechtl's Method on the Qualitative Assessment of General Movements in Preterm, Term and Young infants*. Clinics in Developmental Medicine. London: Mac Keith Press.

Novak I, Morgan C, Adde L, et al. (2017) Early, accurate diagnosis and early intervention in cerebral palsy: advances in diagnosis and treatment. *JAMA Pediatr* 171: 897—907.

Ricci D, Romeo DL, Haataja L, et al. (2008) Neurological examination of preterm infants at term equivalent age. *Early Hum Dev* 84: 751—61.

Romeo DM, Brogna C, Sini F, et al. (2016) Early psychomotor development of low risk preterm infants: Influence of gestational age and gender. *Eur J Pediatr Neurol* 20: 518—523.

WHO Multicentre Growth Reference Study Group (2006) WHO Child Growth Standards based on length/height, weight and age. *Acta Paediatr Suppl* 450: 76—85.

Resources

Cioni G, Mercuri E (2007) *Neurological Assessment in the First Two years of Life. Clinics in Developmental Medicine Series*. London: Mac Keith Press.

Haataja L, Mercuri E, Regev R, et al. (1999) Optimality score for the neurologic examination of the infant at 12 and 18 months of age. *J Pediatr* 135: 153—61.

Hammersmith Neonatal and Infant Neurological Examination Teaching videos. Available at http://hammersmith-neuro-exam.com/videos/#wpforms-21

Heinemann KR, Hadders-Algra M (2008) Evaluation of neuromotor function in infancy — A systematic review of available methods. *J Dev Behav Pediatr* 29: 315—323.

The WHO Child Growth Standards. Available at https://www.who.int/childgrowth/standards/en/

CHAPTER 6

Neurological examination beyond the neonatal period

Colin Kennedy

Key messages

- The taking of the medical history not only guides later examination but also constitutes the first phase of that examination.
- Gaining the confidence of infant and parent during history taking usually secures their cooperation for the examination.
- Flexibility, playfulness, and taking the opportunities offered by the patient are necessary to elicit relevant neurological information in infants.

Common errors

- Towering over the infant.
- Failing to use the neurological examination to localize neurological lesions.
- Overinterpretation of isolated asymmetries, signs found on one examination only, or clinical features of doubtful significance (e.g. tremor of the chin, positive glabellar tap).
- Describing conscious level in vague terms (e.g. semicomatose) rather than as specific degrees of eye opening, verbal, and motor responses.
- Failing to examine brainstem reflex responses in a comatose child.

> **When to worry**
>
> - Unexplained localizing neurological abnormalities, especially if changing over time.
> - Deteriorating conscious level, especially if unexplained.

APPROACHES TO NEUROLOGICAL ASSESSMENT IN INFANCY

The neurological evaluation of young children requires the following.

- A structured validated examination (see Chapter 5). This is applicable to the neonatal period and, in some circumstances, to evaluations in the postneonatal period.

- The assessment of neurodevelopmental milestones using the age-specific functional repertoire of motor patterns and movements.

- The classic, localization-related approach to neurological examination, used in adults and well described in Fuller (2013). The aim is to identify the site of the lesion in the nervous system and narrow the differential diagnosis.

All of these approaches were touched upon in Chapter 5. The approach to apply in any child must reflect the clinical context. A structured neonatal approach would be well suited to, for example, prediction of outcome in a young infant born very preterm, while a classic neurological examination would be well suited to, for example, an 18-month-old with hydrocephalus secondary to a cerebellar tumour.

The sections that follow provide additional guidance on the evaluation of abnormal neurological signs in infants seen in a busy, acute clinical service, including those with a depressed conscious level. See also Plum et al. (2007) and Fuller (2013) for more detailed discussions beyond the scope of this chapter.

THE ROLE OF THE HISTORY

History taking should be aimed at the following:

- *Guiding and focusing the clinical examination* of the infant through eliciting detail of the presenting complaint, previous medical, family, and drug history.

- *Gaining the infant's confidence* and thus increasing his/her tolerance of the subsequent examination, by engaging in a constructive, friendly dialogue with the parent/caregiver. Commencement of the examination as soon as you have entered the room while you are still an unfamiliar adult is less likely to be tolerated by an infant.

- *Providing an opportunity to observe the neurological function* of the infant at a time when the history-giver, rather than the infant, is the prime focus of attention. This may feature important intermittent signs, such as the roving nystagmus of visual impairment, the forced downgaze of hydrocephalus, self-stimulatory behaviour, stereotypies, breath-holding and other abnormal respiratory patterns, or transient posturing (resulting from reflux, central movement disorders, brainstem compression, or other causes). Observation from across the room is a vital component of examination of children of any age, but nowhere is this truer than in the neurological assessment of the infant. *This part of the consultation may, in fact, provide the only examination that is possible in an upset or uncooperative infant.* A warm, bright, comfortable environment with visible, readily available, age-appropriate toys is as important as a reflex hammer.

- *Assessing the infant's social communication* (e.g. eye contact, smiling, playing peek-a-boo) in that part of the consultation when they are least likely to freeze or become upset.

- *Assessing the approach and attitude of caregivers and siblings* to the infant.

NEUROLOGICAL EXAMINATION OF THE INFANT

Acute neurological examination at any age needs to be adapted to the clinical situation to which it is applied. In an adult, an exhaustive neurological assessment of mental state, higher mental functions, the cranial nerves, motor examination, coordination, gait, balance, and sensory examination would take too long and in clinical practice is abbreviated, with detailed evaluation largely confined to confirmation or exclusion of diagnostic possibilities suggested by the history.

A basic principle of localization of lesions in the motor system is the distinction between 'upper motor neuron signs' arising from lesions within the central nervous system (CNS) rostral to the motor neurons (i.e. anywhere in the CNS in the neural pathway above the spinal cord anterior horn cells or cranial nerve motor nuclei) and 'lower motor neuron signs' arising at the level of the motor neuron, peripheral nerve, nerve-muscle junction, or muscle. In adults, the former are classically manifest by weakness, increased deep tendon reflexes, and increased tone and the latter by weakness, decreased reflexes, decreased tone, and muscle wasting. While upper and lower motor neuron signs and the distinction between them are also important in infants, their manifestations are altered, especially in young infants who may, for example, be floppy in association with either upper or lower motor neuron lesions (see Chapter 24).

In infants, the systematic approach of the adult neurological examination should be in the mind of the examiner, but must be applied in the context of the history (as in older patients) and opportunistically in a developmentally appropriate way. Those aspects of the examination that seem most relevant to the history are undertaken first, while examinations likely to lead to loss of the infant's cooperation (e.g. measurement of head circumference in an older infant) are deferred until the end of the examination. The examiner will adapt the examination to make use of the repertoire of action offered by the infant and this will also affect the order in which functions are tested. Where certain functions can only be partially tested, it may be wisest to return to them on another occasion or later in the same consultation, to maintain the infant's cooperation.

In practice, the examination is usually completed in three (or more) iterations: the first during the taking of the history (see above), the second with the infant dressed and comfortable in the care of the mother or other caregiver and the third with the infant undressed. This approach increases the chance that some information is obtained even if the infant's cooperation does not last until the end of the consultation.

A good neurological examination is much easier if we use our own examination tools. These should include, as a minimum, a paper tape measure, brightly coloured visual stimuli, a fully charged ophthalmoscope, and a reflex hammer. A reflex hammer with a soft circular head and a semiflexible plastic handle is more effective than a triangular-headed instrument with a short metal shaft.

Examination during history taking

Dysmorphic features (e.g. Down syndrome, fetal alcohol spectrum disorders; see Chapter 26), should be observed as well as spontaneous movements and posture, alertness, and play with toys, preferably on a comfortable soft floor surface and/or low table.

Examination with infant dressed and held on lap of parent/caregiver

Most information comes from observation and play rather than handling. Handwashing immediately before examination is good practice, not only to decrease the spread of infection but also to increase the confidence of parents in the examiner. Avoid formality, and talk to the infants warmly, expressively, and without inhibition. Make it a game. Do not tower over them but instead get down to their level; be their friend.

Vision and eye movements

Brightly coloured balls are good to stimulate visual tracking; very small, brightly coloured objects can be used as part of assessment of both vision and fine finger movement. A red ring, that can be formed by a single loop in red stethoscope tubing, sometimes elicits visual tracking when a face does not in a neurologically impaired young infant. In the visually 'unresponsive' infant, normal vision with impaired oculomotor control may mimic visual impairment. Distinguishing between these possibilities requires the time and patience to determine whether a visual stimulus is in fact provoking eye movements that are delayed or inaccurate. Hemianopia can often be detected with the examiner behind the child by determining whether a visual stimulus moved by the examiner from the periphery towards the midline in front of the child is more easily seen on one side than the other. An assisting examiner in front of the child may be needed (but may themselves act as a visual distraction, especially for older infants).

Eye movements can almost always be examined in a fully conscious infant and are also of value in coma. Pursuit eye movements may be elicited by the examiner moving about while maintaining eye contact or by moving an interesting age-appropriate toy in the infant's visual field. The pattern of abnormality may be diagnostic, such as restriction of up-gaze in the adducted eye due to the shortened inferior oblique tendon (i.e. trochlear paresis, also known as Brown syndrome), loss of up-gaze with or without forced downgaze ('sun-setting') in hydrocephalus, or may require further investigation, such as in the variable, fatigable paresis of eye movement in myasthenic syndromes. Monocular rapid ocular oscillations (with or without lower frequency head nods during visual fixation) are characteristic of spasmus nutans, usually developmental and self-limiting, but occasionally mimicked by an anterior optic pathway tumour. Opsoclonus ('dancing eye syndrome') consists of conjugate, chaotically variable in direction, high velocity eye movements that are usually accompanied by myoclonus and striking misery in the infant. It is sometimes associated with underlying paraspinal neuroblastoma.

The head-thrusting of oculomotor apraxia is elicited by engaging the child's interest in a visual object that requires a gaze shift. In this disorder, the infant cannot initiate saccadic eye movements and instead achieves change in direction of gaze by moving his/her head in the direction of the visual stimulus of interest, often with a slight overshoot, until the eyes are locked onto the visual stimulus in the new direction of gaze. In this condition, slow rotation of a desk chair in which the mother is seated with the infant on her lap will induce sustained eye deviation in the direction of rotation in place of the normal opticokinetic nystagmus. This may also be elicited by the examiner observing the infant supported under the axillae and rotating on the spot at a moderate rate; or by rotating a striped drum, designed for this purpose, in the infant's visual field. However, these manoeuvres are only needed for infants in whom the question of this diagnosis arises.

Remainder of cranial nerves

Glabellar tap is not helpful in infants but may elicit the striking rigidity of hyperekplexia.

Corneal reflexes   Blowing a short sharp puff of air in each eye is a poor compromise but often the only practicable option in an alert infant.

Facial asymmetry   If mouth droops on one side, consider both facial palsy and absence of the depressor anguli oris muscle ('asymmetrical crying facies') on the side that is *not* drooping.

Lower cranial nerves   These are not formally examined unless a problem with these functions is strongly suggested by specific presentations, such as nasal regurgitation, recurrent aspiration, excessive gagging, or the immobile facies of Moebius syndrome.

Chin tremor   This is often seen in typically developing infants.

Motor systems

Abnormal posture, such as fisting of the flexed, pronated arm, and paucity of movement are vital clues to tone that are observed rather than examined. A number of motor signs may be within the range of typical development when seen in isolation, even though the same sign might indicate motor disorder when seen in combination with other abnormal signs. In infancy, more than at any other age, the presence of unusual motor signs on several examinations at different times is much more significant than their observation on a single occasion. Tremor of the chin is not usually of any diagnostic significance.

Fine finger movements: at the age of 1 year, infants are normally at the right developmental stage to enjoy practising and demonstrating the ability to pick up objects between thumb and forefinger of each hand. Younger infants will often demonstrate ability to reach out for objects, transfer from hand to hand or, later in the first year, show an understanding of the permanence of an object by searching for a block or ball hidden beneath a cup.

Tone may often be inferred by observation of posture and spontaneous movement. Make small amplitude, rapid, shaking non-rhythmical to-and-fro movements of hands and feet by grasping the forearm and calf respectively to assess tone through the degree of wobbliness. This 'quick catch' resistance to rapid movement is a sensitive test for spasticity (i.e. a velocity-dependent increase in tone) and is a manoeuvre that infants find surprisingly acceptable. It is also valuable to evaluate the resistance to passive steady slow movement and to look systematically for contractures or ligament laxity/hyperextension. Reduced axial tone and increased limb tone in early infancy is the most common motor abnormality due to a CNS cause. Reduced limb and axial tone is usually due to a neuromuscular problem but may also be due to a CNS disorder (e.g. Prader–Willi syndrome, see Chapter 24) or connective tissue disorder, and may suggest the need to examine the parents for a hereditary disorder such as myotonic dystrophy or hyperlaxity.

Power is best assessed by spontaneous movements. Attempts to examine formally are often limited and may mislead. A strong hand preference before the age of a year may indicate contralateral weakness. There may be an opportunity to observe the infant's ability to turn around on the floor independently, come up on all fours, and sit with support.

Holding an attractive object above the infant's head may elicit arm abduction and elevation that require anti-gravity power or may bring out a tremor.

Throwing and kicking balls are often popular and useful aspects of examination in the second year.

Running 5 to 10 metres by infants into their mother's arms in a quiet corridor is one of the most informative tests when looking for motor disorders. Running to the examiner, on the other hand, is normally much less attractive to the infant.

Deep tendon reflexes are less likely to mislead if tested in a child who is not apprehensive or upset and so a first assessment may be appropriate before undressing. Further assessment of them after undressing also may be needed, depending on the child and the clinical question. For the ankle jerk, tapping the head of the reflex hammer on the examiner's thumb placed against the plantar surface of the dorsiflexed infant foot is a satisfactory alternative to tapping on the tendon itself.

The younger the infant the wider the normal range and the greater the effect of the child's physiological state of alertness, satiety, comfort, and posture on the test. The influence of primitive reflexes (see 'Completing the examination' section below) may cause asymmetry of deep tendon reflexes in an infant whose head and neck are laterally rotated. Almost any pattern of reflex excitability can be found in a distressed or struggling typically developing infant or in the first few weeks after term. Even the absence of the deep tendon reflexes may occasionally represent difficulty in elicitation rather than true absence. An increased area of elicitation, persistent ankle clonus observed beyond the age of 2 months, and crossed adductor responses observed beyond the age of 8 months are quite likely to be abnormal, but must be interpreted in the light of the state of the child.

Plantar reflexes should be tested with the child supine, head straight, foot at right angles, and toes in neutral position. They are rarely helpful in infancy, but persistent asymmetry may help to confirm hemisyndromes.

Balance and gait

It is usually possible in the second 6 months after term to distinguish specific problems with sitting balance from hypotonia with normal balance and from weakness. In an infant who is walking, the gait may be obviously broad-based or contain minor steps to correct imbalance. The interpretation of tiptoe walking will include evaluation of 'quick catch' resistance to rapid movement and of the deep tendon reflexes.

In the second year, infants will occasionally enjoy games in which the examiner passively extends the infant's leg and pretends to be pushed backwards/toppled over from the squatting position by this. Then the infant does it actively (and laughs at the toppled examiner). When the examiner then becomes less easy to topple, the infant will try quite hard to demonstrate power in leg extension if rewarded by an occasional success in toppling the examiner. This may be useful to demonstrate normal power, for example in a child who is not walking or has an abnormal gait of uncertain type.

Some older infants will allow their upper limb power to be tested by playing 'wheelbarrows' in which they support their weight on their arms with their extended legs supported off the ground by the parent or examiner holding their ankles like the handles of a wheelbarrow. This will only be relevant to address specific questions, usually related to upper limb weakness, in selected infants.

Examination with infant undressed

Reassure the infant by continuing to converse gently. An apprehensive infant may settle and quieten for auscultation if his/her hand is held reassuringly by the examiner.

Inspect for nutritional status and body proportions, bruising or other signs that may indicate abuse, cafe au lait spots, depigmentation, ungual fibromas, spinal dimples, or curvature, and haemangiomas.

Motor examination

Place supine   Observe truncal shape, respiratory movements (e.g. abdominal breathing), and anti-gravity movement. Distinguish floppiness (generalized hypotonia) from weakness plus floppiness to differentiate between floppiness of central or peripheral origin (see Chapter 24).

Place prone   A typically developing infant will show ability to hold head and chest held up by pushing up on arms by 3 months, to sit supported with some head control by 4 months, and to stay for a short while in the sitting position without support by 7 months after term. True independent sitting, including the infant getting in and out of the sitting position by themselves, has an upper age limit of 10 months.

Forward traction   The child is pulled forward by the examiner from supine lying to sitting with the examiner's thumbs grasped by the infant. The head should come forward in line with the trunk by 3 to 5 months. The head may extend behind the line of the trunk ('head lag') either because of low tone or because of an excess of extensor tone (see 'Ventral suspension' below). Asymmetry may imply weakness. Marked extension to standing, on forward traction by the examiner, may imply spasticity.

Ventral suspension   The infant lies prone with the anterior chest supported by the palm of the examiner's hand and the legs and head unsupported. If the legs and head hang near the vertical, this indicates hypotonia. If the head is held horizontal in line with the trunk or extended above the line of the trunk, the child is not displaying hypotonia in this posture. The combination of the latter posture in ventral suspension with head lag in forward traction suggests an excess of extensor tone, such as may be seen in cortico-spinal lesions or dystonia due to basal ganglia dysfunction in, for example, spastic or dyskinetic cerebral palsy.

The motor evaluations listed above constitute a useful minimum motor examination that is usually more informative than examination of the deep tendon reflexes in infancy. Addition of the other elements in the motor examination listed below will be appropriate to some, but not all, clinical contexts.

Axillary suspension The infant is held head up supported by the examiner's hands under the axillae. Slipping through the examiner's hands indicates hypotonia. This position can also be used to test stepping reflexes, which are a good example of reflexes that may be a pleasure to elicit but are of limited diagnostic value in the setting of outpatient evaluations in an acute neurology service.

Primitive reflexes

The Moro reflex (arm extension, followed by arm flexion with extension of the fingers, flexion of the thighs at the hips, often with a cry) may be elicited by several stimuli the most familiar of which is lifting of the head and shoulders slightly off the support surface and allowing the head to drop back about 30 degrees in relation to the trunk. It may be seen up to age 6 months but is usually incomplete after 2 months.

Sucking and rooting reflexes can be useful signs of the state of responsiveness/neurological depression of a young infant and become progressively less relevant through infancy.

The primitive grasp reflex is present in the hands and feet at birth and, if involuntary beyond 3 months, suggests a central motor disorder. Primitive grasp in the hands is assessed at the same time as tone in the 'forward traction' manoeuvre (see above).

The asymmetrical tonic reflex (ATNR) causes the infant to extend the limbs on the side to which the head is turned and flex the contralateral limbs. It is normally maximal at 2 months and gone by 4 months. An obligate ATNR (i.e. one which the infant cannot break out of) is not normal and, like a very active or persistent ATNR, may indicate a dyskinetic central motor disorder. The ATNR imposed by passive turn of the infant's head to the left and then to the right, can also be useful to indicate asymmetry of responses between left and right. Elicitation of the ATNR by head turn also leads to asymmetry of the deep tendon reflexes in typically developing infants who should, therefore, always be examined with their head in the midline.

The downward parachute reflex, in which the arms extend if the infant is grasped firmly under the axillae and moved rapidly headfirst towards the ground, typically develops at around 9 months. Surprisingly, the manoeuvre is rarely upsetting to infants. Asymmetry of this can be a useful sign of a hemisyndrome in a child of around that age who cannot be persuaded to reach for objects.

Completing the examination (undressed or re-dressed as appropriate to the test)

Measurement of the occipitofrontal head circumference, preferably with a non-stretchable paper tape measure, is useful only if plotted on an appropriate head circumference chart. Two or three measurements should be undertaken to check consistency of measurement in situations where the precise circumference is critical, such as monitoring of macrocephaly accompanied by ventriculomegaly (see Chapter 23).

Sensory examination is obviously limited in infancy. It may, nevertheless, be surprisingly easy to establish the dermatomal/root level of a sensory deficit in the context of a deficit at the level of the spinal cord such as occurs in spina bifida.

Examination of other organ systems, length and weight, and special examinations, such as the use of a Wood's light for depigmented patches, can then be undertaken according to the clinical context.

Rolling a white ball may give some idea about infant's perception. Rolling balls is also a good way of persuading infants to reach out, crawl, walk, stoop, and pick up an object; but screening for infants with vision defects should be confined to a history, inspection of the eyes, a properly performed cover test, and recognition of abnormal visual behavior (Hall, Pugh, and Hall, 1982). The cover test involves engaging the infant's visual attention on a near object. A cover is placed over an eye for a short moment then removed while observing both eyes for movement. The misaligned eye will deviate inwards or outwards. The process is repeated on both eyes.

Ophthalmoscopic examination is possible in an even-tempered infant by having a parent cuddle them against their chest so that the infant is looking over the parent's shoulder with chin resting on the parent's shoulder and his/her head gently held still by the parent's hand holding the infant head against the shoulder. An assistant (in sparsely staffed clinics, the other parent can do this) then holds the visual interest of the infant with a suitable glittery or flashing object at a distance of just over a metre. The examiner then uses the ophthalmoscope without touching the child or interfering with the line of vision of the eye not being examined. With severe monocular visual impairment, the infant will object to ophthalmoscopic examination of his/her good eye. Papilloedema and retinal haemorrhages are two physical signs of particular importance in infancy. If these or other important retinal pathologies are suspected before or after the clinical examination, an ophthalmologist should also evaluate the appearances. The use of mydriatics to assist fundoscopy must always be documented in the notes and should be avoided in situations where raised intracranial pressure may become an issue.

Examination of the parents may be crucial in selected cases especially in the differential diagnosis of genetically determined disorders such as familial disorders of head size (e.g. benign external hydrocephalus, see Chapter 23), abnormal fundoscopic appearance (e.g. Drusen mimicking papilloedema, see Chapter 23), phakomatoses (e.g. neurofibromatosis, tuberous sclerosis, see Chapter 26), and hereditary neuropathies or myotonia (see Chapter 24). Siblings may show clinical features of recessive or dominant genetic disorders.

NEUROLOGICAL EXAMINATION OF THE INFANT WITH IMPAIRED CONSCIOUS LEVEL

Only the neurological examination itself is considered here and other aspects of evaluation of the child with an acute encephalopathy are covered in Chapters 14, 17, and 19. The time course of the appearance of brainstem reflexes in infants born preterm is beyond the scope of this chapter.

Conscious level

Precise and reproducible description of a child's vital signs and conscious level is the key to effective communication, early detection of clinical change, and prompt intervention in any child with depressed conscious level. Conscious level is best expressed as a description of eye opening, verbal and motor responses to stimuli (see also Chapters 17 and 19). In infants, the Glasgow Coma Scale (GCS) modified for infants (Chapter 17, Table 17.1) may be used. The GCS also enables conscious level to be expressed as a numerical score, but this score is less informative than a short and specific description of the child's eye opening, verbal and motor responses to stimulation.

Neurological aspects other than conscious level in coma

The clinical findings are substantially dependent on the child's body temperature, blood electrolyte concentrations and on tissue concentrations of drugs, especially those causing sedation or nerve block. The paragraphs below constitute a brief summary. Detailed consideration of the diagnosis of stupor and coma has considerable application to infants but is beyond the scope of this chapter. A good account may be found in Plum et al. (2007).

The pupils may be reactive or non-reactive to light. This should be tested with a bright light from a flashlight or auroscope. Pupillary size and reactivity should both be noted. Reactivity can more confidently be assessed when viewed through the magnifying lens of an auroscope with no earpiece or an ophthalmoscope focused on the pupil rather than the retina and with a separate bright light (rather than the ophthalmoscope light) acting as the stimulus.

Eye movements and vestibulo-ocular reflexes may show diagnostic abnormalities in stuporose infants, such as forced downgaze ('sun-setting') in acute obstructive hydrocephalus (see Chapter 23) or wandering slow conjugate eye movements without corrective saccades in Leigh syndrome (see Chapter 29). Rotation of the head will lead to vestibulo-ocular reflex movement of the eyes relative to the head so that the direction of eye gaze remains unchanged relative to the environment. These are known as Doll's eye movements and may be abolished by sedation. 'Ice-water caloric responses' are a stronger stimulus to the same reflex pathways that are activated by Doll's eye movements, so do not generally need to be tested unless Doll's eye movements are absent. Before testing ice-water caloric responses in an unconscious infant, visualize the tympanic membrane to exclude any contraindications. The child's head should be in the midline at 30 degrees to the horizontal. Ice-cold water in a 10 to 20ml syringe is trickled into the ear for at least 60 seconds. Persistent deviation of the eyes towards the stimulated ear constitutes a normal response in an unconscious individual. An interval of at least 5 minutes should separate testing of the two ears to avoid the risk of persistent cold stimulus on one side masking the response to stimulation of the other side.

Corneal reflexes are tested by touching the eye lateral to the pupil with sterile gauze or similar stimulus. Observe the blink responses in both eyes to stimulation of each cornea.

Nose tapping will induce a marked startle/jerking response to the tip of the nose being tapped in hyperekplexia.

Cough and gag reflex are tested by a spatula to the posterior pharynx and tracheal suction respectively. Hiccups in a newborn infant may be a useful clinical clue to nonketotic hyperglycinaemia.

Reflex motor responses may be elicited by nail bed pressure in the limbs. Withdrawal in the stimulated limb can be the result of reflex response at a spinal segmental level. Stimulation of the sternum leading to limb responses and limb responses to stimulation of other limbs suggest integration of reflex responses at a higher level. Facial grimace (7th cranial nerve) in response to sternal or limb stimuli indicates some functioning brainstem pathways. Pressure upwards and backwards on the supra-orbital ridges can be used to assess brainstem pathways, both by the facial grimace response and by any motor response in the limbs. Any noxious stimuli need to be applied with care in infants to avoid inadvertent tissue injury.

Respiratory response to hypercarbia and the diagnosis of death

Completion of the clinical examination of the brainstem by testing reflex respiratory response to hypercarbia is only required in a few cases. The most common scenario is determination of whether there is a response to hypercarbia after demonstration of unresponsiveness on all other brainstem reflexes. Before testing, inspired oxygen is increased to 100%, arterial blood gas oxygen (PaO_2) is checked, and, where transcutaneous monitoring is in place, correlated with monitored percentage oxygen saturation of haemoglobin. Once saturation levels exceed 95%, the ventilator rate is decreased.

When blood PCO_2 exceeds 6 kiloPascals (kPa), a check is made that PaO_2 exceeds 6kPa, pH exceeds 7.40, and that the blood pressure remains stable. The absence of respiratory response over 5 minutes accompanied by an increase in PCO_2 of at least 0.5kPa constitutes a negative brainstem response to hypercarbia (except with underlying chronic respiratory disorder). Once testing is complete, the ventilator is reconnected to allow a gradual return to normal blood gas concentrations.

Death is a unitary state. In some jurisdictions this is defined as irreversible loss of consciousness accompanied by irreversible loss of the ability to breathe. Death, if thus defined, may be diagnosed either by the combination of prolonged circulatory arrest with absent pupillary response or, in certain circumstances, by the absence of brainstem reflexes. When the brainstem of a child in coma has been damaged to the degree that its integrative functions are irreversibly destroyed, the heart will inevitably stop beating subsequently and death is considered, in some jurisdictions, to have already occurred (Academy of Royal Medical Colleges, 2008). The more recent document relating to the diagnosis of death in infants aged less than 2 months by the Royal College of Paediatrics and Child Health (2015) and a series of related short educational videos on the diagnosis of death in adults, children, and infants may be downloaded free at: www.odt.nhs.uk/deceased-donation/best-practice-guidance/donation-after-brainstem-death/diagnosing-death-using-neurological-criteria/.

Demonstration of the absence of cerebral hemispheric function is deemed by some jurisdictions to be irrelevant to the diagnosis of death and by others to be necessary and to require the use of ancillary tests (electroencephalography, evoked potentials, radionucleotide imaging, and or angiography), but all series show false positive and false negative ancillary tests, especially in young infants.

The diagnosis of death provides the rationale, in an intensive care setting, to consider withdrawal of mechanical ventilation. There must be a known aetiology and there must not be hypothermia, or causative depressant drugs, or any reversible causative circulatory, metabolic, or endocrine disturbance. Additional detail on preconditions for the diagnosis of death (e.g. see Academy of Royal Medical Colleges, 2008) is beyond the scope of this chapter. When these conditions are fulfilled, death may be diagnosed by demonstration of complete unresponsiveness on testing of the brainstem reflexes, as described above, and, in some jurisdictions only, evidence of cerebral unresponsiveness. There is a lower age limit below which the diagnosis of death in this way is not felt to have been sufficiently validated to be applied. This age limit also varies between jurisdictions, but a diagnosis of death on neurological criteria is considered possible over 37 weeks post-gestational age in many countries.

REFERENCES

Academy of Royal Medical Colleges (2008) A code of practice for the diagnosis and confirmation of death. Available at https://www.aomrc.org.uk/reports-guidance/ukdec-reports-and-guidance/code-practice-diagnosis-confirmation-death/

Fuller G (2013) *Neurological Examination Made Easy*, 5th edition. London: Churchill Livingstone.

Gosselin J, Gahagan S, Amiel-Tison C (2005) The Amiel-Tison neurological assessment at term: conceptual and methodological continuity in the course of follow-up. *Ment Retard Dev Disabil Res Rev* 11: 34–51.

Hall S, Pugh AG, Hall DMB (1982) Vision screening in the under-5s. *BMJ* 285: 1096–1098.

Organ Donation & Transplantation (ODT) Diagnosing death using neurological criteria. Directorate of NHS Blood and Transplant (NHSBT) educational resource containing pdfs of the AMRC and RCPCH refs in this list and educational videos. Available at https://www.odt.nhs.uk/deceased-donation/best-practice-guidance/donation-after-brainstem-death/diagnosing-death- using-neurological-criteria/

Plum JB, Saper CB, Schiff ND, Plum F (2007) *Diagnosis of Stupor and Coma*, 4th edition. New York: Oxford University Press

Royal College of Paediatrics and Child Health (2015) The diagnosis of death by neurological criteria in infants less than two months old. Available at https://nhsbtdbe.blob.core.windows.net/umbraco-assets-corp/1354/neurological-death-dnc-guide-final.pdf

CHAPTER 7

Prevention, vaccination, and screening

Jane Williams and Colin Kennedy

Key messages

- Screen only for disorders that meet screening criteria (see Box 7.1).
- Offer universal antenatal screening for fetal infection and Down syndrome.
- Neonatal surveillance and screening includes physical examination, hearing screen, and heel-prick blood tests.
- Prevent neonatal hypothermia and treat neonatal hypoglycaemia or eye infection early.
- Monitor neonatal bilirubin.
- Breastfeeding is best.
- Iron supplementation for high-risk groups (preterm <37 weeks, low birthweight, feeding difficulties).
- Inform families about vaccine safety and immunize systematically.
- Monitor growth on appropriate centile charts.
- Consider screening for anaemia at 9 months, particularly in high-risk groups.
- Protect maternal health and identify early any infant risk factor that could lead to a negative developmental outcome.

Common errors

- Screening without defining precisely the cutoff for a positive screen.

- Screening for target conditions in which the benefit of early diagnosis is doubtful.
- Neglecting the need for counselling before and after screening.
- Overinterpretation of a single late milestone.

When to worry

- Lack of visual fixing or following at 6 to 8 weeks.
- No response to voice at 6 to 8 weeks or risk factors for deafness (syndrome or family history).
- Family history or syndromic features that increase risk of childhood deafness or genetic illness.
- Developmental quotient <70 (i.e. less than 70% of mean reference level).
- Persistent primitive, asymmetric, very brisk, or absent reflexes with abnormal tone.
- Loss of acquired skills.

PRIMARY PREVENTION, SCREENING, AND HEALTH PROMOTION

Although screening and health promotion programmes have been in place for many years in several European and non-European countries, there is still confusion as to what they can and cannot achieve. It is hoped that screening tests will pick out individuals who are at highest risk of having the disorder in question before they become symptomatic and differentiate those who truly have a disorder from those who do not.

It is important to remember that screening is usually not diagnostic testing. Rather, it identifies those at high risk of a given medical condition. When a screening test is positive, the families involved should then be offered the diagnostic test. A screening programme should lead to an improvement in the quality of life of the person and their family. This is an especially important issue in those who screen positive for a target condition, some of whom will be true positives and some false positives (see Glossary at end of this chapter). Families whose child has a false positive result (i.e. who screens positive but does not have the target condition) may be exposed to significant harm, including unnecessary anxiety. The design of screening programmes should be scrutinized by experts and service users offering a wide range of perspectives to guarantee that the positive impact of the test itself outweighs the possible negative effects, including any emotional cost. Screening programmes can be universal, i.e. for the whole population (e.g. measurement of haemoglobin in all pregnant females to detect anaemia), or targeted to high-risk groups (e.g. infants of parents known to be carriers of a genetically inherited condition).

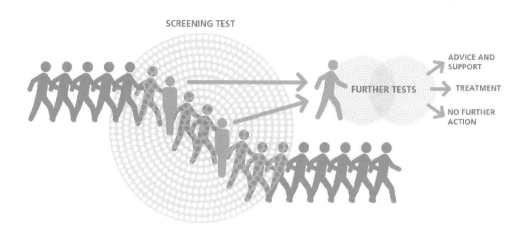

Figure 7.1 Population screening explained. (Reproduced from Public Health England, 2013 courtesy of Public Health England.) A colour version of this figure can be seen in the colour plate section.

Possible benefits of a true positive screen could include the early treatment of a disease so that its adverse effects are minimized or, in the case of prenatal screening, lead to confirmatory tests that show that the fetus has a serious medical condition. This enables a pregnant female to make an informed choice whether or not she wishes to continue with the pregnancy. The success of such programmes must be evaluated on the basis of the proportion of females who feel that they have received enough information and support to allow them to proceed to an informed choice. This is a different criterion from the number of pregnancies affected by the target condition that are terminated. The Wilson–Jungner criteria (Wilson and Jungner, 1968) to evaluate a screening programme, updated in 2003, are shown in Box 7.1.

Information and counselling

The provision of up-to-date information and high-quality/professional counselling and support enables individuals to make the choices that they consider best. It is recommended that:

- females and their partners should feel free to make the decision they feel most appropriate from the options they are given;

- screening and diagnostic tests must only be undertaken with the knowledge and consent of the individual female;

Box 7.1 'Classic' criteria to consider in a screening programme

The condition

- ☑ An important health problem.
- ☑ A simple, safe, precise, and validated screening test.
- ☑ The natural history including from latent to declared disease, should be adequately understood and there should be an early presymptomatic stage.
- ☑ Intervention at the presymptomatic stage should be cost-effective.
- ☑ If carriers of a genetic mutation, as well as cases of the disease, are identified as a result of screening, this impact must be considered.

The test

- ☑ Know the distribution of test values in the target population and agree the cutoff point separating positive from negative screening results.
- ☑ Acceptable.
- ☑ Agree policy on further diagnostic investigation of those with positive results.
- ☑ If testing for mutations, select and provide information to enable interpretation of test results that is appropriate to the subset of mutations screened.
- ☑ An effective treatment or intervention for patients identified and evidence of early treatment leading to better outcome.
- ☑ Evidence-based policies covering treatment.
- ☑ All healthcare providers should optimize care for the condition before participation in a screening programme.

The screening programme

- ☑ Evidence from high-quality, randomized controlled trials that the screening programme is effective in reducing mortality or morbidity.
- ☑ The programme is clinically, socially, and ethically acceptable to health professionals and the public.
- ☑ Benefits of test outweighing harm of test (including psychological harm).
- ☑ 'Value for money'.
- ☑ Agreed plan for monitoring programme.

The treatment

- ☑ Adequate staffing for carrying out programme and treatment.
- ☑ All other options for managing the condition should have been considered.
- ☑ Information from a reliable evidence base available for participants.
- ☑ Anticipate public pressure for widening the eligibility, reducing the screening interval, and increasing the sensitivity of the testing process.
- ☑ If screening is for a mutation, the programme should be acceptable to people identified as carriers and to other family members.

(Wilson and Jungner, 1968)

- for all aspects of antenatal screening, females and their partners must be given verbal information on the screening supported by suitable written or audiotape/audiovisual information, if required;

- for all aspects of antenatal screening, females and their partners should be aware of the risks and benefits associated with each test;

- there should be a policy on how and when females and their partners are given results. Results of specific tests, such as those for fetal abnormality or human immunodeficiency virus (HIV), should be given in person;

- individuals should be informed of all the results of any tests undertaken;

- females should be fully supported and offered access to specialist advice and support if required. This may include counselling or specialist advice for genetic disorders, HIV, or haemoglobinopathy, and/or referral to self-help groups; and

- females should be satisfied with the service offered, this can be audited.

In order to minimize the emotional distress often associated with screening programmes, individuals may be offered accurate and sensitive counselling at the following stages:

- before screening, during which individuals are given the opportunity to make an informed choice about whether or not to have particular tests;

- after screening, during which individuals are given the results of investigations and presented with the options for future action. At this time, support is offered to individuals for decision-making;

- after decision-making, during which information from subsequent investigations is given, support is offered concerning the decision about what action is to be taken, whether this relates to the continuation of a pregnancy or the provision of specialized treatment for a neonatal problem; and

- before a subsequent pregnancy, where parents are helped to make decisions about antenatal diagnostic tests, where available, and cope with the anxiety that often accompanies subsequent pregnancies.

Antenatal screening is undertaken for a number of conditions in the mother and unborn infant. For conditions in the mother, e.g. anaemia and raised blood pressure, treatment is available during the antenatal period to improve her health and, indirectly, that of the infant. For conditions in the infant, the screening test may enable a mother to make an informed choice about continuation of the pregnancy or allow treatment to improve the infant's health to be started as early as possible (see Table 7.1).

Additional important antenatal advice must include avoidance of alcohol or smoking while pregnant and avoidance of nonprescribed drugs before and after delivery.

Screening for maternal disease

Screening for maternal disease involves monitoring pregnancies to try to select pregnant females who, although appearing to be well, have conditions that might be harmful to the unborn infant, (e.g. anaemia, hepatitis B, syphilis, HIV infection, or high blood pressure). Once the condition has been detected, treatment can be started to reduce the effect of the condition on the unborn infant. Immunity to rubella is checked, so that any nonimmune mothers can be offered vaccination with two doses of measles, mumps, and rubella (MMR) vaccine after delivery. If a mother is found to be infected with hepatitis B, then her infant can be immunized soon after birth to reduce the chances of becoming infected.

Screening for abnormalities of the unborn infant

Screening for fetal abnormality is offered to pregnant females as part of routine maternity care. Screening is based on either ultrasound examination, blood tests, or a combination (see Table 7.1).

DELIVERY

It is crucial that delivery is undertaken by a competent birth attendant or midwife and that mother and unborn infant are monitored. High-risk factors for the subsequent health of the infant include maternal ill health, preterm labour, and, for example, unrecognized breech presentation, twins, or other obstetric risk factors.

After delivery it is vital to maintain the infant's body temperature and secure rapid access to a neonatal intensive care unit for those born preterm or manifesting signs of ill health.

Newborn infants are at risk for vitamin K deficiency bleeding (VKDB) caused by inadequate prenatal storage and deficiency of vitamin K in breast milk. A systematic review of evidence to date suggests that a single intramuscular injection of vitamin K at birth effectively prevents VKDB. Oral vitamin K is less effective but 2mg orally at birth and again at 2 to 4 weeks and at 6 to 8 weeks is an alternative to intramuscular injection.

NEONATAL SCREENING

- A detailed physical examination within 72 hours of birth for all infants to exclude visible malformations and examine the eyes for cataracts, the heart for defects,

Table 7.1 Antenatal screening

Gestational age	Screening test	Comments
Preconception		Universal advice cessation of smoking and alcohol consumption. Folic acid prophylaxis of neural tube defects. Targeted advice to females with epilepsy in relation to antiepileptic drug choices, diabetics in relation to control of blood sugar, chronic illness groups.
8—12 weeks	UTI, Rubella, VDRL, HIV, hepatitis B, blood group, Rhesus antibody, FBC, red cell alloantibodies, haemo-globinopathies	
10—14 weeks	USS NIPT	To establish gestational age and screen for more than one fetus
11—13 weeks	USS for nuchal translucency, Beta — HCG, pregnancy associated plasma protein A (Triple test) Screen for Down, Edwards, and Patau syndrome	For females >35 years: positive in 80% infants with Down syndrome
15—20 weeks	(Later bookers) Quadruple test, Detailed USS	Quadruple test detection rate above plus inhibin A for Down syndrome: detects 81% of true cases if screen referral threshold set for false posit-ive rate of 5% for fetal anomalies

UTI, urinary tract infection; VDRL, Venereal Disease Research Laboratory test (blood test for syphilis); HIV, human immunodeficiency virus; FBC, full blood count (maternal for check for anaemia); USS, fetal ultra-sound scan; NIPT, non-invasive prenatal testing: a relatively new technique to detect cell-free fetal DNA from maternal blood in use in some countries to detect Down, Edwards, and Patau syndromes (trisomies of chromosomes 13, 18, and 21 respectively); HCG, human chorionic gonadotrophin.

the hips for dysplasia, the testes for cryptorchidism, and the skin and sclera for jaundice.

- Hearing screening in the first few weeks of life for all infants.

- Heel-prick test: a very small quantity of blood is taken from the infant's heel between 5 days and 8 days after birth. Currently, all infants in the UK are tested for congenital hypothyroidism, cystic fibrosis, sickle-cell disorders, and six inborn errors of metabolism: phenylketonuria, medium-chain acyl-CoA dehydrogenase deficiency (MCADD), maple-syrup urine disease, isovaleric acidaemia, glutaric aciduria type 1, and homocystinuria (pyridoxine unresponsive). The conditions for which neonatal screening is undertaken vary by country. In November 2016, the Recommended Universal Screening Panel (RUSP) of the relevant USA Federal Advisory Committee included 34 core conditions and 26 secondary conditions (document available at www.hrsa.gov).

- Monitoring of jaundice and a programme to check bilirubin levels. This is crucial in preventing kernicterus.

INFANT SCREENING AND HEALTH PROMOTION AFTER THE NEONATAL PERIOD

Universal screening by physical examination of infants subsequent to the neonatal period vary between countries and should exclude prolonged jaundice. In the UK, it is undertaken at 6 to 8 weeks. More than one post-neonatal examination in the first 6 months in infants born at term who are typically developing at post-neonatal discharge has been shown to provide very little additional net benefit. Outlines of universal and targeted testing are given in Table 7.2.

Table 7.2 Health promotion programme: what to include and risk factors

Population to which programme applies	
Universal	**High-risk groups in whom additional targeted actions may be needed**
Health and development reviews at birth, day 1, 6 weeks, and 1 year	Maternal illness, e.g. diabetes, depression, other maternal mental health problems
Immunizations	

Maintenance and promotion of health and well-being
    Reduce parental smoking
    Keep safe
    Dietary advice (mother and infant)
    Promote breastfeeding
    Prevention of sudden infant death (safe sleeping)
	Infant born preterm
	Parental or familial genetic disease
	Maternal alcohol and drug use
	Poor-quality housing
	Poverty
	Single parent
	Domestic violence

Promote parenting and child bonding
    Maternal mental health
    Involve fathers	

Growth monitoring

The weight, length and head circumference of all infants should be measured and plotted sequentially on a standardized growth chart (see Appendix 1) at birth and at intervals over the first year of life. Accurate and calibrated tools for measuring weight and length are essential. A single point on a growth chart is less useful than serial measurements.

Developmental surveillance

It is usual to examine an infant in the first 24 hours of life to look for any obvious structural abnormalities or features that may indicate congenital problems with developmental consequences. In the majority in whom no abnormality is found, the child will be offered routine review of developmental progress at the ages shown below.

It is recommended in many countries to review a child's development routinely as follows:

Universal

- Newborn infant examination (see above).

- Examination at 14 days to exclude jaundice. If jaundice is present, the blood concentration of bilirubin should be measured. Beware the early-discharged jaundiced infant who is feeding poorly.

- 6- to 8-week check, including retinal 'red reflex' response to light.

- Before 1 year; consider haemoglobin check in high-risk groups (e.g. preterm).

- At approximately 18 months.

Targeted

- Infants with known illnesses with developmental consequences (e.g. hydrocephalus or a known chromosomal abnormality) have developmental follow-up to allow early therapy and teacher support.

- Blind or deaf infants usually present with late attainment of developmental milestones and are then found to have a visual or auditory abnormality. Once diagnosed, vigilant developmental follow-up is required and may lead to further investigations to diagnose an underlying cause (e.g. Usher syndrome).

- Infants with known parental genetic illness (e.g. deafness, thalassemia, or sickle-cell disease) will also need relevant targeted screening.

- Infants living in adverse environmental circumstances for optimum growth and development, including domestic violence situations or parental drug abuse.

- Children born preterm: up to 50% of infants born preterm show early neurodevelopmental impairment and are at higher risk of an atypical neurodevelopmental outcome, cerebral palsy, autism, attention deficit disorders, and sensory problems. If developmental impairment is suspected, more formalized testing may be required with appropriate referral.

Developmental screening tests

Identifying a measurement to assess developmental prognosis reliably is not easy. Various screening tests have been validated. Each has inherent difficulties when applied to a population, not least in relation to the practicalities of assessing development in a child's local circumstances (see Chapter 5).

The most commonly used specific tests include the DENVER II test and the Clinical Adaptive Test/Clinical Linguistic and Auditory Milestone Scale, which is heavily language-orientated. There are also tests reliant on parent or teacher questionnaires, such as the Parents' Evaluation of Development Inventory. More detailed assessments of children's developmental performance in comparison to reference ranges for typically developing infants include the Griffiths Mental Development Scales and Bayley Infant Neurodevelopmental Screen.

Personal knowledge of the spectrum of development in typically developing infants (see Chapter 5) is crucial in a neurological examination and will facilitate early detection of preschool children who are late at achieving developmental skills, either generally or in one domain of development.

INFANT DIET AND IRON DEFICIENCY ANAEMIA

Iron deficiency anaemia (IDA) is the most common nutritional deficiency worldwide. Severe or prolonged iron deficiency can cause IDA. Data on the prevalence of IDA in infants 6 to 12 months are sparse and among infants born at term younger than 1 year the prevalence of IDA is low, but high-risk groups include infants born preterm and low-birthweight infants with prolonged neonatal stays in hospital. The risk of IDA is increased if infants are fed on non-iron-fortified milks. Breast milk is the nutrition of first choice. Even though it has less iron per 100ml, it is by far the best source of iron, as well as having many other nutritional advantages. Continuation of breastfeeding for at least the first year of life, while introducing complementary iron-rich foods from 6 months of age, and iron supplementation for infants born preterm and low-birthweight infants are also advised. Age-specific recommended haemoglobin levels are shown in Table 10.4.

Universal screening for IDA

Although studies from several countries show associations between iron deficiency and adverse growth, cognitive, or neurodevelopmental outcome, a US Preventative Services Task Force has concluded that the current evidence is insufficient to assess the balance of benefits and harms of universal screening for IDA in children aged 6 to 24 months.

Targeted screening for IDA

Targeted screening of haemoglobin and/or haematocrit at 9 to 12 months of age and then again 6 months later in groups at high risk of IDA has been recommended by the American Academy of Family Physicians. Screening for iron deficiency anaemia in infants born preterm should occur at 4 months of age and at 9 to 12 months of age.

VACCINATION

Vaccination is one of the greatest breakthroughs in modern medicine. No other medical intervention has done more to save and improve quality of life. Vaccines work by making the body produce antibodies to fight disease without actually infecting it with the disease. If the vaccinated person then comes into contact with the disease itself, their immune system will recognize it and immediately produce the antibodies they need to fight it.

Newborn infants are already protected against several diseases, such as measles, mumps, and rubella (MMR), for a few weeks or months because antibodies have passed to them from their mothers via the placenta if the mother has had exposure to the illness or immunization herself. This is called passive immunity. Passive immunity against MMR may last up to 1 year, which is why the MMR vaccination is given to children just after their first birthday.

The fact that smallpox has been eradicated in the world is an example of the success of vaccination. A more recent example is the 99% reduction in cases of Meningococcus type C infections in the UK among those aged less than 20 years, since 1999, when it added a novel type C vaccine (not shown in Table 7.3 below) to its vaccination schedule. Mortality from this disease has also plummeted from 78 deaths among under-18s in the UK in 1998 compared to only two deaths over a 12-month period in 2011 and 2012. Similar success will also be maintained for the complications of poliovirus and of measles virus if vaccination coverage is sustained at very high levels. Vaccinations additional to those in Table 7.3 will vary by country. In the UK they include rotavirus vaccination at age 8 weeks and 12 weeks; meningococcus B and pneumococcus vaccinations at 8 weeks, 16 weeks, and 12 months; and haemophilus influenzae and meningococcus C vaccinations at 12 months. Certain regions or high risk populations warrant particular mention, e.g. Japanese encephalitis vaccine, a yellow fever vaccine or typhoid and meningococcus vaccines, the list lengthens and is subject to population need and scientific evidence.

Table 7.3 Main vaccine doses, intervals, and routes of administration

Vaccine	Time of vaccination	Dose	Route	Site
INFANTS				
BCG	At or as soon as possible after birth	0.1mL (0.05mL until 1 month of age)	Intradermal	Left upper arm
Hepatitis B	At birth or as soon as possible within 24 hours	0.5mL	Intramuscular	Antero-lateral side of mid-thigh
OPV-0	At birth or as soon as possible within first 15 days	2 drops	Oral	Oral
OPV 1, 2, and 3	At 6, 10, and 14 weeks	2 drops	Oral	Oral
DPT 1, 2, and 3	At 6, 10, and 14 weeks	0.5mL	Intramuscular	Anterolateral side of mid-thigh
Haemophilus Influenza b	At 6, 10 and 14 weeks or 2 or 3 doses and booster 6 months after last	0.5 mL (combination)	Intramuscular	Upper arm
Pneumococcal (Conjugate)	At 6,10 and 14 weeks or 2 primary doses and booster at 9-18 months of age	0.5mL	Intramuscular	Upper arm
Hepatitis B 1, 2, and 3	At 6, 10, and 14 weeks	0.5mL	Intramuscular	Anterolateral side of mid-thigh
Rotavirus	2- 3 doses depending on product with DTP	1.5mL	Oral	Oral
Measles	9 completed months, 12 months (give up to 5 years if not received at 9—12 months)	0.5mL	Subcutaneous	Right upper arm
Rubella	9 completed months with measles or 12 months	0.5 mL	Subcutaneous	Upper arm
CHILDREN				
DPT booster	16—24 months	0.5mL	Intramuscular	Anterolateral side of mid-thigh
OPV booster	16—24 months	2 drops	Oral	Oral
DPT booster	5—6 years	0.5mL	Intramuscular	Upper arm
Tetanus toxoid	10 years and 16 years	0.5mL	Intramuscular	Upper arm
Rubella	Adolescent girls	0.5mL	Subcutaneous	Upper arm
HPV	Two doses (female)	0.5mL	Intramuscular	Upper arm

BCG, bacille Calmette—Guérin; OPV, oral poliovirus vaccine; DPT, diphtheria, pertussis, and tetanus; HPV, Human papilloma virus.

(Reproduced from WHO, 2019. Licence: CC BY-NC-SA 3.0 IGO. Refer to http://www.who.int/immunization/documents/positionpapers/ for table and position paper updates.)

Vaccine hesitancy arises partly as the success of vaccination programmes causes the public memory of the devastating effects of vaccine-preventable illnesses (e.g. poliomyelitis, measles encephalitis) to fade. Public attention is then focused on the unwanted effects of vaccination. Unfounded allegations of the adverse effects of vaccine arise partly for this reason and partly because such a high percentage of the population have experienced vaccination, that very rare coincidental events that are unrelated to vaccination (e.g. autism, unexpected sudden death, multiple sclerosis) may be misattributed to it. Parents' understandable deep concern for the health of their children may be increased by 'bad science', maladministration of vaccination programmes, misreporting by the media, uninformed passive objectors, conspiracy theorists, or alternative lifestyle parents who have built their own theories about vaccination and rely on herd protection from vaccinated children around their own children. The downloadable WHO 'Vaccine safety and false contraindications to immunization' training manual is freely available and highly recommended (WHO, 2020).

Among the most common conditions *incorrectly* considered to be contraindications are diarrhoea, minor upper respiratory tract illnesses (including otitis media) with or without fever, mild or moderate local reactions to a previous dose of vaccine, current antimicrobial therapy, and being in the convalescent phase of an acute illness. Vaccination is also *not* contraindicated by a family history of seizures *nor* by the presence of a stable, long-term, neurological condition (e.g. a cerebral palsy, well-controlled seizures, or early developmental impairment). Vaccination with diphtheria, tetanus, and whole cell pertussis vaccine should be deferred in the presence of a progressive neurological disorder (e.g. infantile spasms, uncontrolled epilepsy, or progressive encephalopathy), in order to avoid misattribution of any adverse consequences of these neurological disorders to coincidental vaccination. Previous severe allergic reaction to the vaccine contraindicates repeat vaccination.

SCREENING FOR HEARING LOSS

It is recommended that all infants have a hearing screen performed as soon as possible after birth, ideally in the neonatal period, to detect permanent childhood hearing loss (PCHL) and facilitate an early intervention to amplify hearing. It is important to stress that any method used is only a screen and must be followed by an evaluation of hearing before any diagnosis is made.

Otoacoustic emission screening test

The otoacoustic emission (OAE) test is commonly used as the neonatal screening test for hearing. It works on the principle that a healthy cochlea will emit a faint sound, the OAE, detectable by a microphone in the outer ear, when stimulated with a repeated clicking sound presented through a small earpiece containing both a loudspeaker and recording microphone. This test can be done with no equipment other than the earpiece and a small computer to average the OAEs occurring a few milliseconds after the click. A normal recording is associated with normal cochlear hair-cell function and this typically reflects normal hearing.

This is a simple and quick test but can have a relatively high false positive rate in the first 24 hours of life due to amniotic fluid in the ear canal. If this happens the test is usually repeated. OAE detection is a test of cochlear function and will not detect auditory neuropathy, also known as auditory dyssynchrony, a rare cause of hearing impairment in which the impairment is in transmission of signals from the cochlea to the brain. If the infant fails again, an automated auditory brainstem response test (AABR; see below) and full assessment are arranged.

The automated auditory brainstem response test

The AABR test works by recording brain activity in response to sounds. An infant may be sleeping naturally or may have to be sedated for this test. Older, cooperative children may be tested in a silent environment while visually occupied. Earphones are placed in or on the infant's ear. Usually click-type sounds are introduced through the earphones and the electrical responses to the sounds in the auditory pathway are measured with scalp electrodes. The computer-averaged electrical response is compared with a stored template of a normal auditory brainstem response test. If the recorded and template responses are similar to one another the test is classified as a pass and if dissimilar as a 'refer'. This test has the advantage that it screens the entire hearing pathway from ear to brainstem, but disadvantages include the need to apply scalp electrodes and for the infant to be asleep during the test.

Distraction hearing test

In this test, a child (developmental range 6–8 months) will sit on a carer's lap while one tester stands behind making sounds and someone else stands in front to distract the child with a visual stimulus, which is then removed, and to watch the child's reaction to the sounds. This test is a good indicator of a general hearing problem if the test is carried out properly, but most infants screening positive at this age will prove to have temporary conductive losses. Furthermore, several studies have found unacceptably high false negative results in infants with permanent hearing loss. Both tester and distractor need to be well trained for this screen to perform it adequately and its use is now confined only to those for whom OAE and/or AABR screening is not available.

HEARING IMPAIRMENT

Epidemiology

Hearing impairment is the most prevalent sensory deficit in the human population. There are two main groups: sensorineural hearing loss and conductive hearing loss. In the child aged less than 1 year, the former is the main concern but the latter is much more prevalent, especially between the ages of 6 months and 12 months when screening leads to detection of many cases of conductive nonpermanent loss for each case of sensorineural hearing loss.

Levels of hearing are described by looking at average air-conduction thresholds; that is, the additional intensity of sound, relative to the normal hearing threshold, required at frequencies of 0.5, 1, 2, and 4Hz to reach the threshold level of audibility in the affected individual. The degree of impairment may be summarized as the average threshold across these four frequencies (Table 7.4).

Table 7.4 Sound intensity relative to normal required to reach hearing threshold level

Hearing loss	Additional sound intensity relative to normal required to reach hearing threshold level
Normal hearing	≤ 15 dB
Mild	15–39 dB
Moderate	40–69 dB
Severe	70–94 dB
Profound	≥ 95 dB

Bilateral PCHL that is of moderate or greater severity leads to well-documented impairment in the development of language and related skills and this impairment can be reduced by universal newborn infant screening, justifying the introduction of such screening programmes (Kennedy et al. 2006). The evidence that the benefit exceeds the risk of harm and justifies the cost of newborn infant screening is less secure for lesser degrees of hearing impairment.

In individuals affected by bilateral moderate or greater PCHL, the impairment will be moderate in approximately 50%, severe in 25%, and profound in 25%. Most cases of permanent hearing loss of this degree are congenital and should be detected soon after birth, but some children present later, either because their hearing loss is acquired (e.g. after meningitis) or because the condition is late-onset and/or there is a progressive increase in severity over time.

High-risk groups for hearing impairment may have:

- a family history of hearing loss;

- extremely preterm birth;

- congenital infection;

- severe neonatal jaundice;

- craniofacial syndromes;

- visual impairment;

- bacterial meningitis or viral encephalitis;

- children with developmental impairments;

- head injury with base-of-skull fracture or auditory symptoms; and

- prolonged use of ototoxic drugs (including oncological drugs).

Sensorineural hearing loss: aetiology and management

The prevention of hearing loss is an important public health issue. Preventative measures include immunization against MMR and bacterial meningitis, effective management of neonatal jaundice, reduction of environmental noise pollution, and education of young people on the long-term risks of high-volume noise from electronic devices (e.g. personal music systems). The aetiology of childhood sensorineural hearing loss has changed in the new millennium in those European countries with an immunization schedule. Fewer cases are now attributed to childhood infections such as mumps, measles, meningitis, or congenital rubella. In other parts of the world the prevalence of these infections is still a major causative factor in sensorineural hearing loss.

The successful implementation of vaccination programmes would have a major impact on decreasing the numbers of affected children.

Where immunization programmes are in place, the importance of genetic causes has now increased, with approximately 50% of cases now being attributed to single-gene mutations. The most common genetic cause of sensorineural hearing loss is non-syndromic or isolated deafness, with no other recognizable features, which may arise at multiple different chromosomal loci. In deafness due to the connexin family of genes, responsible for up to 70% of cases of deafness in European populations, the faulty gene is situated at a single locus on chromosome 13q and results in abnormal recycling potassium ions because of defective gap junctions in cochlear hair cells. In Usher syndrome there are 10 possible genes involved which code for myosin.

There may be a clear environmental determinant, such as congenital cytomegalovirus, but in other cases genes and the environment interact to cause deafness. For example, carriers of the mitochondrial mutation A1555G in *12srRNA* are predisposed to deafness caused by aminoglycosides. The use of this group of antibiotics should be avoided if there is a family history of aminoglycoside-induced deafness.

The best outcome for sensorineural hearing loss is dependent on early detection and early intervention to maximize hearing. The early years offer an enhanced opportunity for better functional outcome, perhaps because of the sensitive period for language development in the central nervous system at this age. Children who lose their hearing ability after having learned to talk usually retain speech. Addressing educational, social, and family issues in conjunction with amplification of residual hearing is essential for optimum prognosis.

Treatment options include education of families regarding communication with the affected child and hearing aids, which can be fitted before 6 months of age. Children with profound loss are often suitable for cochlear implantation at specialized centres.

VISION IMPAIRMENT

Visual development

For the first 4 to 6 weeks of life eye movements are relatively imprecise and slightly jerky, although some ability to fixate on a visual stimulus is often apparent. Poor fixation after 2 months of age is pathological. Accurate smooth pursuit eye movements and central fixation then develop and by 2 to 3 months of age the infant has learned to follow the movement of small objects accurately (Table 7.5).

Infants frequently have variable eye alignment with approximately 70% manifesting transient small, variable squints (esotropia or exotropia) but by 2 to 3 months this will have resolved and developing infants will have established normal alignment (orthotropia).

Table 7.5   Early visual development

Birth to 2 months	2—6 months	3—4 years
Short-lasting fixation, some jerky movements and mild esotropia or exotropia allowed	Accurate fixation Smooth eye movements	Visual acuity 6/9

Definition of blindness

Blindness is defined as a corrected visual acuity in the better eye of less than 3/60 or a central visual field loss to less than 10° around the point of central vision. This is equivalent to the ability to identify script 60mm in size at a distance of 3m. However, this definition immediately raises difficulties in childhood because accurate measurement of visual acuity in children can be difficult for multiple reasons.

Epidemiology

Data are scarce but Scandinavian registers suggest that visual impairment (visual acuity <6/18) affects 8 in 100 000 children each year, but it has been estimated that 500 000 children worldwide become blind each year. In developing countries this is associated with significant mortality from the most common causes, measles infection and vitamin A deficiency.

Prevention of blindness

Primary prevention of blindness can include:

- immunization of the mother against infective disease, for example rubella,

- treatment of sexually transmitted disease or HIV of the mother,

- genetic counselling for those with relevant genetic illness, and

- health education with regard to adverse effects of alcohol, drugs, and X-ray or irradiation exposure in pregnancy, safe food preparations, and avoidance of exposure of pregnant females to potential sources of toxoplasmosis (e.g. from cat litter).

Secondary prevention of blindness can include:

- treatment of disease, for example meningitis,

- early identification of ophthalmia neonatorum,

- prenatal diagnosis on serology and consideration of termination if pregnancy is affected, and

- early identification and treatment of, for example, congenital glaucoma.

Tertiary prevention of blindness can include:

- surgery on cataract, and

- iridectomy for ophthalmia neonatorum.

Causes of neonatal blindness include:

- blurred retinal image (e.g. cataract),

- retinal disease (e.g. toxoplasmosis, retinitis of prematurity, vitamin E deficiency),

- optic nerve disease (e.g. optic nerve hypoplasia, coloboma),

- cortical blindness (e.g. secondary to hydrocephalus or other structural anomaly); in many countries this has become the most common cause of childhood blindness,

- neurogenetic/degenerative disease (e.g. Leber congenital amaurosis), and

- delayed visual maturation; this is a more common cause of poor visual attentiveness in infancy and if not associated with seizures or any other central nervous system defect may be followed by normal visual function in later childhood.

CONCLUSION

Screening has significant differences from other clinical practice as it offers to help apparently healthy individuals to make better informed choices about their health. There are risks involved in screening and it is important, therefore, that individuals have realistic expectations of what a screening programme can deliver. Although screening may have the potential to save lives or improve quality of life through the early diagnosis of serious conditions, it is not a foolproof process. As such, although screening may reduce the risk of developing a condition or its complications, it cannot offer a guarantee of protection against that condition nor, of course, against other conditions and while a positive screening test can bring benefits, it can sometimes cause harm.

'Routine management' of children judged to be at high risk of neurodevelopmental impairments is, in some instances, targeted screening. The potential of such clinical practice for benefit or harm should be considered against the criteria for screening (see Box 7.1) rather than against the criteria that might be regarded as reasonable in the context of management of an identified medical condition or illness.

A vaccination schedule embedded in a screening and health promotion programme is crucial to the enhancement of population health.

REFERENCES

Kennedy CR, McCann DC, Campbell MJ, et al. (2006) Early life detection of permanent hearing loss and subsequent language. *N Engl J Med* 354: 2131–2141.

Public Health England (2013) *NHS population screening explained guidance.* Available at https://www.gov.uk/guidance/nhs-population-screening-explained

Siu AL, US Preventive Services Task Force (2015) Screening for iron deficiency anemia in young children: USPSTF Recommendation Statement. *Pediatrics* 136: 746–752.

US Preventive Services Task Force Evidence Syntheses (2015) *Screening for iron deficiency in childhood and pregnancy.* Report No.: 06-0590-EF-1. Rockville, MD: Agency for Healthcare Research and Quality.

Wang M (2016) Iron deficiency and other types of anemia in infants and children. *Am Fam Physician* 93: 270–278.

WHO (2020) *Vaccine Safety and False Contraindications to Vaccination. Training Manual.* World Health Organization. Available at https://www.who.int/immunization/documents/position-papers/en/

Wilson JMG, Jungner G (1968) *Principles and Practice of Screening for Disease.* WHO Chronicle. Public health papers No 34. Geneva: World Health Organization. Available at https://apps.who.int/iris/bitstream/handle/10665/37650/WHO_PHP_34.pdf?sequence=17

Resources

Dutton G, Bax M (2010) *Visual Impairment in Children due to Damage to the Brain.* Clinics in Developmental Medicine series. London: Mac Keith Press.

NHS (2019) Why vaccination is safe and important. Available at https://www.nhs.uk/conditions/vaccinations/how-vaccines-work/

NHS (2019) NHS vaccinations and when to have them. Available at https://www.nhs.uk/conditions/vaccinations/nhs-vaccinations-and-when-to-have-them/

Preece PM, Riley EP (2011) *Alcohol, Drugs and Medication in Pregnancy: the Outcomes for the Child.* Clinics in Developmental Medicine series. London: Mac Keith Press.

Public Health England (2012) Newborn blood spot screening programme: support publications. Available at https://www.gov.uk/government/collections/newborn-blood-spot-screening-
programme-supporting-publications#blood-spot-screening-information

Sharma A, Cockerill H (2014) *Mary Sheridan's From Birth to Five Years: Children's Developmental Progress*, 4th edition. Abingdon, Oxon: Routledge.

WHO Multicentre Growth Reference Study Group (2006) WHO Child Growth Standards. *Acta Paediatrica Supplement*, 450. Available at https://www.who.int/childgrowth/standards/en/ (growth charts are reproduced in Appendix 1).

WHO (2019) WHO recommendations for routine immunization. Available at https://www.who.int/immunization/documents/positionpapers/en/.

CHAPTER GLOSSARY

False negative result   A negative result is present as is the condition.

False positive result   A positive result is present but the condition is not.

Negative result (on a screening test) This is a result which indicates that an individual is at low risk of a condition.

Positive predictive value   The proportion of people with a positive test result who have the condition.

Positive result (on a screening test) This is a result which indicates that an individual is at high risk of a condition.

Screening programme   This includes screening, diagnosis, and the management of a condition.

Screening test   This is a test that is designed to identify those individuals who are at a high enough risk of having a particular disorder to warrant the offer of a diagnostic test. A screening test may be a procedure, such as a blood test, or it may be the asking of a question, such as 'How old are you?'

Sensitivity of a screening test   This refers to the ability of the test to detect those who have a condition accurately. A highly sensitive test has a sensitivity approaching 100%. The consequence of a test that lacks sensitivity is that individuals are informed that they do not have a condition when in fact they do (this is known as a false negative result).

Specificity of a screening test   The ability of the test to identify those who do not have the condition accurately. A highly specific test has a specificity approaching 100%. The consequence of a test that lacks specificity is that an individual is informed that they have a condition when in fact they do not (this is known as a false positive result).

Surveillance   Health surveillance is a system of ongoing health checks. In some countries the term health promotion is now being used more frequently.

CHAPTER 8

Cranial imaging

Brigitte Vollmer and Harriet Joy

Key messages

- Structural imaging of the brain allows assessment of normal anatomy and brain maturation as well as the effects of disease on the brain parenchyma.
- When making a request for neuroimaging, formulate a clear question to be answered. Incidental findings are common and usually do not explain the reported symptoms. They can cause confusion to doctors and stress to families if their reporting is not managed well.
- To aid accurate reporting, provide the radiologist with details of medical history, clinical findings, and results of laboratory investigations to tailor imaging optimally to the individual case.

Common errors

- Imaging the brain for moderate early developmental impairment with normal head size and in the absence of abnormal neurological signs
- Relying on ultrasound alone for interpretation of changes in brain parenchyma.

When to worry

- No imaging available for a patient with acute undiagnosed neurological illness.

NEUROIMAGING PRINCIPLES

Ultrasound is very useful in infants with an open fontanelle. No radiation is involved, and it is easily performed at the bedside. Serial cranial ultrasound scans are an essential part of routine neonatal intensive care (Ecury-Goossen et al. 2015).

Main indications

- Imaging of intracranial haemorrhage or periventricular white matter abnormalities in the infant born preterm (initial diagnosis and monitoring by serial scanning).

- Initial imaging of infants born at term with neonatal encephalopathy (hypoxic-ischaemic changes, focal infarction) but this should be followed by magnetic resonance imaging (MRI).

- Imaging of macrocephaly for hydrocephalus.

- Detection of intracranial calcification.

Practical requirements

- Cranial ultrasound should be performed according to a standard protocol and include, as a minimum, coronal and sagittal/parasagittal standard views.

- It should be performed serially to evaluate changes in brain pathology.

- Images should be stored so that they are available for review.

Limitations/disadvantages

- Imaging of posterior fossa abnormalities is limited.

- View of the cerebral convexities and extra-axial spaces is limited.

- In preterm brain injury, ultrasound is good at detecting cystic focal lesions but not sensitive for diffuse white matter injury.

Transcranial Doppler ultrasound is used to assess cerebral blood flow and can also be used when the fontanelle is closed.

Skull radiography is useful in the investigation of craniosynostosis (Figure 8.1) and in assessing for fractures in the evaluation of trauma. It remains part of the recommended skeletal survey undertaken in cases of suspected physical abuse.

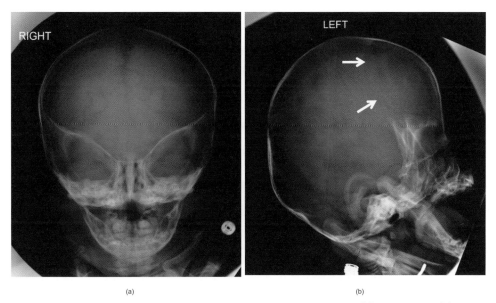

Figure 8.1 Craniosynostosis of coronal sutures and brachycephaly. (a) Frontal and (b) lateral plain skull films of a 4-month-old infant. The coronal sutures are not visible as they have already fused (arrows point to where they should be). Resultant alteration of skull growth causes the brachiocephalic appearance of the skull (shortened in the anteroposterior dimension).

Computed tomography (CT) is an X-ray-based imaging modality. For many indications, CT has been replaced by MRI. However, it remains important because it can be performed quickly and is sensitive and specific for detection of acute intracranial haemorrhage (see Table 18.1), so may be useful in an emergency setting. Secondary low density tissue changes (oedema, ischaemia, infarction) may be identified as well.

CT remains helpful in detection of intracranial calcification and shows bone structures well, so is useful in searching for fractures. Updated guidelines on the investigation of suspected physical abuse in children were published by the Royal College of Radiologists in 2018. These recommend that CT of the head should be undertaken in all children with suspected physical abuse under 1 year of age, and in those older than 1 year with external evidence of head trauma or with abnormal neurological symptoms or signs (see www.rcr.ac.uk/publication/radiological-investigation-suspected-physical-abuse-children).

Contrast enhanced images, using an iodinated contrast medium given intravenously, can be useful in the diagnosis of infection. Intravenous administration of contrast is also required in *CT venography (CTV)* in which the scan is timed to be acquired when the contrast medium is in the venous phase following injection. It can be helpful in suspected venous sinus thrombosis when appearances on MRI are equivocal.

Main indications for CT

- Acute trauma and suspected physical abuse (detection of haemorrhage and fractures).

- Searching for intracranial calcifications (Figure 8.2).

- Diagnosis and evaluation of craniosynostosis.

- Diagnosis of venous sinus thrombosis(see Figure 17.4a2, d3, and f in Chapter 17).

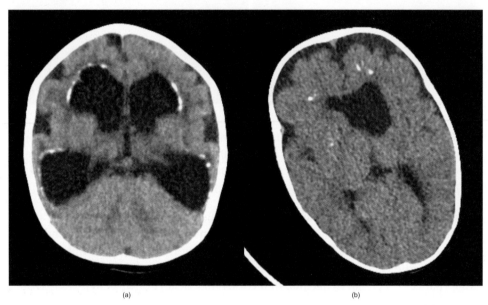

(a)   (b)

Figure 8.2 Intracranial calcification. Calcification is seen as very high density on CT. (a) The small high density foci on the margins of the lateral ventricles along with ventriculomegaly are due to congenital cytomegalovirus infection in this case. (b) Small punctate high density foci within cerebral white matter may be seen in other congenital infections.

Limitations and disadvantages

- MRI is superior to CT in defining parenchymal abnormality and is more accurate in detection of subacute and chronic intracranial haemorrhage.

- CT delivers a dose of radiation to the brain and surrounding structures and there is a slight increase in lifetime cancer risk from this exposure (Matthews et al. 2013).

- Therefore, when CT is required, all efforts should be made to keep the radiation dose as low as possible to achieve a diagnostic study.

Structural MRI is based on the principles of nuclear magnetic resonance. MRI uses a magnetic field (in a clinical setting typically 1.5 or 3 Tesla) to align the magnetization of some atoms in the body, then uses radiofrequency fields to alter the alignment of this magnetization systematically. This causes the nuclei to produce a rotating magnetic field detectable by the scanner and information from this is recorded to construct images of the scanned area of the body. It does not involve radiation and the main advantage of structural MRI is that it can show different tissue contrasts (T1-weighted [T1-w] T2-weighted [T2-w], spin density, diffusion, and flow) in multiple planes (sagittal, coronal, and axial).

Main advantages of structural MRI

- MRI is the most useful imaging modality for assessment of central nervous system (CNS) anatomy, maturation, and pathology.

- It is superior to CT except for imaging of acute haemorrhage, calcification, and bone structures.

- In neonates, MRI provides more detailed information than cranial ultrasound. It is useful in distinguishing pathologies that mimic hypoxic-ischaemic encephalopathy (HIE) (e.g. infection, metabolic disorders, venous infarction, and malformations).

- In HIE, it can also demonstrate patterns of brain injury which help with the timing of injury and prediction of outcome.

Limitations and disadvantages of MRI

- MRI takes time and requires the patient to lie still for at least 20 minutes.

- Movement artifacts are a common problem and degrade image quality.

- Metallic objects cause artefacts and can heat up and cause tissue damage.

- Standard MRI sequences do not depict calcification well.

Practical issues in MRI

- Newborn infants can, in the majority of cases, be scanned in natural sleep ('feed and wrap').

- With infants beyond 3 months of age, sedation or general anaesthesia is often required for MRI.

- MRI is noisy, so hearing protection is utilized (earplugs and infant earmuffs).

- Cardiorespiratory function needs to be monitored during scanning.

Keep the following in mind for MRI in infants:

- MRI protocols need to be tailored to the clinical question and take into account that the brain continues to develop during early infancy and childhood.

- In the first 2 years of life water content of the brain decreases and myelination increases, which results in T1 and T2 shortening, altering signal intensity. Therefore, modifications of sequences are necessary to achieve optimal soft-tissue contrast between normal and pathological structures.

- Before the age of 6 months myelin maturation is best evaluated on T1-w images, while after 6 months until about 2 years T2-w images are more useful. Myelination appears complete on T1-w images by the age of 1 year, but not until around 2 years on T2-w images.

- During myelination there is a time period where grey matter and subcortical structures are isointense, which means that subtle grey matter features, such as migration abnormalities, are difficult to visualize. This occurs at different ages on different sequences.

- Interpretation of MRI in infancy, particularly in the neonatal period, should be done by an experienced person who is familiar with the normal structural features of the developing brain, the range of abnormalities that can be seen, as well as the effect of time from injury to appearance on the images. It is important to consider perinatal and postnatal clinical details for correct interpretation of imaging findings.

Common MRI sequences are useful for the following:

- T1-w images (Figure 8.3ai) are used largely for assessment of anatomy, for evaluation of the extent of myelination in the early months, and when myelination is complete, this sequence is useful for assessing grey/white matter differentiation. It can also be useful for detecting subacute blood products, fat, and some calcification, which are seen as high signal intensity on T1-w images.

- T1 inversion recovery (T1 IR) images (Figure 8.3aii) are useful for assessment of myelin maturation, and beyond 1 year of age are excellent in assessing grey/white matter differentiation, so they are particularly useful in looking for cortical malformations.

- T2-w images (Figure 8.3aiii) are good for detecting 'pathology' such as infection, inflammation, and tumours, which often appear bright on T2-w images.

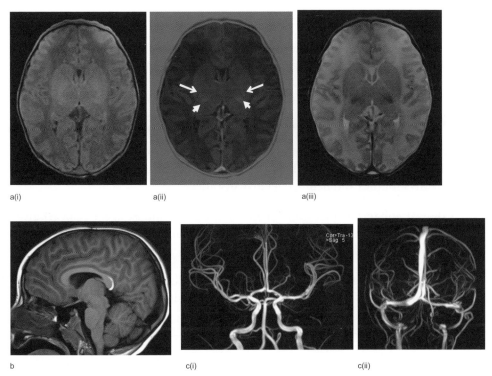

a(i) a(ii) a(iii)

b c(i) c(ii)

Figure 8.3 Examples of different MRI sequences. (a) Normal images: Axial images at the level of the basal ganglia in an infant born at term (i) T1-w, (ii) T1 IR — there is evidence of myelin within the posterior limb of the internal capsules (arrows) and in the ventrolateral nucleus of the thalami (small arrows), (iii) T2-w.

(b) T1-w image: Fat or lipid is of high signal on T1-w images, such as is seen in a lipoma associated with the splenium of the corpus callosum (arrow).

(c) Vascular imaging: (i) MRA and (ii) MRV. Maximum intensity projection reformatted images show flow in the major intracranial arteries and dural venous sinuses respectively.

- T2-fluid-attenuated inversion recovery (FLAIR) suppresses cerebrospinal fluid (CSF) signals and is, therefore, useful for assessment of myelinated white matter close to CSF spaces (e.g. gliosis in periventricular regions); however, it is not a particularly useful sequence for imaging in young infants.

- Diffusion weighted imaging (DWI) is based on the Brownian motion of water and can quantify the extent to which water diffuses freely within tissues. Apparent diffusion coefficient (ADC) maps are calculated from the DWI and give a quantitative measure of the amount of diffusion, reflecting water mobility within the brain. 'Diffusion restriction' (i.e. decrease in water diffusivity) is seen as high signal on diffusion images with corresponding low ADC and is found with a number of pathologies. The main application of this sequence is early identification of ischaemic events (before they are readily visible on T1-w and T2-w images), but it is useful in identification of infection (encephalitis, cerebritis, abscess) as well, and diffusion restriction will be seen in some subacute haemorrhages.

- T2*-w gradient echo imaging is sensitive to field inhomogeneity caused by some blood products, which produces a striking decrease in signal intensity. This effect is even more pronounced in the newer, more detailed sequence, susceptibility weighted imaging (SWI). Brain iron deposition can also be detected on this sequence and a similar but less pronounced effect may be seen with calcification. These sequences are, therefore, useful in imaging vascular malformations and trauma in particular, but SWI now has a wider application in the investigation of leukodystrophies and neurogenerative disorders.

- Contrast enhancement with a gadolinium-based contrast agent (GBCA) given intravenously is useful in the imaging of inflammation, acute infection, tumours, neurocutaneous disorders, and vascular disorders.

- 3D or volumetric sequences are increasingly employed. The images acquired can be reformatted so that they can be assessed in multiple planes.

Imaging protocols

A combination of T2-w images in two planes along with T1-w images in two planes (or a volume T1-w sequence) is a good basic imaging protocol. The acquisition of thin contiguous images and/or volumetric sequences is recommended. DWI is also frequently acquired. Additional sequences such as SWI or post-contrast T1-w images can then be added, depending on the clinical question. In infants under 6 months, axial T1-w images (either standard T1-w or TIR) should be included for assessment of myelination.

Suggested basic MRI protocols

Basic MRI protocol — child under 6 months	Basic MRI protocol — child 6 months–2 years
Axial T2-w	Axial T2-w
Axial T1 IR	Coronal T2-w
Coronal T2-w	Volume T1-w (or standard T1-w in two planes)
Volume T1-w	DWI
DWI	

MRI, magnetic resonance imaging; IR, inversion recovery; DWI, diffusion weighted imaging.

Magnetic resonance angiography (MRA) and magnetic resonance venography (MRV) (Figure 8.3c) are non-invasive (no intravenous contrast agent) and allow quick imaging of the large arteries and veins. They are useful in looking for arteriovenous malformations, arterial stenosis or occlusion, and venous sinus thrombosis. However, in the neonatal period interpretation of MRV can be difficult because of slow flow in the sinuses.

NEUROIMAGING IN CLINICAL SETTINGS

Neonatal encephalopathy

Neonatal encephalopathy (NE) is a clinically defined syndrome of acutely disturbed neurological function in the term infant (see Chapter 14). It is manifested by difficulties with respiration, depression of tone and reflexes, alteration of consciousness, and often seizures. Causes include:

- diffuse cerebral injury (hypoxic-ischaemic insult);

- focal cerebral injury (arterial ischaemic stroke, infarct secondary to venous thrombosis, primary intracerebral haemorrhage);

- metabolic disorders;

- infection;

- drug exposure (not discussed in this chapter);

- CNS malformations.

Cranial ultrasound is useful for initial rapid evaluation, for example to detect haemorrhage, oedema, or infarct (Salas et al. 2018). Early CT can exclude haemorrhage in areas more difficult to visualize with ultrasound. However, it has to be kept in mind that CT exposes the infant to radiation and should only be considered if they are not able to undergo an MRI (e.g. clinically unstable, contraindication to MRI).

A framework for practice for perinatal neuroimaging was published by the British Association of Perinatal Medicine in 2016 (www.bapm.org/resources/33-fetal-neonatal-brain-magnetic-resonance-imaging-clinical-indications-acquisitions-and-reporting). It advises MRI as the imaging modality of choice in NE. It concludes that MRI is useful in aiding the prediction of neurological and neurodevelopmental outcome in newborn infants with HIE, and imaging between 5- and 14-days postpartum is recommended.

Neonatal seizures

There are multiple causes to be considered in a newborn infant with seizures (see Chapter 16), and many of the differential diagnoses overlap with causes of NE. Any neonate with seizures should undergo imaging and the principles outlined above apply with regard to the application of different imaging modalities. However, MRI has been shown to demonstrate the cause in most neonatal seizures. It is also helpful in predicting outcome, with lack of a major abnormality on MRI being associated with a low probability of recurrent seizures or neurodevelopmental impairment (Osmond et al. 2014).

Postneonatal epileptic seizures

Neuroimaging in infants with epilepsy is important in those who develop the condition before the age of 2 years and in those with focal seizures (Gaillard et al. 2009). It may also be helpful in those in whom the epilepsy classification is in doubt.

- Imaging is predominantly performed to detect cortical abnormalities and the imaging modality of choice is MRI.

- The acquisition of thin contiguous images and/or volumetric sequences is recommended.

- The best imaging sequence for demonstrating an abnormality will depend on the extent of myelin development and maturation and, as mentioned previously, there is a time period during this process when differentiation of grey matter and subcortical white matter becomes more indistinct, making delineation of a cortical malformation less certain.

- CT should only be considered where no MRI is available to exclude gross structural abnormality. CT may also be useful in situations where there is suspicion that acute illness may be causing the seizures.

Trauma (postnatal)

Accidental head injury can lead to epidural, subdural, subarachnoid, and parenchymal haemorrhage. In head trauma from suspected physical abuse, the most common location is subdural. The UK Royal College of Radiologists give the following recommendations on imaging of head injury in this scenario (www.rcr.ac.uk/publication/radiological-investigation-suspected-physical-abuse-children).

- CT is the imaging modality of choice for the quick and initial assessment of traumatic brain injury, particularly in looking for acute haemorrhage, and in assessing for skull fractures (Figure 8.4).

- MRI is useful for assessing the extent of parenchymal injury in more detail. It should be undertaken at days 2 to 5 post-trauma in those in whom the CT demonstrates abnormality due to trauma, or in those with abnormal neurological symptoms or signs, regardless of whether the CT performed shows abnormality or not.

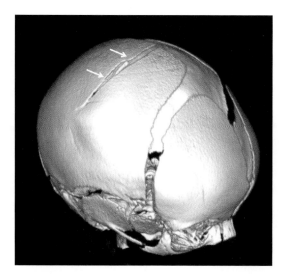

Figure 8.4 Skull fracture. Volume rendered 3D reformat of the skull showing a mildly diastased linear right parietal bone fracture in a 12-day-old infant who had fallen from his parent's arms. The coronal and lambdoid sutures are of normal width for this age.

- When head MRI is undertaken, MRI of the whole spine should also be obtained, as spinal ligamentous injury and spinal subdural haemorrhage are far more frequent following an abusive insult than accidental trauma.

- If imaging shows parenchymal injury MRI should be repeated 2 to 3 months after the trauma to obtain prognostic information, which may aid clinical management.

Macrocephaly, including hydrocephalus

Macrocephaly is due to either a large brain, or large spaces around or within the brain. Causes of macrocephaly are described in Chapter 23.

- In the neonatal period, ultrasound is a good tool for initial evaluation and monitoring of ventriculomegaly.

- CT or MRI is necessary for more detailed investigation of underlying causes following initial evaluation with ultrasound.

- MRI is the method of choice for detailed evaluation of structural brain abnormalities that may cause hydrocephalus (Figure 8.5a) (e.g. aqueduct stenosis, obstruction by a tumour, previous intraventricular haemorrhage), and for assessment of parenchymal abnormalities that may cause a large brain (Figure 8.5b) (see Chapter 23).

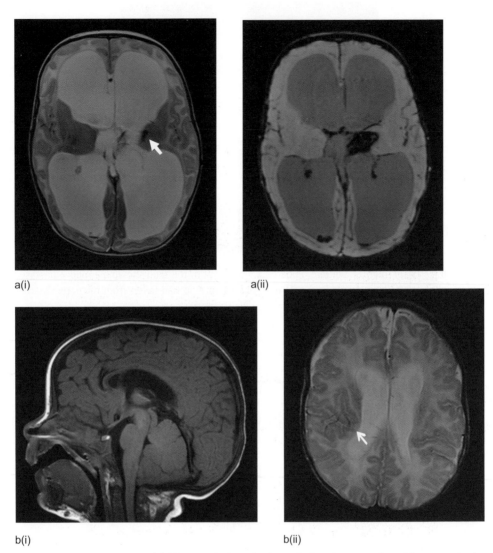

a(i)

a(ii)

b(i)

b(ii)

Figure 8.5 Macrocephaly.(a) Macrocephaly — hydrocephalus due to perinatal intraventricular haemorrhage: (i) Axial T2 image showing markedly enlarged lateral and third ventricles. A tiny focus of low signal is seen in the left caudothalamic groove. This appears much larger on the equivalent SWI (ii) with evidence of haemosiderin staining also seen in the occipital horns and related to choroid plexus within the lateral ventricles. Intraventricular haemorrhage is the likely cause of the hydrocephalus.

(b) Macrocephaly — brain overgrowth in a 2-year-old female with macrocephaly-cutis marmorata. (i) The midline sagittal T1 image shows frontal bossing related to the macrocephaly, and overgrowth of the cerebellum with cerebellar tonsillar ectopia. (ii) Axial T2 image showing ventricular enlargement and abnormal cortex with polymicrogyria in the right posterior perisylvian region (arrow).

Microcephaly, including congenital infections

The aetiology of microcephaly is diverse (see Chapter 22). Primary microcephaly has heterogeneous genetic origins (Figure 8.6a). Secondary microcephaly is caused by acquired lesions or pathological processes that affect the developing brain in the first years of life and result in volume loss/atrophy (Figure 8.6b). Neuroimaging plays an important role in identifying possible underlying causes and in differentiating acquired microcephaly from genetic types of microcephaly.

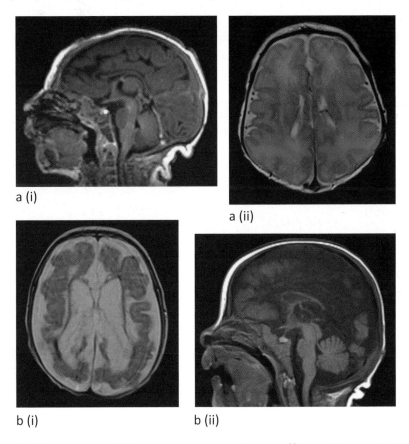

a (i)

a (ii)

b (i)　　　　　　b (ii)

Figure 8.6 Microcephaly. (a) Microcephaly from genetic cause: (i) The midline sagittal T1 images shows relative reduction in the size of the calvarium compared to facial structures. (ii) Axial T2 image showing the relatively simple gyral pattern without formation of many secondary sulci in this infant born at term.
(b) Microcephaly as the sequela of an acquired insult: (i) Axial T2 image showing marked increase in ventricular size and in the volume of the CSF resulting from profound cerebral volume loss due to perinatal hypoxic-ischaemic insult. (ii) Midline sagittal T1 image showing thinning of the corpus callosum, secondary to significant white matter volume loss.

- Structural brain abnormalities such as malformations, hypoxic-ischaemic lesions, postinfective lesions, and CNS abnormalities in metabolic disorders are best visualized with MRI (see relevant sections below).

- CT is sensitive in the detection of calcifications, such as may be seen in many congenital infections. These frequently lead to microcephaly. Radiological signs of some congenital infections are summarized in Table 8.1.

Table 8.1 Radiological signs of congenital infections

Infection	Findings in CT and/or MRI
Toxoplasmosis	Calcifications in basal ganglia, periventricular white matter, and cortical grey matter Ventriculomegaly
Cytomegalovirus	Calcifications in periventricular white matter Neuronal migration abnormalities such as polymicrogyria and lissencephaly Delayed myelination and glial scars in white matter Cerebellar hypoplasia
Rubella	Calcifications in periventricular white matter, basal ganglia, cortical grey matter Ventriculomegaly Delayed myelination Diffuse areas of increased signal on T2-w images
Syphilis	Cerebral infarcts Meningeal enhancement (on contrast-enhanced images)
HIV	Calcifications in periventricular white matter and basal ganglia Brain atrophy, ventriculomegaly Signs of progressive leukoencephalitis with demyelination possible

The 'floppy' infant

The diagnostic approach for the 'floppy' infant depends on whether there is a suspected central origin for the hypotonia or whether the clinical signs point towards a peripheral cause (see Chapter 24). In the majority of infants, the origin is central and for these infants neuroimaging should be part of the diagnostic process.

- In the neonatal period, ultrasound can be used for initial assessment of gross structural abnormalities, such as the presence of haemorrhage or features of hypoxic-ischaemic injury. Most of the disorders outlined in the section on NE can be associated with 'floppiness'.

- MRI is the method of choice, particularly beyond the neonatal period, for detection of structural abnormalities, signs of neurodegenerative or metabolic disorders, ischaemic injury, infection, or trauma.

Early developmental impairment

(see Chapter 26)

- Moderate developmental impairment without other clinical features is not an indication for neuroimaging. Severe or profound impairment is an indication for neuroimaging. If there are clinical signs such as abnormal head size, dysmorphic features, abnormal findings on neurological examination, or epilepsy, neuroimaging is likely to be helpful in establishing the cause.

- MRI is the imaging modality of choice and the basic protocol outlined at the beginning of this chapter should be used.

- CT is preferable for visualization of calcification that is associated with, for example, congenital infections.

- Delayed myelination (identified on MRI) is a nonspecific feature observed in many children with developmental impairment of any cause.

IMAGING APPEARANCES OF DISEASE

Diffuse cerebral injury: perinatal hypoxic-ischaemic insult

Following a hypoxic-ischaemic insult (see Chapter 14), different injury patterns may be seen, involving both grey and white matter. Patterns of brain injury also differ between infants born at term and born preterm and in this section only the infant born at term is considered.

Ultrasound is useful in the initial evaluation, which, depending on the severity of the insult, may show the following:

- brain swelling;

- diffuse hyperechogenicity, loss of sulci and fissures, slit ventricles ('fuzzy brain');

- increased echogenicity in the thalami (and relative hypoechogenicity of the caudate nuclei);

- early haemorrhage in primary ischaemic areas that have subsequently become hyperaemic.

Structural MRI can provide more detailed delineation of the injury, particularly when looking at subcortical structures and for parasagittal cortical injury. Diffusion MRI depicts abnormality at an earlier stage than conventional MRI sequences and should be performed within 1 week of birth for early identification of ischaemia. MR spectroscopy (MRS) may also be useful in early imaging of HIE, but further discussion is beyond the scope of this chapter (for a review of MRS in neonatal HIE, see e.g. Robertson et al. 2014).

Hypoxic-ischaemic injury has characteristic appearances on conventional T1-w and T2-w imaging (Figure 8.7b) that depend on the severity and duration of the insult as well as the stage of brain development:

- Central injury with thalami, basal ganglia (mainly putamen), hippocampi, brainstem, and corticospinal tract involvement (posterior limb of the internal capsule); typically seen after an acute hypoxic-ischaemic insult.

- Parasagittal cortical injury and subcortical white matter injury ('watershed injury') with relative sparing of the central grey matter structures (basal ganglia, thalami, brainstem), usually bilateral; seen following a prolonged partial hypoxic-
ischaemic insult.

The timing of MRI depends partly on the reason for imaging, i.e. whether MRI is performed to aid in diagnosis or in prediction of outcome.

- On T1-w and T2-w images, lesions are obvious 1 to 2 weeks from the time of the insult and imaging at this time is useful in aiding prediction of outcome (mainly motor outcome).

- However, in order to clarify the diagnosis, or help with clinical management, earlier imaging may be required.

- It is important to keep in mind that on T1-w and T2-w imaging performed within a week of the likely insult, subtle abnormalities may not be readily visible. However, diffusion restriction due to ischaemic injury can be shown on DWI within hours after the insult and can last for approximately 7 days (Figure 8.7a), by which time abnormality will be more evident on T1-w and T2-w images (Figure 8.7b).

Focal cerebral injury

This includes focal cerebral injury (see Chapter 18) due to arterial ischaemic stroke, infarct and/or haemorrhage secondary to venous thrombosis, and primary intracerebral haemorrhage.

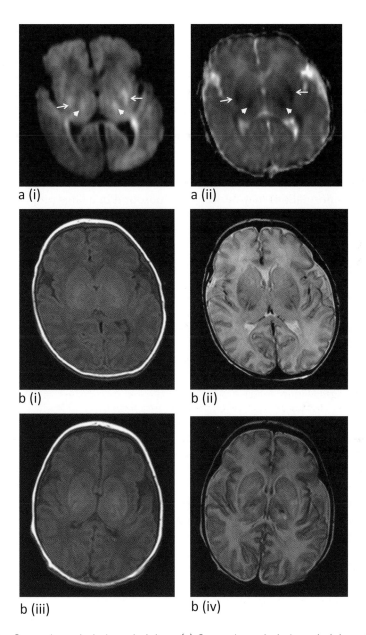

Figure 8.7 Severe hypoxic-ischaemic injury. (a) Severe hypoxic-ischaemic injury: DWI at day 4. (i) DWI and (ii) corresponding ADC map showing bilateral areas of restricted diffusion in the posterior putamina (arrows) and the ventrolateral nucleus of the thalamus (small arrows), and also in the optic radiations.

(b) Severe HIE — T1 and T2 imaging at days 4 and 14: Minimal change is seen in the basal ganglia and thalami on (i) axial T1 and (ii) axial T2 images on day 4 post-perinatal hypoxic-ischaemic insult, but on a repeat scan at day 14, there is now (iii) more faint T1 high signal than expected and (iv) patchy T2 high signal in the posterior basal ganglia and lateral thalami.

On ultrasound, focal cerebral injury may be seen as a hyperechogenic focus. MRI is the imaging modality of choice in neonatal focal cerebral injury.

- In addition to conventional T1-w and T2-w sequences and DWI, vascular imaging with MRA and/or MRV should be included for detection of abnormalities in the large arteries and the deep venous system and major dural venous sinuses.

- In most cases, MRA should not only include the brain but should also cover the neck.

Arterial ischaemic stroke (AIS) involves middle cerebral artery territory in the majority of cases, and abnormalities may be seen on ultrasound in a large proportion of cases, particularly when it is performed 3 or more days after the onset of symptoms (Cowan et al. 2005). Early findings include areas of increased echogenicity with a normal pattern of gyri and sulci. Subsequently, the affected regions become more hyperechoic and better defined, and there is loss of grey/white matter differentiation.

MRI can delineate the extent of the parenchymal injury and help with prognosis. The appearance of the infarct evolves over time (Dudink et al. 2009).

- In the acute phase the area of infarction may be difficult to visualize on T1-w and T2-w images but may be seen as loss of grey/white matter differentiation with increased signal in the affected cortex on T2-w images and decreased signal on T1-w images (Figure 8.8a).

- In the acute phase DWI is extremely useful because the infarct is seen as high signal on the diffusion weighted images and low signal on the ADC map consistent with restricted diffusion, caused by cytotoxic oedema.

- A few days after the event there is a decrease in signal intensity on diffusion weighted images and an increase in ADC values (due to the development of necrosis, cell lysis, and cell shrinkage, resulting in an increase in extracellular space and increased water diffusion).

- The area of injury becomes less obvious on diffusion weighted images towards the end of the first week after the insult; however, by this time lesions are clearly seen on T1-w and T2-w images, with T1 high signal and T2 low signal within affected cortex apparent at this time.

In most cases of *venous sinus thrombosis*, the superior sagittal sinus is affected, with the transverse sinuses and then the straight sinus the next most frequently involved. Associated lesions, such as thalamic or intraventricular haemorrhage and parenchymal haemorrhagic infarction, are frequently seen.

- High frequency ultrasound may identify venous sinus thrombosis, the adjacent area of increased echogenicity in the parenchyma and the secondary associated

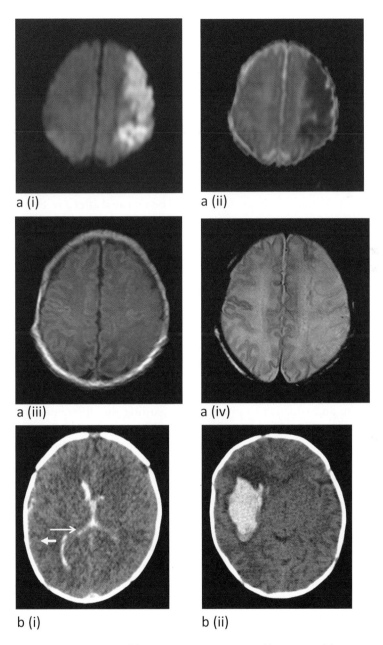

Figure 8.8 Focal cerebral injury. (a) Acute ischaemic stroke: (i) DWI and (ii) corresponding ADC map showing restricted diffusion in a large part of the left MCA territory. The affected cortex shows decrease in signal on T1 (iii) and increase in signal on T2 (iv) making it less easy to distinguish from the signal returned by white matter.

(b) Location of acute haemorrhage on CT: (i) As well as intraventricular haemorrhage in the lateral and third ventricles (arrow), a small volume of surface blood is shown, likely subarachnoid in location (small arrow). (ii) A large acute haematoma is visible as an area of high density in the right basal ganglia.

lesions. However, ultrasound has poor sensitivity for cerebral infarction and should not be used for the primary detection of venous sinus thrombosis and delineation of the extent of injury. Doppler ultrasound can detect absent or reduced flow in the superficial venous sinuses.

- If MRI is not easily available, ultrasound with Doppler and/or CT venography should be considered.

- However, MRI with MRV is the method of choice for diagnosis of venous sinus thrombosis and any associated injury. MRV will show lack of flow in the involved venous sinus with lack of normal flow void seen on conventional sequences. DWI will identify ischaemic tissue. MRI should be repeated after a week to check there is no thrombus propagation, and again after 2 to 3 months to assess recanalization of the vessel.

Primary intracranial haemorrhage, which accounts for up to a third of intracranial bleeding in infants born at term, can be solitary or multifocal.

- Ultrasound will demonstrate the presence and extent of a haemorrhage.

- CT readily identifies the presence and location of subdural, subarachnoid, and parenchymal acute haemorrhage (Figure 8.8b).

- MRI is helpful in more detailed characterization of location and extent of the lesion, and superior to ultrasound regarding the differentiation between a primary parenchymal haemorrhage and non-haemorrhagic infarction. If there is an underlying arteriovenous malformation (which should be suspected in the absence of birth trauma or coagulopathy), MRI with MRA is helpful in its detection after the initial oedematous phase.

CNS infection (see Chapter 19)

Although meningitis is identified through a clinical and laboratory-based diagnosis, neuroimaging is useful in the evaluation and monitoring of infants who respond poorly to treatment and it is essential for early diagnosis of encephalitis. It is important to remember that the imaging appearances, potential complications (common in neonatal meningitis), and clinical course can differ in neonates from those seen in older children (Schneider, 2011). Contrast-enhanced imaging is useful with both CT and MRI in providing more detailed information.

Imaging for bacterial meningitis

- Cranial ultrasound aids the management of neonatal meningitis and serial examinations at the bedside can monitor the progression of complications. Initial signs of meningitis are widened echogenic sulci. Intraventricular strands attached to the ventricular surface and thickened ependymal with increased echogenicity are signs of ventriculitis. Additional complications, such as parenchymal changes, subdural collections, and ventricular dilatation can also be assessed. Postinfective changes include ventricular dilatation, parenchymal cysts, and periventricular calcification (Gupta et al. 2017).

- CT provides information on oedema severity, the location of any obstruction to CSF flow (causing hydrocephalus), areas of infarction, and can detect an abscess or subdural collection. In the longer term, ventricular dilatation (due to atrophy or hydrocephalus), the development of cysts, or brain atrophy can also be visualized.

- MRI provides more detailed information about the abnormalities that are seen on CT. DWI will show ischaemic lesions earlier and more effectively than CT, and helps to differentiate subdural effusion from subdural empyema; the contents of an empyema will show restricted diffusion and the periphery will enhance, these features are not present with a simple subdural effusion. Debris showing restricted diffusion on DWI and ependymal enhancement are features suggestive of ventriculitis. See, for example, Figure 8.9(a) for DWI and ADC maps in group B streptococcus meningitis.

Imaging for encephalitis

- MRI is very useful for the early diagnosis of encephalitis since it will show patchy signal abnormalities in white matter on T1-w and T2-w images and changes on DWI before CT becomes abnormal.

- All three imaging modalities (ultrasound, CT, MRI) are suitable for visualizing progression of abnormalities to multicystic encephalomalacia, but MRI is the most useful modality for detection and delineation of parenchymal injury.

Neonatal herpes simplex virus (HSV) encephalitis is more frequently due to HSV-2 (rather than HSV-1) and a more diffuse distribution of brain abnormalities is seen with no particular predilection for the temporal lobes (Figure 8.10a). Bilateral but asymmetrical temporal lobe predominant abnormality is more typical in in HSV-1 infection and is seen in older infants and children. Enteroviruses and parechoviruses are also a cause of intracranial infection in the neonatal period. Parechovirus infection can cause a distinctive abnormality on MRI with areas of diffusion restriction radiating through white matter from the periventricular zone out into deep and subcortical areas (Figure 8.10b). The long-term sequelae of this infection results in periventricular gliosis and volume loss, akin to the appearances seen with white matter disease of prematurity.

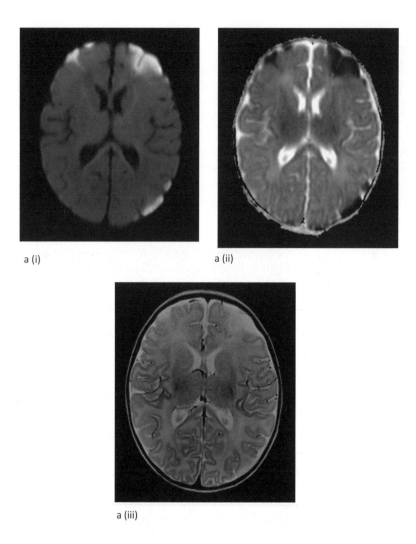

a (i)   a (ii)

a (iii)

Figure 8.9 Imaging for bacterial meningitis. (a) Superficial infarcts in group B streptococcus meningitis: (i) DWI and (ii) ADC map showing restricted diffusion in superficial areas of the cerebral hemispheres in a 3-week-old infant with proven group B streptococcal meningitis. (iii) The affected cortex is of high signal and is indistinguishable from adjacent white matter on the corresponding axial T2 image.

Metabolic and degenerative disorders

Inherited metabolic disorders (see Chapter 15) may present with NE, but acute meta-bolic derangement in the neonate may also cause neurological dysfunction, such as that found in kernicterus (bilirubin-induced neurological dysfunction; BIND) and hypo-glycaemia.

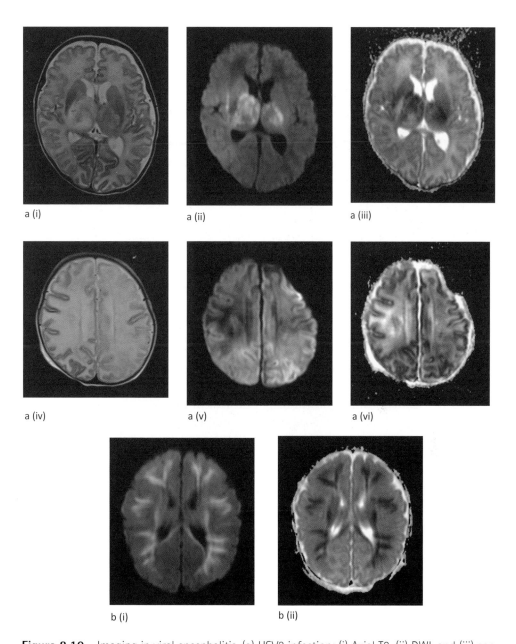

Figure 8.10 Imaging in viral encephalitis. (a) HSV2 infection: (i) Axial T2, (ii) DWI, and (iii) corresponding ADC map show involvement of the thalami bilaterally but asymmetrically and more extensively through the superior aspect of the left frontoparietal region (iv–vi).
(b) Parechovirus: (i) DWI and (ii) corresponding ADC map show the typical radiating pattern of diffusion restriction which is seen in cerebral white matter in parechovirus encephalopathy.

In kernicterus

- Ultrasound can show increased echogenicity in the basal ganglia and white matter.

- Lesions develop with age on MRI, the most frequent abnormality being increased signal on T1-w images in the globus pallidus, which also occurs less frequently in other regions such as the thalami, hippocampi, substantia nigra, and dentate nuclei. Later in infancy signal changes in these regions are mainly seen on T2-w images, along with volume loss. Diffusion MRI does not seem to be useful in this diagnosis.

In hypoglycaemia

- Ultrasound can show patchy areas with increased echogenicity in white matter.

- The typical pattern of injury consists of abnormal signal on T2-w MRI in the occipital and parietal regions. Haemorrhage, middle cerebral artery territory infarction, basal ganglia and thalamic abnormalities, and cortical injury have also been described. On DWI, restricted diffusion is seen in affected regions.

MRI is the imaging modality of choice for the diagnosis of early-onset metabolic and degenerative disorders of the brain. (Figure 8.11) The minimum imaging protocol includes the standard MRI protocol as outlined in the section 'Neuroimaging principles', with the addition of FLAIR images. Enhanced T1-w images (following the intravenous administration of a GBCA), SWI, and MRS may also be helpful. It is beyond the scope of this chapter to cover in detail the imaging features of the individual early-onset disorders. However, it is important to consider the following points in order to attempt to narrow the diagnosis based on imaging characteristics:

- Decide which structure is affected primarily: cortical grey matter, basal ganglia, white matter, or both grey and white matter.

- In assessment of white matter, is there delayed myelination or hypomyelination? It is important to know the pattern of myelination in the typically developing brain so that delayed myelination is not confused with hypomyelination. Hypomyelination can be diagnosed if there is an unchanged pattern of deficient myelination on two MRIs at least 6 months apart in a child older than 1 year (van der Knaap and Wolf, 2010).

- Are the abnormalities focal, multifocal or confluent? In leukodystrophies (genetic disorders) abnormalities are mainly bilateral and confluent, whereas in acquired disorders they are often multifocal and asymmetric in location.

- Localization: is the abnormality distributed in the frontal, parieto-occipital, periventricular, or subcortical regions, with or without involvement of the posterior fossa, or a diffuse cerebral abnormality?

- Are there other specific brain abnormalities such as cysts, small haemorrhages, calcium deposits, or megalencephaly?

- Using such a 'pattern-recognition' approach will help to achieve a specific diagnosis in a large proportion of patients (Schiffmann and van der Knaap, 2009).

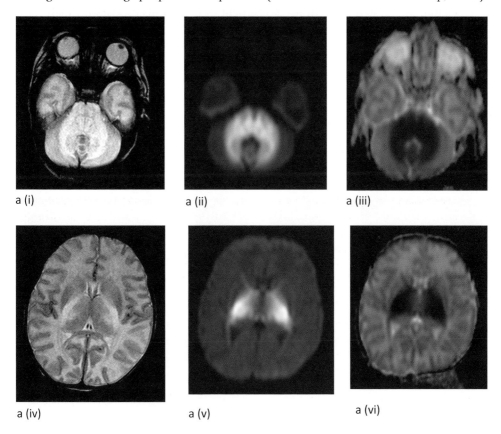

a (i)

a (ii)

a (iii)

a (iv)

a (v)

a (vi)

Figure 8.11 Metabolic disorders. (a) Metabolic disorders — maple syrup urine disease (MSUD). A 13-day-old neonate with hypotonia and seizures: (i), (ii), and (iii) at the level of the brainstem with (iv), (v), and (vi) at the level of basal ganglia: very symmetrical areas of abnormal high T2 signal and corresponding restricted diffusion. The patient was found to have MSUD.

CNS malformations

Here, malformation refers to morphological abnormalities of the CNS that date from the embryonic or fetal period, regardless of the underlying mechanism. One way of categorizing CNS malformations is according to the three phases of CNS organogenesis: (1) neurulation, formation and closure of the neural tube, (2) prosencephalation, development of the forebrain, and (3) histogenesis, proliferation and migration of neurons.

- MRI is the best imaging modality, particularly for cortical malformations, although ultrasound and CT may provide useful information (Figure 8.12).

- A sagittal plane image (or a volume scan that can be reformatted to include the sagittal plane) is important for assessment of the corpus callosum, which functions as a 'marker': if there is a malformation of the corpus callosum it is imperative to search for other associated CNS malformations.

- High-resolution MRI may be necessary for the diagnosis of disorders of histogenesis (e.g. polymicrogyria).

- Identification of abnormal patterns of grey matter, such as those suggestive of neuronal migration defects, becomes easier after myelination is complete. It is, therefore, sometimes necessary to wait until the age of at least 2 years before such malformations can be confirmed.

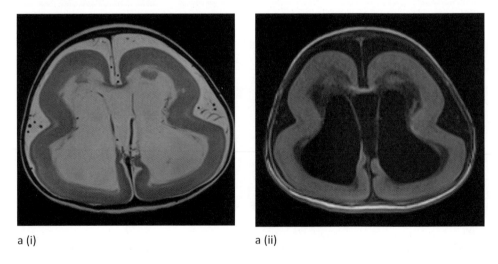

a (i)   a (ii)

Figure 8.12 Cortical malformation. (a) Cortical malformation — lissencephaly: (i) axial T2 and (ii) axial T1 images in a 21-month-old child. The cerebral hemispheres are smooth, lacking the normal gyral formation, with a thick band of grey matter signal intensity.

REFERENCES

Cowan F, Mercuri E, Groenendaal F, et al. (2005) Does cranial ultrasound imaging identify arterial cerebral infarction in term neonates?*Arch Dis Child Fetal Neonatal Ed* 90: F252—F256.

Dudink J, Mercuri E, Al-Nakib L, et al. (2009) Evolution of unilateral perinatal arterial ischemic stroke on conventional and diffusion-weighted MR imaging. *AJNR Am J Neuroradiol* 30: 998—1004.

Ecury-Goossen GM, Camfferman FA, Leijser LM, Govaert P, Dudink J (2015) State of the art cranial ultrasound imaging in neonates. *J Vis Exp* 2: e52238.

Gaillard WD, Chiron C, Cross JH, et al. (2009) Guidelines for imaging infants and children with recent-onset epilepsy. *Epilepsia* 50: 2147—2153.

Gupta N, Grover H, Bansal I et al. (2017) Neonatal cranial sonography: ultrasound findings in neonatal meningitis-a pictorial review. *Quant Imaging Med Surg* 7: 123—131.

Matthews JD, Forsythe AV, Brady Z, et al. (2013) Cancer risk in 680,000 people exposed to computed tomography scans in childhood or adolescence: data linkage study of 11 million Australians. *BMJ* 346: f2360.

Osmond E, Billetop A, Jary S, Likeman M, Thoresen M, Luyt K (2014) Neonatal seizures: magnetic resonance imaging adds value in the diagnosis and prediction of neurodisability. *Acta Paediatr* 103: 820—826.

Robertson NJ, Thayyil S, Cady EB, Raivich G (2014) Magnetic resonance spectroscopy biomarkers in term perinatal asphyxial encephalopathy: from neuropathological correlates to future clinical applications. *Curr Pediatr Rev* 10: 37—47.

Salas J, Tekes A, Hwang M, Northington FJ, Huisman TAGM (2018) Head ultrasound in neonatal hypoxic-ischemic injury and its mimickers for clinicians: a review of the patterns of injury and the evolution of findings over time. *Neonatology* 114: 185—197.

Schiffmann R, van der Knaap MS (2009) An MRI-based approach to the diagnosis of white matter disorders. *Neurology* 72: 750—759.

van der Knaap MS, Wolf NI (2010) Hypomyelination versus delayed myelination. *Ann Neurol* 68: 115.

Schneider J (2011) Neonatal brain infections. *Pediatr Radiol* 41(Suppl 1): S143—S148.

Resources

British Association of Perinatal Medicine (2016) Fetal & Neonatal Brain Magnetic Resonance Imaging: Clinical Indications, Acquisitions and Reporting. Available at https://www.bapm.org/resources/33-fetal-neonatal-brain-magnetic-resonance-imaging-clinical-indications-acquisitions-and-reporting

Govaert P, deVries LS (2011) *An Atlas of Neonatal Brain Sonography*, 2nd edition. Clinics in Developmental Medicine series. London: Mac Keith Press.

Rutherford M (2001) MRI of the Neonatal Brain. Philadelphia: Saunders Ltd.

The Royal College of Radiologists (2017) The radiological investigation of suspected physical abuse in children. Available at https://www.rcr.ac.uk/publication/radiological-investigation-suspected-physical-abuse-children

CHAPTER 9

Neurophysiology

Bernhard Schmitt and Varsine Jaladyan

Key messages

- A normal electroencephalography (EEG) does not exclude epilepsy.
- Sleep EEG provides additional information.
- Interpretation of EEG requires knowledge of the patient's clinical condition during the EEG recording.
- 80% to 90% of neonatal seizures are 'EEG-only', i.e. only recognizable on EEG.
- Consider video-EEG monitoring or amplitude integrated EEG (aEEG) in neonates at risk.

Common errors

- Mistaking immaturity in neonates for burst-suppression or discontinuity.
- Mistaking age-specific normal EEG patterns for an EEG abnormality.
- Mistaking artefacts, drug effects, or noncerebral causes for an EEG abnormality.

When to worry

- Isoelectric or low voltage EEG.
- Burst-suppression pattern.
- Prolonged periodic discharges.
- Lack of sleep cycles and lack of responsiveness on stimulation.

- Hypsarrhythmia.
- Electrographic seizures.

PREREQUISITES

Qualification of the persons involved

Electroencephalographer

Special electroencephalography (EEG) training and experience in neonates and infants is an essential prerequisite. The risk of misinterpretation and doing harm is considerable. The electroencephalographer should know when and when not to perform EEG. For this reason, this chapter does not include electromyography (EMG) or nerve conduction velocity (NCV) studies within its scope. When these studies are contemplated, clinicians are strongly advised to liaise with an expert neurophysiology service experienced in undertaking such studies in infants. Those with limited expertise or experience frequently misinterpret the results of EMG and NCV in this age group.

EEG technician

Electrode montage (see Figure 9.1) and EEG recording in neonates and infants need a high level of training, experience, patience, and empathy. Cooperation with nurses or parents and attention to hygiene, particularly on intensive care, is mandatory.

Environment and condition of the patient

The recording of EEG in intensive care is a challenge, even for well-trained EEG technicians. Technical artefacts produced by machines and monitors must be reduced as far as possible. In the EEG laboratory the atmosphere should be quiet and relaxed. The infant should be warm and well fed and the nappy/diaper changed. To avoid the need for drugs to induce sleep, the time of the EEG recording should be scheduled to the usual sleep time and infant's sleeping routine should be considered. Interference with the infant during the recording should be avoided.

Technical aspects

The International 10−20 System and the standard montages are used. In neonates and infants with small heads the number of electrodes can be reduced to Fp1, Fp2, T3, T4, C3, C4, O1, O2, Cz (see Figure 9.1) and ear (A1, A2) or mastoid (M1, M2) (Kuratani et al. 2016).

In neonates, additional polygraphic recordings are necessary to assess accurately the infant's state during the recording. For recording eye movements (electro-oculography,

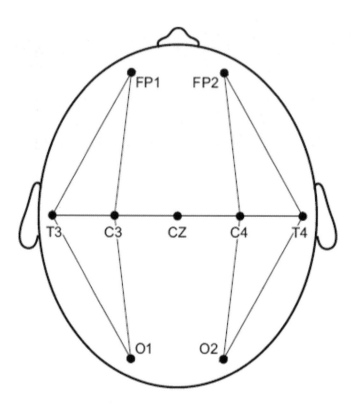

Figure 9.1 Electrode map and neonatal bipolar montage

EOG), one electrode is placed 0.5cm above and slightly lateral to the outer canthus of one eye (E1) and another 0.5cm below and slightly lateral to the outer canthus of the other eye (E2) and linked either to each other (E1-E2) or to the ear or mastoid E1 to A1/M1 and E2 to A1/M1 (or E1-A2/M2, E2-A2/M2). Muscle movements are recorded by submental EMG 1 to 2cm from the midline and the heart rate (electrocardiography, ECG) by electrodes placed on both arms or the praecordium. A respirogram can be recorded by abdominal or thoracic strain gauges, impedance pneumogram, or airway thermistors.

Electrode impedances of less than 5 kohms can usually be obtained, although higher impedances may be allowed to avoid excessive abrasion of the skin. Marked differences in impedances among electrodes should be avoided. For filter settings and amplification see Table 9.1. Digital EEGs should be registered with a sampling rate of 256Hz. In neonates, all sleep stages should be recorded, which will take at least 60 minutes. Synchronized video recording is helpful for the interpretation of seizures and EEG abnormalities. In neonates at risk, video-EEG monitoring or amplitude integrated EEG (aEEG) of at least 24 hours should be considered because of the high prevalence of electrographic (EEG-only) seizures in this population.

Table 9.1 Technical parameters in the EEG and polygraphic recording of neonates

Para-meter	Trans-ducers	Electrode placement	Amplifica-tion	Filters	
				Time constant (high-pass)	Low-pass
EEG	Silver cups	Fp1, Fp2, C3, C4, T3, T4, O1, O2, Cz (Fz, Pz)	7—10µV/mm	0.3s (0.5Hz)	70Hz
EOG	Silver cups	0.5cm 1 × above and 1 × below the lateral outer canthus of the eyes	7µV/mm	0.3s (0.5Hz)	30—70Hz
EMG	Silver cups	Submental 1—2cm from midline	3µV/mm	0.1—0.03s (1.6—5Hz)	70—120Hz
ECG	Dispos-able ECG electrodes	Precordial or both arms	200µV/mm	0.3—0.1s (0.5—1.5Hz	35—70Hz
Respira-tion	Strain gauges	2cm above umbilicus	10µV/mm	1s (0.15Hz)	15Hz
	Thermis-tors	Nasal, buccal (airflow)			

Information and documentation

Reliable interpretation of EEG requires clinical information about the patient and the conditions during recording. As a minimum, the following information should be carefully documented:

- Medical history: family history, pregnancy, birth (Apgar score, umbilical arterial pH), birthweight, head circumference.

- Postmenstrual age (PMA) = weeks from the first day of the last menstrual period. Preterm is <37 weeks PMA, term is ≥37 weeks PMA.

- Postnatal age at time of recording.

- Conditions during recording: vigilance (sleep, awake, drowsy), eyes closed or open, movement (including abnormal eye movements), breathing, artificial ventilation, responsiveness, skin condition (oedema, haematoma), deformations of the skull, etc.

- Hypothermia: duration and depth, induced or spontaneous.

- Time interval from the acute event (seizure, hypoxic-ischaemic event, etc.).

- Drugs, including dosage.

- Movement or other care given during the recording, technical and other artefacts.

- Seizures or abnormal movements.

Steps to interpret the EEG

- Background activity (continuity, symmetry, synchrony, amplitude, responsiveness to stimulation, sleep/wake cycle, EEG elements, variability, spatial organization).

- Is the EEG activity age appropriate?

- Epileptiform activity (ictal and interictal)?

NORMAL EEG

Neonates

The EEG shows dynamic changes between 26 weeks and 44 weeks PMA that parallels brain maturation. Every PMA has typical EEG features which allow determination of PMA with an accuracy of ±2 weeks.

Continuity: discontinuous activity (tracé discontinue; see Figure 9.2) is the characteristic EEG pattern at less than 30 weeks PMA. Bursts of activity alternate with inactivity. The interburst intervals (IBI) (inactivity between the bursts) decrease from <60s at 24 to 27 weeks PMA to <26s at 28 to 29 weeks PMA (Table 9.2). After 30 weeks PMA discontinuity occurs only in non-rapid eye movement (NREM) sleep and falls to <10s at 34 weeks PMA. Beyond 34 weeks PMA inactivity is replaced by low voltage activity (tracé alternant), which persists until term and disappears before 46 weeks PMA.

Variability describes spontaneous EEG changes in frequency, continuity, or voltage and is increasingly apparent by 28 weeks PMA and well established by 30 to 31 weeks PMA. *Sleep/wake cycles* can be recognized at later than 30 weeks PMA by more continuous activity during rapid eye movement (REM) sleep. After 38 weeks PMA, six sleep states are defined:

- REM 1: continuous delta, theta, and alpha activity (40–100μV).

- NREM 1: continuous high-amplitude (50–150μV) delta activity mixed with low-amplitude theta and beta waves.

- NREM 2: tracé alternant (synchronous high-amplitude delta/theta waves alternating with low-amplitude fast activity).

- REM 2: low-amplitude activity (20−50µV) with intermingled alpha-waves.

- Indeterminate sleep: activity between sleep states.

- Awake: continuous diffuse central theta waves (20−50µV), occipital delta waves (20−50µV), central high-amplitude theta waves lasting 1 to 3s, irregular alpha/beta activity (<30µV).

REM sleep is the first and dominating sleep state until birth and lasts up to 20 minutes. After 42 to 43 weeks PMA, NREM replaces REM sleep as the first sleep state and the proportion of REM decreases. Sleep spindles become obvious after 44 weeks PMA.

Reactivity of EEG is demonstrated when there is an obvious cerebral EEG response (frequency, continuity, voltage) to external stimulation. Reactivity first appears at 30 to 32 weeks PMA. Tactile stimulation causes generalized desynchronization or voltage changes after 30 weeks PMA.

Delta waves (100−300µV or more) are dominant at >24 weeks PMA and are uni- or bilaterally synchronous. Occipital delta waves become longer after 28 weeks PMA. Frontal delta-rhythms are obvious in REM sleep at 36 to 37 weeks PMA.

Delta brushes are delta waves with spindle-like fast activity (8−24/s, 10−25µV) superimposed on the ascending part of the wave. They occur after 28 weeks PMA, are dominant in REM sleep at 31 to 32 weeks PMA and in NREM sleep after 33 weeks PMA. After 35 weeks PMA they become less and disappear in the first weeks of life.

Theta-waves are often sharply contoured. Between 24 weeks and 40 weeks PMA (max 28−32wks) they occur uni- or bilaterally over the temporal regions (temporal saw-tooth waves). STOPs (sharp theta on the occipitals of infants born preterm) are sharp theta rhythms over the occipital areas.

Spikes are transients, clearly distinguished from background activity, with pointed peak and a duration from 20 to <70ms. The main component is generally negative relative to other areas. Amplitude is variable.

Sharp waves are transients, clearly distinguished from background activity, with pointed peak and duration of 70 to 200ms. The main component is generally negative relative to other areas; amplitude is variable. Spikes and sharp waves occur after 30 weeks PMA, become more frequent at 32 to 34 weeks PMA, and decrease after 35 weeks PMA. High-amplitude (50−200µV) uni- or bilateral *frontal sharp transients* occur later than 35 weeks PMA and persist in NREM sleep after 38 weeks PMA. They disappear by the age of 8 weeks.

Infants

- *Posterior dominant rhythm*, apparent during wakefulness over the posterior region after eye closure, increases from 2 to 3/s at age 2 months to 3 to 4/s at 4 months, 5/s at 5 months and 6 to 7/s at 1 year. However, this maturation shows distinct variability. Blockade by eye opening is detectable after age 4 months.

- *Shut-eye waves* are bilateral high-amplitude (100–200µV) biphasic transients over the occipital region provoked by eye blinking. They occur after age 6 months.

- *Lambda waves* (occipital positive, sawtooth-like waves <50µV) are provoked by visual exploration and are visible from birth.

- *Photic driving* is detectable at low-frequency photic stimulation (4–7Hz) after age 3 to 4 months.

- *Drowsiness* is characterized by slowing and voltage increase of background activity. Between age 6-months and 24-months central beta activity increases during the transition from wake to sleep.

- *Sleep:* REM sleep decreases from 50% at birth to 30% at age 1 year. Centromedian vertex waves become apparent after age 3 months and K-complexes after age 6 months. Rhythmic 13 to 15/s sleep spindles appear after age 4 weeks. In the first 6 months they are most numerous and their duration increases up to 10s. Most of them occur asynchronously. After age 6 months spindle duration decreases to less than 1s at age 6 years. Awakening is characterized by voltage attenuation in the first 3 months of life and by more and more serial frontal delta/theta waves after 3 months.

ABNORMAL EEG

Neonates

EEG abnormalities can be divided into acute and chronic, as follows.

- Temporary changes reflect recent or ongoing disturbances of the brain. They are characterized by: (1) significant increase in discontinuity, (2) reduction of alpha, theta, or beta activity, or (3) voltage attenuation (moderate <50µV, distinct/extensive <20µV).

- Persistent changes reflect brain injury in the past. They are characterized by: (1) abnormal or delayed maturation, (2) abnormal organization (deformed or abnormal quantities of theta/delta waves or delta brushes), or (3) increased sharp-wave activity.

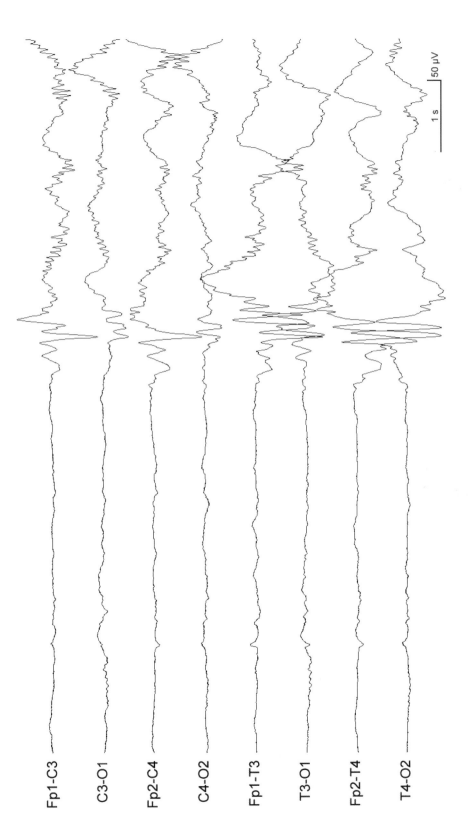

Fp1-C3

C3-O1

Fp2-C4

C4-O2

Fp1-T3

T3-O1

Fp2-T4

T4-O2

1 s

50 µV

Figure 9.2 Tracé discontinue: interburst-interval up to 10s. Preterm 29 weeks PMA

Table 9.2 Maturation of EEG

Weeks PMA	24–27	28–29	30–31	32–34	35–37	38–42	>42
Longest duration of burst	60s	160s	Continuous activity awake and in REM-sleep				
Longest IBI	<60	<26s	8–18s	4–10s		<6s	
Activity in IBI	TD	TD	TD	TD/TA	TA	TA	TA
Sleep states	Not detectable		3 states: awake, REM, NREM		4 states: awake, 2 REM, 1 NREM	6 states: awake, 2 REM, 2 NREM, undetermined sleep	
Synchrony of bursts	88%	100%					
Delta brushes		X	XXX	XXX	XX	X	
			REM>NREM		NREM>REM		
Temporal saw-tooth waves	X	XXX	XXX	X	X	X	
Frontal sharp transients					X	X	X
Multifocal spike waves			X	XX	XX	X	X

PMA, postmenstrual age; REM, rapid eye movement; IBI, interburst interval; TD, tracé discontinue; TA, tracé alternant; NREM, non-rapid eye movement; X, occur; XX, occur often; XXX, occur regularly.

EEG activity can improve or normalize in the follow-up period after an abnormal EEG, but this does not exclude later neurological problems. Background activity and seizure burden (electroclinical and electrographic seizures, status epilepticus) are the most useful predictors of outcome.

Maturation: extrauterine and intrauterine brain maturation follow the same speed and sequence. The EEG activity is immature when the pattern is more than 2 weeks behind the age-appropriate level. Criteria for immaturity are inadequate sleep cycles, prolonged IBIs, and localization and occurrence of delta brushes. Immaturity is a risk factor, but does not exclude typical development.

Excessive discontinuity denotes abnormally discontinuous tracings with bursts that contain some normal patterns separated by IBIs that are too prolonged and/or periods of EEG activity that are voltage depressed for PMA. Age-appropriate IBI are given in Table 9.2, however, absolute limits do not exist.

Burst-suppression pattern is characterized by bursts (1−10s) of high-amplitude synchronous theta/delta activity mixed with spike and sharp waves alternating with isoelectric or very low-voltage (<5−15μV) activity. The pattern does not vary during the EEG recording, persisting during both wakefulness and sleep, and is not influenced by stimulation. After 34 weeks PMA, burst suppression can be easily distinguished from tracé alternant. Before 34 weeks it is difficult to distinguish PMA from tracé discontinue. Intoxication (i.e. by barbiturates or lithium) has to be excluded. Burst-suppression is the typical EEG pattern of early infantile epileptic encephalopathy (EIEE) or Ohtahara syndrome and early myoclonic epilepsy (see Chapter 16), but also occurs in other situations.

Lack of EEG variability and reactivity is critical in neonates born preterm and at term. After 30 weeks PMA repeated recordings without sleep/wake cycles indicate poor prognosis. Abnormal sleep architecture is found in neonates of drug-addicted mothers and in neonates with brain malformations or surfactant deficiency disorder (neonatal respiratory distress syndrome).

Asymmetries: voltage differences of more than 25% registered during the whole recording or asymmetrical occurrence of sustained waveforms indicate a local disturbance. Unilateral delta brushes indicate the less abnormal hemisphere in the infant born preterm and the abnormal hemisphere in the infant born at term. Transient voltage asymmetries are normal. The EEG is asynchronous when morphologically similar bursts appear with an interhemispheric time difference of more than 1.5s.

Low-voltage EEG is characterized by amplitudes between 5μV and 25μV, poor variability, lack of sleep cycles, and, in infants born preterm, lack of delta brushes. Technical, toxic-metabolic, and causes external to the brain (e.g. subdural haematoma, scalp oedema, caput succedaneum) should be excluded.

Inactivity is the most severe EEG abnormality in neonates. The term inactivity is more appropriate than isoelectric, because rare bursts of low-voltage activity may occur. Long time constants, maximal amplification, large interelectrode distances, and long-lasting recordings without artefacts are technical prerequisites for this diagnosis. Intoxication, acute hypoxia, hypothermia, or a postictal state should be considered as possible causes. The EEG should be repeated, especially when the inactivity is recorded shortly after a critical event. The diagnosis of death in neonates by neurological criteria do not include EEG criteria in any national jurisdiction.

Spike and sharp waves are found in typically developing infants born at term and infants born preterm. They might be abnormal when they occur unilaterally and frequently. **Positive Rolandic sharp waves** (positive over C3, C4, Cz) are abnormal before 34-weeks PMA or when they occur more than 1 to 2/min. They indicate periventricular leukomalacia but have no epileptic background. **Positive temporal sharp waves** (positive over T3, T4) are abnormal in infants born at term when they appear frequently.

Ictal EEG: Neonatal seizures are classified as clinical-only, electroclinical, or electrographic (EEG-only) seizures. Clinical-only seizures do not correlate with a simultaneous EEG seizure. In electroclinical seizures clinical symptoms are simultaneously coupled with an ictal EEG discharge. Electrographic seizures occur without any clinical correlates and are defined as sudden, abnormal EEG events with a repetitive and evolving pattern, a voltage of $>2\mu V$ and a duration of $>10s$. 'Evolving' is defined as an unequivocal evolution in frequency, voltage, morphology, or location. An interval of at least 10s is required to separate two distinct seizures. The morphology of ictal discharges consists of rhythmic spikes, sharp-waves, or rhythmic beta, alpha, theta, or delta waves. In infants born preterm, rhythmic delta waves are the most common ictal pattern. The onset can be unifocal, multifocal, lateralized, bilateral independent, migrating, or diffuse with asynchronous involvement of all brain regions. Electrographic seizures constitute up to 90% of all neonatal seizures. Focal clonic or focal tonic seizures exhibit focal EEG discharges while generalized myoclonic jerks are associated with generalized bursts. On the other hand, focal myoclonic jerks and generalized tonic movements may exhibit no ictal EEG changes and may be nonepileptic in nature. Subtle seizures occur with and without ictal changes. Apnoea in neonates usually has a nonepileptic aetiology but the rare epileptic apnoea starts with monomorphic alpha/beta activity followed by sharp wave discharges over the temporal region.

Electrographic status epilepticus is defined as uninterrupted electrographic seizures lasting at least 30 minutes or repeated electrographic seizures totalling more than 30 minutes in any 1-hour period.

Brief rhythmic discharges (BRDs) consist of evolving rhythmic patterns of electrical activity that share many characteristics with electrographic seizures but are very brief, with a duration of $<10s$. The significance of these discharges is uncertain. A recent case series showed a similar mortality and neurological disability for infants with BRDs as with seizures.

Periodic patterns are described as uniform waveforms recurring at almost regular intervals without evolution, lasting >10s. They present with different morphologies and focal, bilateral synchronous, bilateral asynchronous, or diffuse localizations. They are of uncertain significance and rare in neonates.

Infants aged 1 to 12 months

EEG abnormalities are divided into two categories: (1) disappearance of normal patterns and (2) appearance of abnormal patterns. Most abnormal patterns are nonspecific and not associated with a specific aetiology. Interpretation should be made only in the context of the patient's history and the clinical and neuroradiological findings.

Abnormal maturation of the posterior dominant rhythm should be diagnosed when the frequency deviates by more than 2/s from the age-appropriate values.

Abnormal background activity should be characterized according to the following criteria:

- Localization: focal, unilateral, generalized.

- Frequency: beta, theta, delta, subdelta activity.

- Continuity: excessive discontinuity, burst-suppression pattern, lack of variability, and responsiveness to stimulation.

- Sleep: absence or abnormality of sleep cycles or sleep patterns.

- Symmetry and synchrony.

- Voltage: asymmetries, high- or low-voltage activity, inactivity, or intermittent voltage depression.

Inactivity, burst-suppression pattern, and low-voltage (<20µV) are the most severe abnormalities. They can indicate severe brain injury. Before drawing conclusions, technical, noncerebral, and drug-related causes have to be excluded, as well as recent acute hypoxic events, seizures, or medical interventions. Other EEG risk factors for poor outcome are lack of fluctuation and responsiveness to stimulation, and lack of sleep cycles in prolonged EEG recordings. Background slowing, even when registered over several days, has no prognostic value and does not exclude normal outcome. Focal abnormal background activity is detected by comparison with the contralateral hemisphere. Over the abnormal hemisphere the activity is often slower; the amplitude, however, might be higher or lower.

Interictal epileptiform activities are focal, multifocal, or generalized spikes, sharp waves, polyspikes, spike and polyspike wave complexes, 3/s spike waves, and slow-spike wave complexes. They should not be confused with artefacts and physiological sharp elements.

Hypsarrhythmia (see Figure 9.3) is characterized by random high-voltage slow waves and spikes. The spikes vary from moment to moment, both in duration and in location. At times they appear to be focal, and a few seconds later they seem to originate from multiple foci. Occasionally the spike discharge becomes generalized. Variations of hypsarrhythmia are those with: (1) increased interhemispheric synchronization, (2) episodes of voltage attenuation, (3) a consistent focus of abnormal discharge, (4) little spike or sharp activity, and (5) asymmetric hypsarrhythmia. The abnormality may be confined to the sleeping record but is apparent in the awake record in most cases. Hypsarrhythmia is the characteristic EEG pattern of infantile spasms (West syndrome).

Ictal EEG patterns can be associated with clinical features or occur without them.

Focal seizures often start with focal desynchronization and very fast low-voltage spiky activity which gradually rises in amplitude and diminishes in frequency. Sometimes only a focal change of frequency is obvious, which gradually becomes slower and involves adjacent electrodes. Focal seizures do not always indicate brain lesions or malformation. In **benign localized epilepsies of infancy**, low-voltage spiky activity evolves from the temporal or parieto-occipital region and spreads to the ipsilateral hemisphere. In **malignant migrating partial seizures**, focal EEG discharges are typically migrating, starting from a cortical area and remaining localized or spreading to contiguous regions whereas others develop independently in different areas of the same or the opposite hemisphere. Three different ictal patterns can be distinguished: (1) rhythmic focal spikes or sharp alpha-theta activity over the Rolandic region; (2) polymorphic theta-delta activity over the temporo-occipital region; and (3) initial flattening or small discharge of fast polyspikes in one hemisphere.

Spasms: the ictal EEG pattern of infantile spasms (West syndrome) consists of: (1) a high amplitude positive-vertex slow wave or a generalized slow wave or sharp-and-slow-wave complex, (2) sometimes followed by variable voltage attenuation, and (3) a fast spindle-like activity (14−16/s) which can precede the slow wave. The spasms usually occur in clusters. Before the first spasm, hypsarrhythmia is often replaced by a mixture of irregular middle-amplitude faster frequencies. This 'relative normalization' of background activity usually persists until the end of the cluster.

Myoclonic seizures are characterized by generalized irregular spike/polyspike waves. They occur in benign myoclonic epilepsy and in Dravet syndrome and can sometimes be provoked by photic stimulation.

Atypical absence seizures show regular and irregular 2 to 3.5/s spike waves, for example in Dravet syndrome.

Tonic seizures exhibit desynchronization with almost flat EEG and fast, very low-voltage activities which may gradually increase in voltage and decrease in frequencies.

Tonic-clonic seizures: fast rhythmic spikes (tonic phase) which become discontinuous with rhythmic spike or polyspike waves (clonic phase).

Periodic EEG patterns are usually not associated with epileptic seizures. The term includes several patterns of more or less continuous, repetitive, rhythmical monomorphic waves, and often indicates severe ongoing brain disease.

AMPLITUDE INTEGRATED EEG OR CEREBRAL FUNCTION MONITORING

Amplitude integrated EEG (aEEG) allows continuous assessment of brain function in critically ill neonates and is an indispensable diagnostic tool on neonatal intensive care units. It is widely available, easy to install, and allows interpretation by non-electroencephalographers. Focal seizures can be missed because of the reduced number of electrodes. Brief seizures may be overlooked in the time-compressed aEEG trend and artefacts may be mistaken for seizures. The aEEG is usually recorded from two pairs (C3-P3, C4-P4) of electrodes, amplified and passed through an asymmetrical bandpass filter that suppresses activity below 2Hz and above 15Hz. The signal is displayed on a semi-logarithmic scale at slow speed (6cm/h). The original EEG tracing is continuously displayed separately.

Assessment of aEEG background

- Continuous normal voltage pattern: continuous trace with a voltage 10 to 25µV (up to 50µV).

- Discontinuous normal voltage pattern: discontinuous trace, low voltage predominantly >5µV.

- Discontinuous background pattern (burst suppression): periods of low voltage (inactivity) intermixed with bursts of higher amplitude.

- Continuous background pattern of very low voltage ($\leq$5µV).

- Very low voltage, mainly inactive tracing with activity <5µV (flat trace).

Sleep/wake cycling is characterized by semi-periodic variation in bandwidth. Broadening of the bandwidth represents the discontinuity of quiet sleep, narrowing represents the more continuous activity during wakefulness or active sleep.

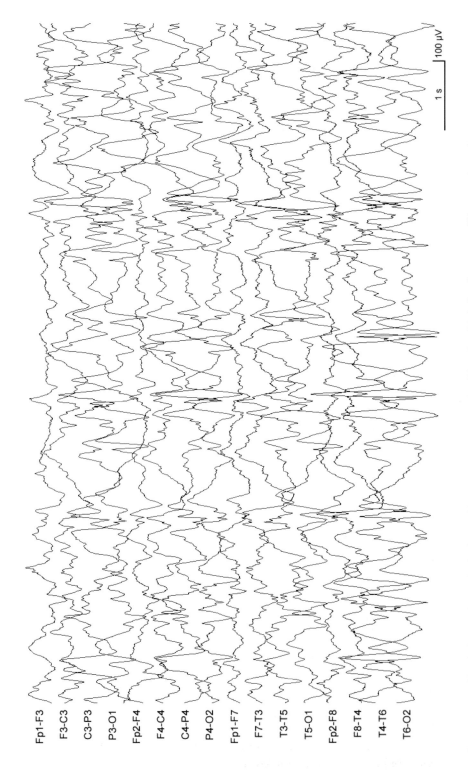

Fp1-F3
F3-C3
C3-P3
P3-O1
Fp2-F4
F4-C4
C4-P4
P4-O2
Fp1-F7
F7-T3
T3-T5
T5-O1
Fp2-F8
F8-T4
T4-T6
T6-O2

1 s

100 μV

Figure 9.3 Classic hypsarrhythmia during waking state on a 5-month-old male with infantile spasms (West syndrome)

Neonatal seizures are characterized in aEEG as a transient, sharp rise in the lower margin of the bandwidth often accompanied by a smaller rise in the upper margin, with narrowing of the bandwidth (see Figure 9.4). Neonatal status epilepticus can present as a 'saw-tooth pattern' or as a continuous increase of the lower and upper margin.

WHEN TO DO EEG OR AEEG?

Neonates

- Continuous video-EEG monitoring of at least 24 hours is recommended for all neonates at risk. In neonates with seizures, EEG monitoring should be continued for a 24-hour period of no seizures. In view of resource issues, aEEG is an alternate modality for monitoring newborn infants at risk.

- Standard video-EEG of 60 minutes is useful for a detailed analysis of age-appropriate or abnormal EEG patterns and is necessary for confirmation of findings obtained from aEEG monitoring.

In infants

Continuous video-EEG monitoring is recommended in infants:

- with suspected subclinical seizures (i.e. under treatment with antiepileptic drugs);

- with ambiguous paroxysmal events;

- with hypsarrhythmia, but no obvious infantile spasms; and

- in all critically ill children on ICU (at least 24h). EEG monitoring should be continued for a 24-hour period of no seizures.

Video-EEG awake and asleep should be performed in infants:

- with suspected seizures (including infantile spasms); and

- with acute encephalopathies.

WHEN NOT TO DO EEG

Inappropriate questions and overuse of EEG may do harm by overinterpretation of harmless abnormalities found by chance and unrelated to the present neurological problem. EEG should, therefore, be avoided in the following:

- Benign neonatal sleep myoclonus. Diagnosis can be made by history alone.

- Early developmental impairment as an uncomplicated clinical problem: the diagnostic yield of EEG is very low, approximately 1%.

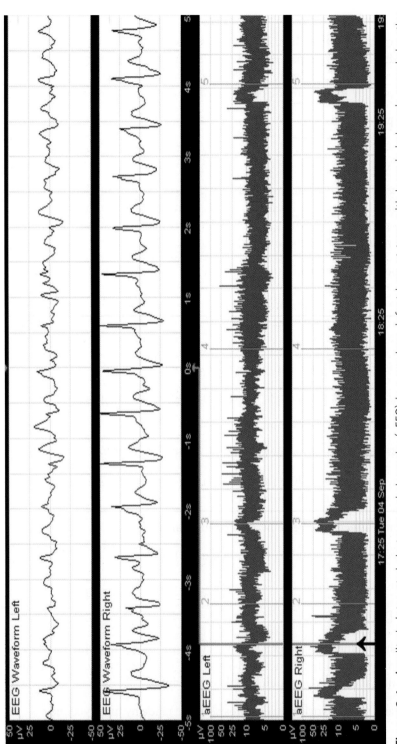

Figure 9.4 Amplitude integrated electroencephalography (aEEG) in a newborn infant born at term with hypoxic-ischaemic encephalopathy and seizures. Lower 2 lines: amplitude integrated aEEG over 3 hours. Line 4, arrow and grey line: transient sharp rise in the lower margin of the bandwidth accompanied by a smaller rise in the upper margin, with narrowing of the bandwidth and in line 2 the respective original right hemispheric epileptiform discharge.

- Febrile seizures: EEG results have no therapeutic implications.

- Breath-holding spells are caused by an immature autonomic nervous system. They are nonepileptic, benign, age-limited, and have an excellent prognosis. Diagnosis can be made by history alone.

- Hyperekplexia, characterized by pronounced startle responses to tactile or acoustic stimuli and hypertonia, is a dysfunction of glycine neurotransmission. EEG is normal and does not provide any additional information.

- Shuddering attacks (benign myoclonus of early infancy) are a benign condition. Diagnosis is based on descriptive history and video review. The attacks are not associated with EEG abnormalities.

- Mild head trauma: if there are no seizures, EEG is not informative and has no therapeutic consequences.

- 'Cranial hypertension' — if indeed such a thing in neonates and infants exists in any context other than intracranial hypertension in the setting of acute encephalopathy or obstructive hydrocephalus causing excessive head growth, depressed conscious level, vomiting, or forced downgaze (sunsetting) — cannot be diagnosed by EEG.

- Hydrocephalus: EEG does not contribute to diagnosis.

- Headache cannot be diagnosed at this age. If suspected by abnormal behaviour of the infant, EEG is — as in older children and adults — not contributory to the underlying diagnosis.

REFERENCES

Kuratani J, Pearl PL, Sullivan L et al. (2016) American Clinical Neurophysiology Society Guideline 5: Minimum technical standards for pediatric electroencephalography. *J Clin Neurophysiol* 33: 320–323.

Resources

Abend NS, Wusthoff CJ, Goldberg EM, Dlugos DJ (2013) Electrographic seizures and status epilepticus in critically ill children and neonates with encephalopathy. *Lancet Neurol* 12: 1170–1179.

André M, Lamblin MD, d'Allest AM, et al. (2010) Electroencephalography in premature and full-term infants. Developmental features and glossary. *Neurophysiol Clin* 40: 59–124.

Caraballo RH, Fontana E, Darra F, et al. (2008) Migrating focal seizures in infancy: analysis of the electroclinical patterns in 17 patients. *J Child Neurol* 23: 497–506.

Hellström Westas L, de Vries LS, Rosén I (2008) *Atlas of Amplitude-Integrated EEGs in the Newborn*, 2nd edn. London: Informa Healthcare.

Hrachovy RA, Frost Jr JD, Kellaway P (1984) Hypsarrhythmia: variations on the theme. *Epilepsia* 25: 317—325.

Nagarajan L, Palumbo L, Ghosh S (2011) Brief electroencephalography rhythmic discharges (BERDs) in the neonate with seizures: their significance and prognostic implications. *J Child Neurol* 26: 1529—1533.

Okumura A, Watanabe K, Negoro T, Hayakawa F, Kato T, Natsume J (2007) Ictal EEG in benign partial epilepsy in infancy. *Pediatr Neurol* 36: 8—12.

Petersen I, Eeg-Olofsson O (1971) The development of the electroencephalogram in normal children from the age of 1 through 15 years. Non-paroxysmal activity. *Neuropadiatrie* 2: 247—304.

Shewmon DA (1990) What is a neonatal seizure? Problems in definition and quantification for investigative and clinical purposes. *J Clin Neurophysiol* 7: 315—368.

Stockard-Pope JE, Werner SS, Bickford RB (1992). *Atlas of Neonatal Electroencephalography*, 2nd edn. New York, Raven Press.

Tsuchida TN, Wusthoff CJ, Shellhaas RA, et al. (2013) American Clinical Neurophysiology Society Standardized EEG Terminology and Categorization for the Description of Continuous EEG Monitoring in Neonates: Report of the American Clinical Neurophysiology Society Critical Care Monitoring Committee. *J Clin Neurophysiol* 30: 161—173.

van Rooij LG, de Vries LS, Handryastuti S, et al. (2007) Neurodevelopmental outcome in term infants with status epilepticus detected with amplitude-integrated electroencephalography. *Pediatrics* 120: 354—63.

Watanabe K, Hara K, Miyazaki S, Hakamada S, Kuroyanagi M (1982) Apneic seizures in the newborn. *Am J Dis Child* 136: 980—4.

Watanabe K, Hayakawa F, Okumura A (1999) Neonatal EEG: a powerful tool in the assessment of brain damage in preterm infants. *Brain Dev* 21: 361—372.

CHAPTER 10

Biochemical and haematological testing

Valerie Walker and Mary Morgan

Key messages

- Biochemistry tests are a supportive diagnostic tool.
- Use tests selectively to address specific questions.
- Interpret results within the clinical context.
- Check the reference range used by your laboratory.

Common errors

- Inappropriate samples.
- Inappropriate reference ranges.
- Ignorance of test limitations.

When to worry

- Acute encephalopathy.
- Intractable seizures resistant to conventional treatment.
- Hypotonia, dystonia, and/or movement disorders.
- Progressive loss of skills.
- Multisystem disorders with neurological abnormalities.
- Macrocephaly or microcephaly with neurological abnormalities.

Biochemical tests are among the tools used to diagnose a neurological disorder. They can be very helpful when considered in the clinical context along with the evidence acquired from other investigations. They must be used selectively because of the size and small blood volume of neonatal patients, and because the tests for rare disorders have restricted availability and are expensive. Good reference range data for neonates and infants are sparse. They should encompass the rapid changes in biochemical indices as the infants develop. Tables 10.1 to 10.3 present ranges for tests selected for their relevance for neurological investigations; they are far from comprehensive. They were compiled from ranges used in Southampton, UK, and from published sources accessible on the internet. It is important to be aware that different analytical methods frequently produce different values. It is therefore essential to apply the ranges provided by the laboratory undertaking the tests when interpreting results.

CEREBROSPINAL FLUID ANALYSES

Although neurological disorders are associated with widespread biochemical disturbances within the central nervous system (CNS), we can get only a very limited view of them. Because it bathes the brain, analysis of cerebrospinal fluid (CSF) is often more useful than analysis of blood or urine, and an increasing number of metabolites are measured in CSF.

Cerebrospinal fluid is produced primarily by filtration from plasma across the blood–CSF barrier with a small contribution by active secretion. The choroid plexuses are the principal source, with a contribution from the ependymal lining.

Constituents and significance of abnormalities

Proteins

More than 80% of proteins in CSF originate from plasma by ultrafiltration through the walls of capillaries in the meninges and choroid plexuses. The remainder are from the brain and cells in the CSF. Protein concentrations are higher in lumbar CSF than in ventricular fluid and many are around 200 times lower than in serum. After concentration of CSF, a band of transferrin-lacking sialic acid (β-transferrin; tau protein; note that this is distinct from Alzheimer-related tau protein) is a normal finding. Total protein concentrations are high in the neonate, due to increased capillary permeability, but generally fall to adult levels by 3 months of age (Table 10.1).

Table 10.1 Lumbar CSF reference ranges

Constituent	Reference ranges	Comments
Volume (ml)	Infants: 40—60; young children: 60—100	
White blood cells (cells/ml)	Infants: preterm 0—25, term 0—22; Post-neonatal infants <5	
Protein (mg/l)	0—1 month term 600—2000; preterm 500—2500; VLBW <3700; 1—3 months: 200—600; >3 months: 100—400	Ranges influenced by analytical method
Glucose (mmol/l)	1—4 weeks: term and preterm mean 3.0 (range 1.5—5.5); 4—8 weeks 1.7—5.6; 2—6 months 2.0—5.6	Varies with blood glucose; may take up to 4 hours to equilibrate
Albumin: CSF/serum albumin index (mg/g)	<9 BBB intact; 9—14 slightly, 14—30 moderately, and 30—100 severely impaired; >100 complete breakdown	
Amino acids (μmol/l)	Alanine 15—60, phenylalanine 6—40, glutamine 231—940, taurine 6—62, glycine 3—19, threonine 12—178 Serine: 1 week: 43—74; 1 month 38—66	Blood contamination invalidates the results
Amine neurotransmitters (nmol/l)	Aged 0—0.2y: 5HIAA 208—1159, HVA 337—1299; HVA/5HIAA ratio 1.0—3.7	Special collection protocol; freeze at bedside
Bilirubin (umol/l)	Neonates 0.7—7.5; higher in preterm; older: not detectable	High in neonates with severe hyperbilirubinaemia
α-fetoprotein (AFP) (KU/l)	After 1 month <2; may be detectable in typically developing neonates	Check for leaky BBB with CSF/serum albumin index
Lactate (mmol/l)	<2.1	

Table 10.1 (continued)   Lumbar CSF reference ranges

Constituent	Reference ranges	Comments
β2-Microglobulin (mg/l)	2—3	Check for leaky BBB with CSF/serum albumin index
Neuron-specific enolase (μg/l)	<10	Check for leaky BBB with CSF/serum albumin index
Pipecolic acid (nmol/l)	9—120	
Pterins (nmol/l)	Aged 0—0.2y: tetrahydrobi-opterin 40—105; neopterin 7—65	Special collection protocol; freeze at bedside
Pyridoxal phosphate (nmol/l)	<30 days ≥26; 30 days to 1y ≥14	Special collection protocol; freeze at bedside
Pyruvate (μmol/l)	70—140	Special collection protocol; restricted value-see text

VLBW, very low birthweight; CSF, cerebrospinal fluid; BBB, blood—brain barrier; β-HCG, β-human chorionic gonadotropin, 5HIAA 5-hydroxyindole acetic acid (5-hydroxytryptamine metabolite); HVA, homovanillic acid (dopamine metabolite).

CSF proteins are raised for the following reasons:

- Increased transudation of plasma proteins across an impaired blood—brain barrier (BBB) due to inflammation associated with bacterial or viral meningitis or encephalitis, brain tumours, intracerebral haemorrhage, trauma, and mechanical obstruction of CSF circulation. Its severity can be demonstrated by analysis of albumin in paired CSF and serum samples.

- Local production of gamma globulins within the CNS. Although mixtures of immunoglobulins, these show restricted heterogeneity and may appear as distinct bands on electrophoresis. It is assumed that they are products of a small number of B-cell clones. They are classed as oligoclonal bands if there are two or more bands, shown to be IgG, which are not found in paired serum. To demonstrate local production of IgG, albumin and IgG are analysed in paired CSF and serum samples to calculate the IgG index. This excludes or corrects for leakage through a defective BBB (Table 10.1), although there may be false positive and false negative results.

Disorders with intrathecal IgG synthesis and oligoclonal bands include multiple sclerosis (more than 90% if clinically definite), subacute sclerosing panencephalitis (SSPE; 100%), viral encephalitis (35%), meningitis (including cryptococcal, 33%), neurosyphilis (55%), systemic lupus erythematosus, Guillain—Barré syndrome, sarcoidosis, and tumours. The likelihood of these disorders varies widely with geographical situation and age.

Glucose

The glucose concentration in CSF is regulated by facilitated diffusion across the blood–CSF barrier. In neonates, concentrations in newly secreted CSF may approach 80% that of plasma. Thereafter, they are around 60%. This fraction may fall in the presence of hyperglycaemia because of saturation of glucose transport. Paired blood and CSF samples are essential for interpretation and, in general, the blood sample should be obtained immediately before the procedure for lumbar puncture. However, equilibration between plasma and CSF glucose may take up to 4 hours, and the ratio is less reliable during states of metabolic flux.

Causes of low CSF glucose include: hypoglycaemia; most, but not all, cases of pyogenic bacterial and tuberculous meningitis; around half of cases of fungal meningitis; a minority of cases (<5%) with viral meningitis (including mumps); neurosyphilis; Lyme disease; meningoencephalitic mumps; leukaemic, lymphomatous, or carcinomatous infiltration; subarachnoid haemorrhage; neurosarcoidosis; systemic lupus erythematosus; and the rare inherited deficiency of glucose transporter 1 (GLUT1) of the brain.

Lactate and pyruvate

The CSF concentrations of lactate and pyruvate largely reflect production from CNS glycolysis. Inflammatory, malignant, and red blood cells in the leptomeninges or subarachnoid space are other possible sources. At physiological pH, lactate is ionized and crosses the BBB slowly. CSF levels are, therefore, independent of serum lactate if the barrier is intact. CSF lactate is analysed to investigate for defects of the respiratory chain or tricarboxylic acid cycle or deficiencies of pyruvate dehydrogenase (PDH), pyruvate carboxylase, or biotinidase (which recycles biotin from carboxylases).

Causes of raised CSF lactate include spurious increases due to blood contamination from traumatic lumbar puncture or delayed analysis if the CSF cell count is raised. True increases may be due to thiamine deficiency, inherited defects of pyruvate metabolism, the respiratory chain, and tricarboxylic acid cycle; bacterial meningitis; brain trauma and/or ischaemia; intracranial haemorrhage; brain abscess; cerebral leukaemia; or lymphomatous or carcinomatous infiltration of the leptomeninges. Usually when the plasma or CSF lactate is raised the lactate/pyruvate ratio is also increased. Because pyruvate is unstable, its analysis requires careful sample collection procedures. It is usually enough to measure lactate only. The lactate/pyruvate ratio is helpful, however, in investigations of an inherited lactic acidosis if PDH deficiency is suspected. If lactate is raised, a normal ratio (approximately 20) is consistent with PDH deficiency. In respiratory chain defects the ratio is increased (≥25).

Amino acids

Causes of abnormal CSF amino acid concentrations include generalized increases due to breakdown of the BBB, for example severe hypoxia-ischaemia; autopsy samples (generally uninterpretable); intracranial haemorrhage; bacterial meningitis; or cerebral abscess.

Glutamine detoxifies ammonia in the brain and CSF concentrations are high normally. Concentrations of the other amino acids are much lower, due partly to restricted entry from blood and partly to active transport from CSF to blood by carrier-mediated mechanisms. Glutamine is increased in inherited urea cycle defects and the hyperammonaemia of hepatic encephalopathy.

Glycine is increased, with a high paired CSF/plasma glycine ratio, in nonketotic hyperglycinaemia. Glycine, threonine, histidine, and taurine are variably increased, and arginine decreased, in pyridox(am)ine 5'-phosphate oxidase (PNPO) deficiency.

Serine is low in the serine biosynthetic defect, 3-phosphoglycerate dehydrogenase deficiency.

Phenylalanine concentrations are high, with low tyrosine, in poorly controlled phenylketonuria.

Neurotransmitters and related metabolites

Dopamine, 5-hydroxytryptamine (5HT), noradrenaline, and their metabolites homovanillic acid (HVA), 5-hydroxyindoleacetic acid (5HIAA), and 3-methoxy-4-hydroxyphenylethylene glycol respectively, do not readily cross the BBB. They are actively transported out of the CSF. CSF concentrations are assumed to reflect changes in the brain, particularly of the striatum, which can discharge neurotransmitters into adjacent ventricular fluid. These compounds, together with **biopterins** needed for their biosynthesis, are measured in CSF for diagnosis of inherited defects causing dystonia or severe seizures. After a hypoxic-ischemic episode, 5HIAA, HVA, and tetrahydrobiopterin may virtually disappear from the CSF and **neopterin** is often increased (Hyland, 2006). Causes of abnormal neurotransmitters and their metabolites include inherited tyrosine hydroxylase deficiency, aromatic L-amino acid decarboxylase deficiency, defects of biopterin metabolism, poorly controlled phenylketonuria, and Menkes disease (causes severe copper deficiency).

Other CSF metabolites in neonatal seizure and/or encephalopathic disorders

A range of metabolites in CSF can now be analysed to aid diagnosis of severe neonatal seizures or encephalopathies, including pyridoxine-dependent seizures due to antiquitin deficiency, **pyridoxal phosphate** and **cerebral folate deficiency**, and **per-oxisomal disorders**.

Tumour markers

The malignancies most likely to be found in the CNS are primary brain tumours, brain metastases, lymphomas, and leukaemia. Identification of **tumour cells in CSF** is the most specific test, short of biopsy, however, it is insensitive, detecting only some tumours which involve the leptomeninges or lie close to the ventricles, but not deep-seated primary malignancies. It may be difficult to identify tumour cell origins or to differentiate them from inflammatory cells. β-**Human chorionic gonadotropin (β-HCG)** and α-**fetoprotein (AFP)** are valuable when measured together for diagnosis of germ-cell tumours of gonadal or extragonadal origin (excluding dysgerminomas). Neither is normally expressed in the brain.

β-HCG must be measured in paired blood and CSF samples to correct for spillover from high blood levels. A serum/CSF ratio of less than 60:1 strongly suggests intracranial germ-cell tumour. A low ratio may precede radiological evidence of metastases. Causes of intracranial HCG synthesis include primary choriocarcinoma, malignant teratoma, embryonal carcinoma and pineal germ-cell tumour, metastatic teratomas, or tropho-blast tumours.

AFP is produced by yolk-sac elements. The CSF/albumin index should be measured (see above) to correct for increased blood−CSF barrier permeability. AFP may be detectable in neonatal CSF because of high serum levels (Table 10.2) and the permeable BBB. Causes of intracranial AFP synthesis include primary or metastatic germ-cell tumours.

Table 10.2 Blood reference ranges

Constituent	Reference ranges	Comments
Acid/base: hydrogen ions (nmol/l)	38−48	
pH	7.35−7.42; neonates 7.32−7.42	
Bicarbonate (mmol/l)	22−27; neonates 17−25	
Base excess (mmol/l)	−4 to +4	
Anion gap (mmol/l) = $[Na^+]-([Cl^- + HCO^{3-}]$	7−16	
Alanine (μmol/l)	0−1 week: 108−448; 1−4 weeks: 116−376	

Table 10.2 (continued)   Blood reference ranges

Constituent	Reference ranges	Comments
Albumin (g/l)	Neonates 28—44; then 35—48	Lower in neonates born preterm; ranges vary with method
α-fetoprotein (KU/l)	At birth: 50 000—150 000; 4 weeks: 1500—2500; 8 weeks: 50—100; 10 weeks: 6—12; from 3 months: 3—8	Higher in neonates born preterm; plasma half-life approx. 5 days
ALT IU/l	6—40	Method-dependent
Ammonia (μmol/l)	Neonates: healthy <110; sick <180; if >200 metabolic disease strong possibility; from 1 month: healthy <40; if >80 metabolic disease strong possibility	Must reach the laboratory within 15 minutes
AST IU/l	1—7 days: 20—98; 8—30 days: 16—69	Method dependent
Total bilirubin (μmol/l)	Neonates up to 10 days: <200μmol/l; 14—28 days: <50; (conjugated <20μmol/l); from 1 month <18μmol/l (conjugated <10%)	Higher in neonates born preterm
Total calcium (mmol/l)	Neonates 0—5 days: 1.95—2.65; then 2.15—2.55	
Ionised calcium (mmol/l)	1.13—1.32	
Caeruloplasmin (mg/l)	1—30 days: 33—275; 1—4 months: 150—560	Ranges vary with method
Carnitine (μmol/l)	total: 20—65 free: 25—50; 20—55*	*Ranges differ among laboratories
Chloride (mmol/l)	95—110	
Cholesterol (total; mmol/l)	1—30 days: 1.4—4.0	

Table 10.2 (continued) Blood reference ranges

Constituent	Reference ranges	Comments
Copper(μmol/l)	0—6 months: 3—11; then 12—26	
Cortisol (nmol/l)	0—5 days term: 54—839; preterm: 73—562; at 30 days: 55—64 >500: adrenal insufficiency excluded; >600: good response to stress	No diurnal rhythm until around 6 weeks; random levels often low — do synacthen test if deficiency suspected
C-reactive protein (mg/l)	<10	
Creatine kinase (IU/L)	In first 2 weeks possibly ≥3 times higher than normal paediatric ranges, then rapid fall	Peaks at 24—48 hours; ranges vary widely according to analytical method
Creatinine (μmol/l)	0—2 days: 40—100; 3—14 days: 30—65; 14 days—3 months: 10—60; 3—6 months: 10—50; 6 months—1 year: 10—60	
Glucose (random) (mmol/l)	3.5—5.5	Hypoglycaemia: ≤2.5mmol/l
Glutamine (μmol/l)	0—1 week: 198—886; 1—4 weeks: 178—670	
γ-GT (γ-glutamylamino transferase) (IU/l)	1-30 days: 16-148	Method dependent
Glycine (μmol/l)	0-1 week 101-317; 1 to 4 weeks 20-356	

Immunoglobulins g/l	IgG	IgA	IgM
0—2 weeks:	5.0—17.0	0.01—0.08	0.05—0.20
2—6 weeks:	3.9—13.0	0.02—0.15	0.08—0.40

Constituent	Reference ranges	Comments
Lactate (mmol/l)	<2.1	
Lactate/pyruvate ratio (mmol/mmol)	<20 or >25 abnormal	Special collection protocol; restricted value- see text

Table 10.2 (continued) Blood reference ranges

Constituent	Reference ranges	Comments
Lead[whole blood] (µmol/l)	<0.5	Lead is transported in erythrocytes
Magnesium (mmol/l)	0.74—1.03	Ranges vary with method
Osmolality (mmol/kg water)	275—295	
Phenylalanine (µmol/l)	Term: 38—137; preterm: 98—213	
Phytanic acid (µmol/l)	0—4 months ≤10; pristanic/phytanic acid ratio ≤0.35	
Pipecolic acid (µmol/l)	<1 week 0.55—10.8; >1 week 0.54—2.46	
Potassium (mmol/l)	3.5—5.0	Often higher due to poor-quality samples
Pristanic acid (µmol/l)	0—4 months ≤1.0	
Total protein (g/l)	1—30 days: term 41—63; preterm 36—63	
Pyruvate (µmol/l)	1—30 days: 80—150	Special collection protocol; restricted value- see text
Serine (µmol/l)	0—1 week: 62—206; 1—4 weeks: 60—240	
Sodium (mmol/l)	Term 7—31 days: 132—142	
Free thyroxine (pmol/l)	Term 1—3 days: 26—68; preterm 0—7 days: 6—61; up to 1 year: 7.5—30	
Thyroid-stimulating hormone (mU/l)	0—48 hours: 2.5—66; 3 days—1 month: 0.5—10; 1 month—5 years: 0.7—8.5; preterm after 7 days: 0.8—12.0	Ranges vary with method

Table 10.2 (continued) Blood reference ranges

Constituent	Reference ranges	Comments
Urate (µmol/l)	Neonates: 120—340; 1—12 months: 80—390	
Urea (mmol/l)	1.0—5.0	
Very-long-chain fatty acids (µmol/l)	C26:0/C22:0 ratio ≤0.023; ≤0.025; ≤0.028* C24:0/C22:0 ratio ≤1.10; ≤1.15*	*Cutoff ratios differ among laboratories
Blood volume (ml/kg)	At birth: 61—100 (mean 78); then gradual fall to adult values: 53—87 (mean 71)	May be higher in neonates born preterm
Plasma volume (ml/kg)	Term neonates: 39—72; infants: 40—50; older children: 30—54	

γ-GT, γ-glutamyl transpeptidase; ALT, alanine aminotransferase; AST, aspartate aminotransferase.

β2-**Microglobulin** is synthesized by all nucleated cells and, in high concentrations, by activated T-lymphocytes. Measurement of the CSF/albumin index corrects for increases in blood—CSF barrier permeability. Causes of increased intracranial synthesis include CNS lymphoma and leukaemias. An increase may predict relapse (note: this is nonspecific; CNS infection may also increase levels).

Inorganic ions

Measurement in CSF has little practical value. CSF potassium and total and ionized calcium are lower than in plasma, and magnesium is higher. Their concentrations are regulated largely by choroid plexus transport mechanisms and do not vary with plasma levels. CSF sodium reflects plasma levels.

Haemoglobin and bilirubin

After the first month of life, normal CSF is crystal clear, with no red cells or detectable bilirubin. In typically developing infants born preterm and some neonates born at term without evidence of intracranial bleeding, CSF bilirubin (mostly unconjugated) is increased and the fluid appears yellow (xanthochromic). This is correlated with serum bilirubin levels and largely explained by hyperbilirubinaemia and increased permeability of the blood—CSF barrier to proteins.

Following haemorrhage into the subarachnoid space, red blood cells undergo lysis and phagocytosis. Liberated oxyhaemoglobin is converted *in vivo* into bilirubin in a time-dependent manner. Negative brain computed tomography does not exclude subarachnoid haemorrhage. Visual inspection of the CSF supernatant fluid for xanthochromia

Table 10.3   Ratios of metabolite concentrations to plasma concentrations in CSF

Constituent	Reference ratio	Comment
Albumin: CSF/serum albumin index (mg/g)	<9	To test whether the BBB is intact; refer to Table 10.1
Glycine: CSF/plasma ratio	<0.04; neonatal nonketotic hyperglycinaemia >0.09–0.25; atypical forms 0.06–0.09	Blood contamination invalidates test; valproate therapy may increase the ratio
Glucose: CSF/ plasma ratio (mmol/mmol)	Fasting 0.65 ±0.1; ratio <0.46 is consistent with GLUT1 deficiency	Take the blood sample first. Typically developing neonates sometimes have a low ratio- repeat test
β-HCG: serum/CSF ratio	>60	Ratio <60 indicative of intracranial germ-cell tumour
IgG index	0.30–0.70; >0.70 suggests intrathecal IgG synthesis	CSF IgG × serum albumin/serum IgG × CSF albumin. False positives and negatives occur
β2-Transferrin (desialated transferrin; mg/l)	3–5	Collect a paired plasma to exclude a genetic transferrin variant

BBB blood brain barrier; GLUT1, glucose transporter 1; β-HCG, β-human chorionic gonadotropin.

is insensitive and should not be used. Examination of CSF for blood cannot distinguish between an *in vivo* haemorrhage and a traumatic tap. In these cases, the most appropriate investigation is analysis by spectrophotometry to look for oxyhaemoglobin and its product bilirubin, in CSF collected more than 12 hours after the acute event. For interpretation, results are also required for serum bilirubin and serum and CSF protein levels. Most positive cases have increases in both oxyhaemoglobin and bilirubin, but increased bilirubin alone is more likely after an interval of several days.

Subarachnoid haemorrhage is unlikely if results are negative and further investigation (e.g. cerebral angiography) is not indicated. Results from patients with hyperbilirubin-aemia or CSF protein of more than 1000mg/l must be interpreted cautiously.

CSF rhinorrhoea

The best indication that nasal fluid contains leaking CSF is finding β2-transferrin in the fluid. In the CNS up to around 30% of transferrin is converted to β2-transferrin by the removal of its sialyl group by neuraminidase. The desialylated protein is identifiable by electrophoresis. It is not present in serum. Rarely, genetic mutations code for abnormal forms of transferrin that masquerade as β2-transferrin on electrophoresis. Detection of 'β2-transferrin' in serum reveals the defects and prevents misdiagnosis of CSF leakage. If this test is not available, the presence of glucose will differentiate CSF from nasal mucus.

Specimens for biochemistry tests

Results of biochemical tests from inappropriate samples may provide misleading information and lead to incorrect management. Special requirements are needed for the tests listed below. Refer to the clinical sections of this book for investigation protocols. Analysis of samples for DNA and collection of skin and tissue biopsies requires informed written parental consent.

Blood

Acylcarnitines and carnitine: these may be analysed from blood spotted onto filter paper or separated plasma or serum.

Amino acids (plasma): if possible, collect at least 4 hours after food or from infants just before a feed. Plasma should be separated within 4 hours and stored at −20°C. Delayed separation causes spurious abnormalities.

Ammonia: plasma concentrations rise rapidly after venesection. Free-flowing blood should be collected into ethylene-diamine-tetra-acetic acid (EDTA) or lithium-heparin (check with local laboratory) in an ammonia-free tube, transported to the laboratory within 15 minutes, preferably on water ice, and separated as soon as received in the laboratory. If not analysed immediately, plasma may be stored for up to 4 hours at 4°C. Causes of spurious increases: delayed separation, haemolysis, struggling during venesection.

Lactate: plasma concentrations rise rapidly after venesection. If not measured on a blood gas analyser, samples must be separated within 15 minutes. Causes of spurious increases: delayed separation, haemolysis, venous obstruction with a tourniquet, struggling and crying during venesection, breath-holding.

Lead: more than 95% of blood lead is in red blood cells; hence whole blood and not plasma is analysed. Samples must be collected into EDTA or heparin and not centrifuged.

Pyruvate: pyruvic acid is very unstable, and blood must be collected into perchloric acid at the bedside following strict protocols and centrifuged under refrigeration. Analysis is required only exceptionally.

Red cell enzymes (e.g. for deficiencies of galactose-1-phosphate uridyl-transferase [GAL-1-PUT; GALT] or glutathione synthetase): samples should not be collected until 3 months after blood transfusion.

White cell enzymes (e.g. for lysosomal storage disorders): at least 7ml of blood (absolute minimum 5ml) is required, even from very small infants, to extract and wash enough cells for analysis. Whole-blood samples must be delivered to a specialist laboratory within 24 hours at room temperature and hence should not be collected before weekends or public holidays.

Urine

Amino acids, organic acids, orotic acid, glycosaminoglycans (mucopolysaccharides), α-aminoadipic semialdedehyde (α-AASA, for pyridoxine dependency), purines, pyrimidines, creatine, and other metabolites are analysed on random urine samples that are not faecally contaminated. A bag urine sample is preferred. If this proves difficult, unsoiled urine collected into a cotton wool ball may be the only option. Urine thus sampled is drawn into a syringe and transferred into a sterile container. Samples should be stored at -20°C until analysed. Fluids should not be increased to induce a diuresis. Bacterial contamination and very dilute samples cause spurious results. It is essential to obtain urine for analysis at presentation of an acutely ill child even if the sample is of poor quality. If transport to the laboratory is delayed, samples should be refrigerated (4°C if overnight; -20°C if longer).

Sulphite: A dipstick test (Merckoquant Sulfite Test) can be used as a rapid screen for increased sulphite (in molybdenum cofactor or isolated sulphite oxidase deficiency). Because sulphite is unstable, urine must be tested within minutes of voiding or frozen immediately if this is not possible. False negatives occur even with fresh samples. Urine analysis of sulphocysteine is the definitive test if these disorders are strongly suspected.

CSF

Bilirubin and oxyhaemoglobin spectrophotometry to investigate for subarachnoid haemorrhage with a negative brain scan: CSF samples are collected 12 hours or more after the acute event in sequence for (1) glucose and protein, (2) microbiology, and (3) spectrophotometry. The third sample must be protected from light and sent immediately for analysis. Blood is collected simultaneously for bilirubin and protein analysis. Causes of spurious results: samples collected too early, delayed analysis, interpretive difficulties if there is hyperbilirubinaemia, or CSF protein exceeds 1000mg/l.

Glycine analysis for suspected nonketotic hyperglycinaemia: CSF must be clear since blood contamination makes the result uninterpretable (glycine in plasma is normally 10–20 times higher than in CSF). A paired blood sample must be taken for glycine analysis to calculate the CSF/plasma ratio. Causes of spurious results: blood contamination, treatment with valproate.

Glucose analysis: paired blood and CSF samples are needed for interpretation. If the test is to exclude inherited deficiency of the GLUT1 glucose transporter, samples should be collected after a 4 to 6 hours fast when nonictal, and blood should be collected first to minimize a stress-induced increase in plasma glucose.

Lactate: samples must either be analysed immediately at the bedside, using, for example, a blood gas analyser, or reach the laboratory within 15 minutes of collection. Causes of spurious results: delayed analysis, especially if CSF is contaminated with blood, white blood cells are increased, or tumour cells are present..

Neurotransmitters: because there is a lumbosacral gradient, samples must be collected in a standardized volume fraction following protocols provided by the referral laboratories. The samples must be frozen immediately after collection (at the bedside) in solid carbon dioxide or liquid nitrogen.

Serine analysis for serine biosynthesis defects: paired plasma and CSF samples are needed and analysed for amino acids.

Tissue biopsies

Skin: local anaesthetic is injected or applied to the skin of the forearm, upper leg or armpit and the skin cleaned carefully. A 3mm full-thickness punch biopsy is taken with a full aseptic technique and placed in tissue culture fluid for fibroblast culture. If the culture medium is not available, the biopsy may be stored overnight at 4°C (not frozen) either in an empty sterile container or in sterile saline, according to instructions from the local tissue culture laboratory. Fibroblasts can often be cultured from skin taken 2 or 3 days after death and autopsy biopsies should be taken if indicated (with prior consent).

Muscle: biopsies should be undertaken in collaboration with the muscle histopathologist so that samples are collected and processed appropriately for histology, histochemistry, electron microscopy, and biochemical analyses. The tissue for biochemistry must be frozen at the bedside in solid carbon dioxide or liquid nitrogen.

Liver: a biopsy should be obtained if possible when nonketotic hyperglycinaemia is diagnosed, and in a very small number of inborn errors involving enzymes expressed only in liver when mutation analysis is not an option, or if mitochondrial depletion is likely. One or two good needle biopsy cores are transferred to sterile containers and frozen immediately at the bedside in solid carbon dioxide or liquid nitrogen. An additional core is needed for histology and electron microscopy if required and should be stored as directed by the histopathologist. If open biopsy is undertaken, $1cm^3$ of tissue should suffice.

HAEMATOLOGY INVESTIGATIONS

Full blood count

Fully automated cell counters provide a result for haemoglobin, total leukocyte count with differential, and platelet count. Normal age-related reference ranges need to be applied as these are different from adult values. Spurious results may arise due to blood sampling (often difficult in small children with poor venous access), hence it is essential to correlate the clinical findings with the laboratory result. (See Table 10.4 and Table 10.5.

Table 10.4 Normal haematological values in children

Age	Haemoglobin (g/dl)*		Mean cell volume		Mean corpuscular haemoglobin (pg)	
	Mean	−2SD	Mean	−2SD	Mean	−2SD
Birth (cord blood)	16.5	13.5	108	98	34	31
1—3 days (capillary)	18.5	14.5	108	95	34	31
1 week	17.5	13.5	107	88	34	28
2 weeks	16.5	12.5	105	86	34	28
1 month	14.0	10.0	104	85	34	28
2 months	11.5	9.0	96	77	30	26
3—6 months	11.5	9.5	91	74	30	25
0.5—2 years	12.0	10.5	78	70	27	23
2—6 years	12.5	11.5	81	75	27	24
6—12 years	13.5	11.5	86	77	29	25
12—18 years:						
Female	14.0	12.0	90	78	30	25
Male	14.5	13.0	88	78	30	25

* To convert g/dL to mmol/L, divide by 1.8.

Table 10.5   Reference ranges for leukocyte counts in children

Age	Total leukocytes		Neutrophils			Lymphocytes			Mono-cytes	
	Mean	Range	Mean	Range	%	Mean	Range	%	Mean	%
Birth	18.1	9.0–30.0	11.0	6.0–26.0	61	5.5	2.0–11.0	31	1.1	6
12 hours	22.8	13.0–38.0	15.5	6.0–28.0	68	5.5	2.0–11.0	24	1.2	5
24 hours	18.9	9.4–34.0	11.5	5.0–21.0	61	5.8	2.0–11.5	31	1.1	6
1 week	12.2	5.0–21.0	5.5	1.5–10.0	45	5.0	2.0–17.0	41	1.1	9
2 weeks	11.4	5.0–20.0	4.5	1.0–9.5	40	5.5	2.0–17.0	48	1.0	9
1 month	10.8	5.0–19.5	3.8	1.0–9.0	35	6.0	2.5–16.5	56	0.7	7
6 months	11.9	6.0–17.5	3.8	1.0–8.5	32	7.3	4.0–13.5	61	0.6	5
1 year	11.4	6.0–17.5	3.5	1.5–8.5	31	7.0	4.0–10.5	61	0.6	5
2 years	10.6	6.0–17.0	3.5	1.5–8.5	33	6.3	3.0–9.5	59	0.5	5
4 years	9.1	5.5–15.5	3.8	1.5–8.5	42	4.5	2.0–8.0	50	0.5	5
6 years	8.5	5.0–14.5	4.3	1.5–8.0	51	3.5	1.5–7.0	42	0.4	5
8 years	8.3	4.5–13.5	4.4	1.5–8.0	53	3.3	1.5–6.8	39	0.4	4
10 Years	8.1	4.5–13.5	4.4	1.8–8.0	54	3.1	1.5–6.5	38	0.4	4

The full blood count (FBC) result includes a value for the red cell indices, mean cell volume (MCV) reflecting the size of the red cells, and mean corpuscular haemoglobin (MCH) indicating the haemoglobin content. These values, in addition to a reticulocyte count, are also helpful in assessing the *cause* of anaemia.

Reticulocytes are immature red blood cells which mature in the bone marrow and then circulate in the blood stream before developing into mature red cells. The number of reticulocytes is an indicator of marrow activity. The value can be used to determine whether a production problem is contributing to the anaemia. In haemolytic anaemias there is a reticulocytosis.

Blood film examination

Indicated for any abnormality in the FBC. A systematic examination of the red cell, leucocyte, and platelet morphology may provide clues to the diagnosis. In thrombocytopenia, the blood film should be reviewed to confirm the low platelet count, as clumping of platelets will give rise to a spuriously low count.

Laboratory investigations for iron deficiency for the following reasons:

- haemoglobin may be low;

- reduced MCV and MCH;

- blood film shows hypochromic, microcytic red cells;

- reduced serum ferritin (ferritin is an acute-phase protein which increases in infection and inflammation) reflects iron deficiency but a normal level does not necessarily confirm iron sufficiency; and

- reduced serum iron with raised total iron-binding capacity (transferrin). Both values can, however, fall with inflammation.

Causes of iron deficiency

Most common causes are (see Figure 10.1):

- inadequate intake:

  o prolonged breast feeding;

  o formula milk without iron fortification;

  o malnourishment;

- increased physiological requirements — rapid growth in early childhood; and adolescence;

- blood loss.

Clinical features of iron deficiency

- tiredness;

- pallor, if anaemic;

- angular stomatitis.

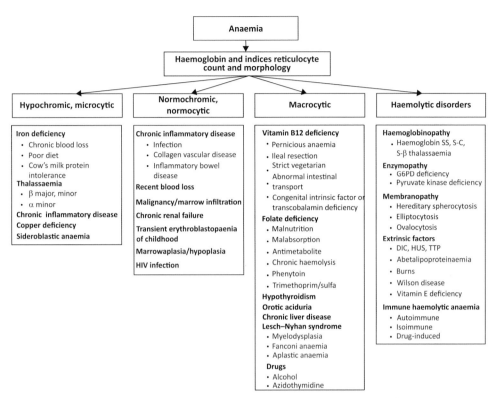

Figure 10.1 Causes of anaemia . DIC, disseminated intravascular coagulation; G6PD, glucose-6-phosphate dehydrogenase; HUS, haemolytic uraemic syndrome; TTP, thrombotic thrombocytopaenic purpura.

Haemolysis

Investigations for haemolysis

- Full blood count and film examination (red cell morphology), reticulocytes.

- Direct antiglobulin test.

- Elevated lactate dehydrogenase.

- Elevated unconjugated bilirubin.

- Reduced haptoglobin.

In haemolytic anaemia, the child may be jaundiced (usually not clinically apparent until 40µmol/l) and have splenomegaly but not always.

Leukocyte abnormalities

Causes of neutrophilia include (see Table 10.5):

- infection;

- inflammation;

- metabolic disturbance;

- neoplasia;

- steroid therapy; and

- myeloproliferative disorders

Causes of lymphocytosis include

- viral infections;

- tuberculosis;

- brucellosis; and

- thyrotoxicosis.

Haemostasis

The coagulation system is immature at birth and even more so in the infant born preterm. Plasma concentrations of coagulation proteins may vary from the adult normal range. Monagle et al. (2006) provide comprehensive age-related normal values for the coagulation proteins in infants born preterm and infants born at term. Blood for coagulation tests is taken into tubes containing a measured amount of citrate which is used as the anticoagulant. The correct amount of blood should be added. Under- or overfilled tubes will cause abnormal results. The laboratory should reject these samples.

Laboratory investigations

Prothrombin time (PT) is a measure of the 'extrinsic system' (Figure 10.2), whereas activated partial thromboplastin time (APTT) is a measure of the 'intrinsic system'. Also measured are thrombin clotting time (or TCT), fibrin degradation products (or D-dimers), and fibrinogen.

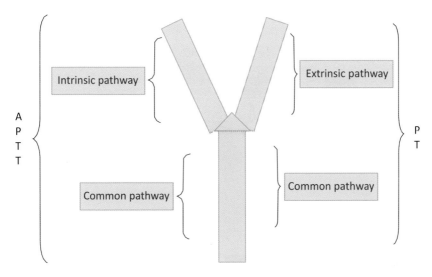

Figure 10.2 Prothrombin time (PT) and activated partial thromboplastin time (APTT)

Coagulation cascade

Prothrombin time measures the vitamin K-dependent coagulation factors (Factors II, VII, IX, and X; see Figure 10.3). PT is prolonged because of:

- sampling error;

- vitamin K deficiency;

- deranged liver function;

- factor deficiency; and

- warfarin (the therapeutic effect is achieved by a reduction in the vitamin K-dependent factors synthesized in the liver).

Vitamin K deficiency may cause haemorrhagic disease of the newborn infant, which can be classified into three patterns depending on the time of onset:

- Early: within 24 hours, serious life-threatening bleeding including intracranial haemorrhage;

- Classic: days 1 to 7, breastfed infants;

- Late: beyond the first week up to 6 months, breastfed infants, usually associated with underlying disorders that compromise the supply of vitamin K.

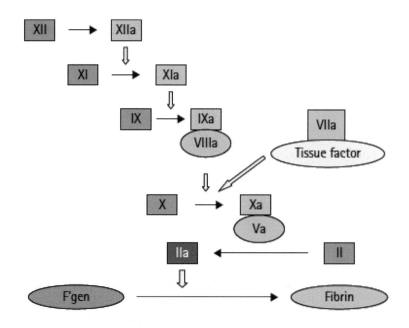

Figure 10.3 The coagulation cascade. F'gen, Fibrinogen

Table 10.6 Vitamin K deficiency

	Early	Classic	Late
Age at onset	<24 hours	Day 1—7	Week 2—6 months
Aetiology	Drugs administered in pregnancy	Inadequate milk intake, low vitamin K in breast milk	Low vitamin K in breast milk, malabsorption of vitamin K (liver and bowel disease)
Frequency without prophylaxis	<5% in high-risk groups	0.01—1.5%	4—10 in 100 000 births
Precautions	Stop or substitute offending drugs	Adequate vitamin K supply by early breast feeding, prophylaxis	Vitamin K prophylaxis recognition of predisposing factors

Intracranial haemorrhaging may occur as well as bleeding from other sites and into vital organs (see Table 10.6).

APTT measures Factors VIII, IX, XI, and XII, and the kallikrein—kinin system. It is prolonged for the following reasons:

- sampling error;

- factor deficiency;

- inhibitor: lupus anticoagulant; and

- heparin.

Caution: even small amounts of heparin in the blood taken from central lines will prolong the APTT. Deficiencies of factor XII, high-molecular-weight kininogen, and prekallikrein result in a prolonged APTT, but do not cause haemorrhaging.

Thrombin clotting time measures the amount and quality of fibrinogen and the rate of conversion of fibrinogen to fibrin. A prolonged thrombin clotting time may indicate a deficiency of fibrinogen (<1g/l) as seen in congenital hypofibrinogenaemia or afibrinogenaemia. It is markedly prolonged in the presence of heparin.

A fibrinogen assay should be included in the basic coagulation screening tests. It is reduced in acquired (disseminated intravascular coagulation, liver dysfunction, increased fibrinolysis) and hereditary (afibrinogenaemia, hypofibrinogenaemia, and dysfibrinogenaemia) coagulopathies. Haemorrhage does not usually occur until the level is less than 1.0 g/l, *unless it is a dysfunctional protein*.

Disseminated intravascular coagulation

Laboratory abnormalities include:

- prolonged PT and APTT;

- thrombocytopenia;

- reduced fibrinogen; and

- raised fibrin-degradation products.

Acquired disorders of coagulation

- Vitamin K deficiency.

- Liver disease.

- Disseminated intravascular coagulation.

- Associated with malignancy.

- Acquired inhibitors: lupus anticoagulant.

- Massive blood transfusion.

Congenital coagulation disorders

- Haemophilia A: deficiency of Factor VIII.

- Haemophilia B: deficiency of Factor IX (Christmas disease).

- Von Willebrand disease Type 1, 2, 3.

- Deficiency of Factors II, V, VII, X, XI, XII, and XIII.

- Dys-/hypofibrinogenaemia.

Factor XIII deficiency

Severe Factor XIII deficiency can result in intracranial haemorrhage. The PT and APTT are normal and a specific factor assay is necessary to make the diagnosis.

Haemoglobinopathy

Haemoglobinopathies are disorders of haemoglobin arising as a result of a disturbance of the globin chain production or a mutation resulting in an abnormal haemoglobin (Hb variant). Thalassaemia syndromes are characterized by diminished or absent production of alpha or beta globin chain synthesis. Alpha thalassaemia occurs in people of African, Mediterranean, South Asian, and South-East Asian origin. Beta thalassaemia is found in the Mediterranean, India, Pakistan, and Africa.

Haemoglobin variants arise as a result of a single amino acid substitution in the alpha or beta globin chains. This results in alteration in the structure of the typical adult haemoglobin. The most common of these are S, C, E, D^{Punjab}. HbS and HbC are found in the Afro-Caribbean population, HbE in the South-East Asian population, and HbD^{Punjab} in the Indian population. The most important of these is sickle haemoglobin found in Africa, the Near East, Mediterranean, and parts of India, which in the homozygous or double heterozygous state can result in a condition characterized by chronic haemolysis and sickle cell crises.

Haemoglobinopathy could be suspected for the following reasons:

- family history;

- hypochromic, microcytic indices not due to iron deficiency;

- target cells on blood film; and

- red cell fragments or sickle cells.

Laboratory diagnosis

- Examination of a blood film.

- Cellulose acetate electrophoresis to identify an abnormal Hb band.

- High-pressure liquid chromatography to identify the various haemoglobins.

- Sickle solubility test which detects the presence of HbS but does not distinguish the hetero- from the homozygous state.

Caution: the majority of haemoglobin at birth is fetal HbF before the switch to adult HbA. Children with a haemoglobinopathy should be referred to a haematologist.

REFERENCES

Hyland K (2006) Cerebrospinal fluid analysis in the diagnosis of treatable inherited disorders of neurotransmitter metabolism. *Future Neurol* 1: 593—603.

Monagle PT, Chan AKC, Massicotte MP, deVeber G, (2006) *Paediatric Thromboembolism and Stroke*, 3rd edn. Hamilton ON: BC Decker.

Resources

Jones CM, Smith M, Henderson MJ (2006) Reference data for cerebrospinal fluid and the utility of amino acid measurement for the diagnosis of inborn errors of metabolism. *Ann Clin Biochem* 43: 63—66.

Oski FA, Brugnara C, Nathan DG (2003) *Nathan and Oski's Haematology of Infancy and Childhood*, 6th edn. Philadelphia: Saunders.

Rennie JM (Ed) (2012) *Rennie and Robertson's Textbook of Neonatology* 5th edn. Churchill Livingstone. London: Elsevier, pp. 1309—1322.

CHAPTER 11

Genetic testing

Geoffrey Woods and Catarina Olimpio

Key messages

- Paediatric neurologists are amongst the biggest users of genetic testing.
- Molecular genetic testing is sometimes the only route to an exact diagnosis or can be the quickest and most expedient method, reducing the need for other investigations.
- Use genetic testing to answer a specific clinical question.
- You do not need to be a molecular geneticist or clinical geneticist to correctly use genetic testing. All relevant background is easy to look up and the test result should be sufficiently explained for you to use it with confidence.
- Read all of the molecular genetic test report; important information is often given in the covering paragraphs.
- Give the laboratory relevant clinical details and let them know how to contact you.
- Involve/use clinical genetics for family testing and discussion of recurrence risk and prenatal diagnosis.

Common errors

- Not requesting a microarray to detect deletions/duplications as well as gene sequencing (e.g. in suspected Pelizaeus-Merzbacher disease, a microarray would detect a causative PLP1 duplication; sequencing would detect point mutations: both tests may be needed).

- Not having as clear a description as possible of the patient's phenotype (this makes interpretation of variants of unknown significance (VUSs) impossible, especially when using panels with many genes, e.g. for intellectual disability).
- Not understanding what questions each type of genetic testing answers (e.g. testing for abnormal methylation in suspected Angelman syndrome will not detect those cases with UBE3A mutations).
- Not consenting patients for the correct genetic test, particularly for the possibility of the test being predictive of disease rather than a carrier test (e.g. in families with Friedreich's ataxia or adrenoleukodystrophy).
- Not discussing the meaning of possible test results when seeking a family's consent to undertake it (e.g. mutation detected – provides a clear-cut answer; normal result – may not mean invalidate a specific clinical diagnosis; VUS detected – will be difficult to interpret).

When to worry

- When you do not understand a genetic report.
- When the genotype does not equate with the phenotype.
- When the inheritance pattern seems wrong for the disease gene found by molecular testing.

INTRODUCTION

Our understanding of the genetic phenotypes seen in paediatric neurology is rapidly expanding, and the use of genetic tests in clinical practice is increasing. The number of genes recognized to cause a phenotype, and also the phenotypes that can be caused by different mutations continue to increase. Seemingly impenetrably complex phenotypes with no easy guides to dissecting heterogeneity can be individually diagnosed with gene panel analysis. Disease prognosis and response to therapy can be predicted increasingly accurately in some conditions. The speed and scope of gene analysis is increasing, and the cost continues to decrease. However, clinicians must remember that the clinical diagnosis always takes precedence over a genetic result.

To use genetic testing most effectively, clinicians need to understand the scope, limitations, and consequences of each genetic test they order. This is the aim of this chapter; but the clinician should also be helped by the molecular genetic report (see Box 11.2 and Figure 11.1) and through contact with the Molecular Genetics laboratory that produced the report or their local clinical geneticists.

Genes are composed of nucleotides. A nucleotide is composed of a 5 carbon-ring sugar molecule, a nitrogenous base, and a phosphate group. The phosphate connects the sugar rings between two nucleotide monomers. Long strings of nucleotide thus form

---

Box 11.1 Test definitions

☑ **Diagnostic:** to confirm the gene mutation(s) causing the patients phenotype. Use: to confirm diagnosis or exact molecular subdiagnosis. It may help management and will confirm, or give, the inheritance pattern of the condition.

☑ **Predictive:** to discover if a clinically unaffected individual has a gene mutation(s) that can cause a known phenotype before it has developed. Use: as in a diagnostic test. Beware of doing such tests without adequate discussion with the parent and patient.

☑ **Carrier test in a recessive disorder:** to discover if a clinically unaffected individual has a single copy of a proven recessive mutation. Use: to confirm that the mutations found in the person's child(ren) are valid; as part of couple testing to tell if they are at risk of having a specific recessive disease. Beware that you are not performing a diagnostic test (e.g. sibling of adolescent with Friedreich's ataxia, or male sibling of a male with X-linked adrenoleukodystrophy).

☑ **Female carrier test in an X-linked disorder:** genetic test to discover if a clinically un-affected individual has a single copy of a proven-linked mutation. Use: to determine if a female is a carrier of the condition and, hence, at 50:50 risk of having an affected male. Beware that you are not performing a diagnostic test, or at least have discussed the possibility, as some X-linked recessive disorders have a phenotype (e.g. carrier female of fragile X mutation can have intellectual disability, or premature ovarian failure).

Box 11.2 What to expect in a genetic report?

☑ Name of the laboratory contact details and the people producing the report.

☑ Date of sample receipt and test report writing.

☑ Reason for testing (summary).

☑ Result stating the definite gene mutation found, or that no mutation has been found.

☑ A description of the molecular genetic test and the methodology used.

☑ A list of all genes tested, and how completely this was performed for each gene.

☑ If relevant, discussion of variants found which may be significant, and what further action should be taken to clarify the situation.

☑ Hopefully, the percentage of mutations detected by the methodology for the phenotype, or the gene tested.

☑ Other tests that should be done for the testing situation (or may be of use in achieving a diagnosis).

---

links through the phosphate groups. Two nucleotide strings can interact, one running in the opposite direction to the other, and so create a double helix. A gene is read

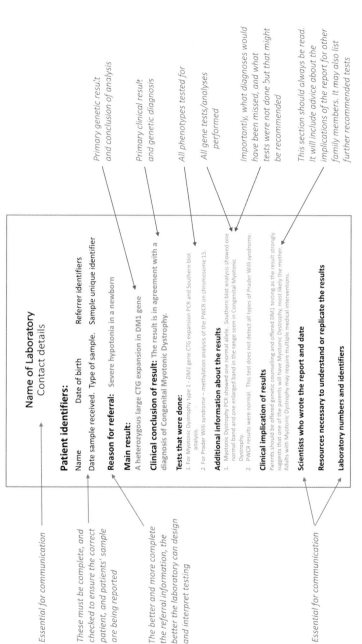

Name of Laboratory
Contact details

Essential for communication

Patient identifiers:

Name   Date of birth   Referrer identifiers
Date sample received.   Type of sample.   Sample unique identifier

These must be complete, and checked to ensure the correct patient, and patients' sample are being reported

Reason for referral: Severe hypotonia in a newborn

Main result:
A heterozygous large CTG expansion in DM1 gene

Primary genetic result and conclusion of analysis

Clinical conclusion of result: The result is in agreement with a diagnosis of Congenital Myotonic Dystrophy.

Primary clinical result and genetic diagnosis

Tests that were done:
1. For Myotonic Dystrophy type 1 – DM1 gene CTG expansion PCR and Southern blot analysis.
2. For Prader Willi syndrome – methylation analysis of the PWCR on chromosome 15.

All phenotypes tested for

Additional information about the results
1. Myotonic Dystrophy PCR showed one normal allele. Southern blot analysis showed one normal band and one enlarged band in the range seen in Congenital Myotonic Dystrophy.
2. PWCR results were normal. This test does not detect all types of Prader Willi syndrome.

All gene tests/analyses performed

Clinical implication of results
Parents should be offered genetic counselling and offered DM1 testing as the result strongly suggests that one of the parents will have Myotonic Dystrophy, most likely the mother. Adults with Myotonic Dystrophy may require multiple medical interventions.

Importantly, what diagnoses would have been missed, and what tests were not done but that might be recommended

Scientists who wrote the report and date

Resources necessary to understand or replicate the results

Essential for communication

Laboratory numbers and identifiers

The better and more complete the referral information, the better the laboratory can design and interpret testing

This section should always be read. It will include advice about the implications of the report for other family members. It may also list further recommended tests

Figure 11.1   An idealized molecular genetic report is shown within the box at the centre of the figure. Report headings are in bold and should all be included on any laboratory result. Comments about the structure of the report are to the left. Clinically relevant comments are to the right. These can often be important for the further management of the case or the family and should always be read.

from only one of the two nucleotide strands. The nitrogenous bases in deoxyribose nucleic acid (DNA) are adenine, guanine, cytosine, and thymine (abbreviated A, G, C, and T respectively). In ribose nucleic acid (RNA), the four bases are A, G, C, and uracil (U). For this discussion, we use the term 'mutation' as any change to the nucleotide composition of a gene, or its surroundings, that causes a disease phenotype — this is what used to be called a 'pathogenic mutation'. Any change to a gene or its surrounding, compared to the reference human genome, is known as a variant. Only a minority of these are 'mutations' while the majority are harmless and should not be reported to you. Some variants will be difficult or impossible to classify as either benign or pathogenic, and these are currently called 'variants of unknown significance' and will be discussed in your report and any action that can be taken to clarify their pathogenicity will be suggested. Laboratories try to avoid reporting 'variants of unknown significance', as this is not clinically useful (Richards et al. 2015).

INHERITANCE PATTERNS

The different Mendelian inheritance patterns are reviewed here. This will then be explored in more depth in some common genetic disorders seen in paediatric neurology practice.

Autosomal dominant

Clinical: conditions with this inheritance pattern can be passed from an affected parent to half (on average) of their children — and this applies to both fathers and mothers. There is often a multigenerational family tree of affected individuals. If the disease is severe it can have occurred for the first time in the affected individual. The condition affects males and females equally and the phenotype varies considerably from person to person (even if they have the same gene mutation).

Genes and mutations: this condition is caused by one mutation/fault/change in a gene on an autosomal chromosome, therefore, not the X or Y chromosomes. Autosomal chromosomes are always paired, and so the 'other' gene has no mutation. To generalize, a dominant mutation can cause disease in two ways: either the 'dose' of the gene is critical (two copies is normal, and increased or decreased gene expression leads to a disease) or the gene fault alters the normal function of the gene, despite the presence of a normal copy of the gene.

Disease examples include *PMP22* hereditary sensory and motor neuropathy and many of the recently emerging causes of severe learning difficulties, which are de novo genetic events such as Dravet syndrome caused by *SCN1A* mutations.

Autosomal dominant with anticipation

Whilst generally rare, this pattern of inheritance deserves special mention because of its occurrence in paediatric neurology practice.

Clinical: in these disorders, which can be dominant or X-linked, the severity of the disorder can vary from generation to generation, and generally become more severe as it is passed down to subsequent generations. The features of the phenotype can become both more severe and also present at an earlier age; some features of the phenotype may only emerge in the most severe cases.

Genes and mutations: in these disorders the mutations are unstable and can change when passed from an affected parent to their affected child. These can be best thought of as stutters in the DNA, either in or close to the gene, the larger the stutter the more severe the phenotype. The stutter is usually a nucleotide triplet repeat in the gene (such as GGC or GAG). For each disorder there will be a range of normal stutter size and disease-causing stutter sizes. The number of stutters can increase, decrease, and remain constant when passed from parent to child; and the pattern of this is disease and sex specific. The correlation between stutter size and phenotype is usually only general, but in some instances can accurately predict the phenotype.

Disease examples include Huntington disease, myotonic dystrophy, and fragile X syndrome.

Autosomal recessive

Clinical: conditions with this inheritance pattern occur in the offspring of unaffected parents (there are rare exceptions, e.g. occasionally in highly consanguineous pedigrees); the recurrence risk for each subsequent child is 1 in 4. The condition affects males and females equally in occurrence and phenotype. The phenotype usually does not vary from person to person (there are very rare exceptions, such as spinal muscular atrophy [SMA] and Smith-Lemli-Opitz syndrome). This inheritance pattern is more common in consanguineous relationships and cultures.

Genes and mutations: this condition is caused by having a mutation/fault/change in each of a pair of genes on an autosomal chromosome (therefore, not the X or Y chromosomes). Recessive mutations are usually either nulls (either the mRNA of the gene is not made, hence no protein, or the protein is made but is not functional) or hypomorphic (meaning that either significantly reduced amounts of mRNA are made or that the proteins' function is reduced below a necessary level). For a gene to cause disease in a recessive manner, then one normal, functioning gene is sufficient for completely typical health. Therefore, in nearly all cases the parents of a child with a recessive disease will each possess one normal and one mutated copy of a gene, are 'carriers', and will not have any features of the recessive phenotype found in their affected child. For many conditions the only way to identify carriers of a recessive disease is by gene sequencing.

Disease examples are the neuronal ceroid lipofuscinoses (Batten disease) and SMA.

X-linked recessive

Clinical: conditions with this inheritance pattern occur in the offspring of unaffected parents; the recurrence risk of inheriting the mutation for each subsequent child is 1 in 4. However, the recurrence risk for the clinical condition affects only males, where the risk is 1 in 2, whereas in females the risk is nil. The phenotype does not vary from male to male in an affected family; this condition is only passed through the female line and female carriers do not have a phenotype (although 10–15% of female carriers of Duchenne muscular dystrophy [DMD] are or will be symptomatic, not because of muscular weakness but because of a possible effect on cardiac function. Currently the recommendation is to assess cardiac function in documented carriers of DMD).

Genes and mutations: this condition is caused by having a mutation/fault/change in a gene on an X chromosome (males have only one X chromosome, and females two X chromosomes). Some carriers of a X-linked recessive disease can be identified by biochemical or brain scans, but always by gene sequencing.

Disease examples are Duchenne/Becker muscular dystrophy and Pelizeus–Merzbacher disease.

X-linked dominant

X-linked dominant inheritance patterns are generally very rare but do occur in a number of conditions seen in paediatric neurology practice, such as Aicardi syndrome and incontinentia pigmentii. The causative mutation is on the X chromosome and in males is generally prenatally lethal, whereas in females the presence of an unmutated gene on the second X chromosome is sufficient to cause disease, but not early lethality.

Mitochondrial (genome)

The majority of mitochondrial diseases are encoded by nuclear genes. This section deals only with mitochondrial disease encoded by genes on the mitochondrial genome within each and all mitochondria in each cell.

Clinical: the inheritance pattern can be difficult to discern as the phenotypes are notoriously variable between and within families. The condition can appear to be either sporadic or if familial will be only passed through the female line because at fertilization the oocyte, but not the spermatocyte, contributes with mitochondria. Thus, in a small family there can be mitochondrial (genome).

Genes and mutations: mutations are in the circular mitochondrial genome, which encodes for 37 genes. The proportion of mitochondria carrying a mutation in each cell can vary from effectively all to almost none. This then leads to the average proportion of affected cells per tissue also varying randomly. This complexity is further increased by

the fact that some mutations are more deleterious than others, and by variation in the sensitivi-
ties and thresholds of different cell types and tissues in different mitochondrial diseases. Multiple tissues may need to be investigated to detect the mutation, and to predict the phenotype. Investigation of an affected individual may need to include biochemical analysis of enzyme function/activity in muscle and, occasionally, also in other tissues.

Disease examples are mitochondrial encephalomyopathy, lactic acidosis, and stroke-like episodes (MELAS) and neurogenic weakness, ataxia, and retinitis pigmentosa (NARP) syndrome.

TYPES OF GENETIC MUTATIONS

Molecular genetic laboratories should only report gene variants they believe to be mutations and so benign and harmless changes should not be reported. All types of mutations can occur in each inheritance pattern. Loss-of-function mutations are nonsense (as long as not in the last two exons of a gene, see below), frame shift deletions (when the number of nucleotides lost is NOT divisible by three), whole gene deletions (but these usually give a less severe phenotype than the other mutations listed here), and functionally-validated (i.e. experimentally 'examined' and proved to be a functional null) missense mutations.

Missense mutations

Missense mutations are nucleotide alterations that cause an amino acid change in the translated protein. They are easy to detect but can be difficult to categorize, especially if occurring in a recessive condition. A minority of missense variants are disease causing 'mutations'. Missense mutations can cause both reduced or loss of function (typically in recessive conditions, but also in dosage-sensitive dominants), or can cause abnormal activity (typically as dominant-negative, i.e. a mutation whose gene product adversely affects the normal, wild-type gene product within the same cell effects in dominant disorders).

Nonsense mutations

Nonsense mutations are nucleotide alterations that cause a premature stop codon to occur (i.e. TAC — encoding for Tyrosine changes to TAG), causing the gene transcription to stop at the prior amino acid. This has two possible consequences: the cell transcription mechanisms senses that the mRNA is incomplete and degrades it so that no protein is produced; or if the nonsense mutation is near the end of a gene, then the protein will still be made but will be shorter than normal. These two possibilities can both have the same effect, or the latter can cause a lesser disease or, rarely, even a different disease phenotype.

Splicing mutations

Most genes consist of exons separated by much larger introns, and splicing is the mechanism by which the exons are joined together to form an mRNA. If this process goes wrong, the effects are almost always deleterious. Point mutations in the underlying DNA or errors during transcription can activate a cryptic splice site in part of the transcript that usually is not spliced. This results in a missing section of an exon. In this way, a point mutation, which might otherwise affect only a single amino acid, can manifest as a deletion or truncation in the final protein. Unless the specific sequence of nucleic acids suggests such a deletion, changes in the sequence may be difficult to interpret without functional studies, thus, splicing mutations can be missed and be difficult to assess. If suspected, the laboratory may suggest further testing of mRNA or using a MiniGene assay.

Small (intra-exon) deletions, duplications, and rearrangements

If these disrupt the 3-nucleotide codon sequence of a gene sequence they can be regarded as a nonsense mutation, otherwise they can be difficult to interpret for the laboratory.

Repeat mutations

Repeat mutations are typically increases in size of triplet repeats within genes (encoding for additional glutamines in a polyglutamine tract or alanines in a polyalanine tract), and of 1, 2, 3, or 4 nucleotides repeats outside of exons. Polyglutamine or polyalanine repeats typically cause neuronal dysfunction and disease by a complex pathophysiology including sequestering of useful proteins and toxic gain of functions. Triplet repeat expansions in the regions of introns before or after a gene cause either gene silencing or reduced transcription. For diseases associated with triplet repeats there is a normal range of numbers of repeats, an abnormal rage of increased numbers of repeats giving rise to disease, and, in some instances, an intermediate range where the disease usually does not occur but the repeat number is likely to increase in size in subsequent generations. To generalize, small repeats can be easily assessed by sequencing (such as the spinocerebellar ataxias), but diseases involving larger numbers of repeats (such as myotonic dystrophy and fragile X syndrome) need other techniques to confirm or assess them, including Sothern blotting and specialized polymerase chain reaction (PCR) methods.

Large deletions, duplications, and intra-gene rearrangements

Deletions and duplications are detected currently by microarrays using DNA-chip technology (and were previously detected by cytogenetic analysis of cells blocked in mitosis). Rearrangements on a large scale can only be detected, currently, by cytogenetic analysis and specialized/rearrangement-specific genetic analysis. On a small scale (within gene) these are currently difficult to detect unless they are within an exon in which case they are easily detected by sequencing. Determination of deletion and 'microdeletions' (those <5Mb in size and only currently detectable by microarrays) depends upon previously published cases and the genes within the deletion. The laboratory issuing the report will interpret the result and reference previous literature. All this will start to change as and when whole genomic sequencing is introduced as it has the potential to detect all deletions, duplications, and rearrangements.

Methylation mutations

Methylation mutations alter the methylation status of cytosines (methylcytosine can be easily produced and has to be changed back to cytosine by cells, if not they are read as thymidine). Typically, cytosine methylation defects are on CpG regions that control gene transcription (epigenetic gene control). As the DNA sequence is not changed, the methylation status of genes needs to be specifically assessed by methylation sensitive assays, which are specific to each gene. Examples of diseases caused by methylation defects are Angelman syndrome and Prader—Willi syndrome.

TYPES OF GENETIC TESTING

Advancing technology is rapidly changing our ability to analyses the human genome. In the past, cytogenetic analysis was achieved through observation of mitosis by microscopy, and we used Sanger sequencing to read genes exon by exon. Then, a plethora of techniques evolved that enabled us to sequence particular mutations of particular genes. Now (i.e. currently in Europe and the USA), cytogenetic analysis is by microchips and massive parallel sequencing. This allows multiple genes in multiple people to be sequenced simultaneously. Added to this has been an accumulating knowledge of genetic disease phenotypes and genotypes, the population frequency of variants in the human genome, and advanced computing techniques to store and analyse results. It is a time of change that should produce far wider availability of targeted genetic testing, better interpretation of results, quicker and cheaper analysis, and an increased usefulness of genetics. Currently genetic testing can be divided into the following types.

Cytogenetics

The analysis of genome scale changes by microarrays (also known as array-CGH), with the rapid and reliable detection of chromosome deletions and duplication, and chromosome mosaicism. The result is a genome-wide assessment for all deletions and duplications. Of note, chromosome rearrangements, such as balanced translocations, insertion/deletions, and ring chromosomes, are not detected by these methods, and so traditional microscopy methods are still in use.

Molecular genetics — single mutation or single gene testing

For many mutations, such as fragile X syndrome, where almost all cases are caused by the same mutation — a triplet repeat expansion — specific PCR-based testing has been perfected to be reliable, cheap, and rapid. Other examples are methylation of specific gene regions (e.g. Prader–Willi syndrome), or the assessment of the number of copies of exons (often called dosage) for genes such as *DMD*. Often these mutations are hard to detect reliably with other methods.

For many genes, such as *SCN1A* (causing Dravet syndrome or lesser epilepsy phenotypes) or *CLN3* (causing juvenile Batten disease), all exons are sequenced, and considerable expertise has been accumulated for the test and interpretation of results. This has resulted in a test which, as far as is possible, is a complete analysis for mutations, e.g. in *CLN3* a 1Kb deletion is a common mutation that could be missed by Sanger sequencing alone.

Molecular genetics for 'gene panels'

For an increasing number of phenotypes multiple genes are known to be the cause. These are increasingly grouped together and analysed concurrently. This has considerable advantages compared to gene-by-gene analysis, and vastly increases the likelihood of a positive result. There are, however, real and potential pitfalls: not all genes will be completely sequenced (as they were previously in single gene analysis), the panels need to be updated to include newly discovered genes and with increasing numbers of genes sequenced, the greater will be the number of variants that need analysis. This has the real risk of leading to erroneous assignment of pathogenicity to a change — especially so when the condition has a poorly defined phenotype, such as severe nonsyndromic intellectual disability or early onset epilepsy. In practice, however, the advantages of gene panels far outweigh the potential disadvantages.

The future: whole genome sequencing

Whole genome sequencing uses a different approach to all other genetic tests — and potentially will detect all types of mutations, cytogenetic, as well as base changes, but it will not detect methylation defects. The sequencing equipment and computational requirements are considerable, but this methodology is being introduced and trialled at present. It has the potential to revolutionize our approach to an affected neonate or child by seeking, in one quick test, all genetic diagnoses that might possibly be the cause of the child's illness. It will, most likely, take over the bigger panel tests, but individual gene and mutation testing will continue for the time being. A potential problem to overcome is to interpret the large number of variants of unknown significance resulting from this very wide genetic search.

A GUIDE IN COMMON CLINICAL SITUATIONS WHERE GENETIC TESTING CAN BE OF USE

Recurrence risks and prenatal diagnosis are in italics.

Autosomal dominant disorders

Dravet syndrome is caused commonly by heterozygous mutations in *SCN1A*. *SCN1A* encodes for a voltage-gated sodium cell membrane channel $Na_V1.1$, which is widely expressed in neurons of the central nervous system (CNS) and is critical for the generation of action potentials. Both over activity and under activity/loss of $Na_V1.1$ cause severe CNS dysfunction. So, finding a:

1. previously validated loss of function mutation which is de novo in the child (i.e. parents do not carry the mutations) means that you have found your diagnosis; *<5% recurrence risk; refer to clinical genetics for evaluation of need for prenatal diagnosis;* or

2. previously validated loss of function or previously reported variant which is also carried by an unaffected parent, first check the parent is not a mosaic (i.e. has less than 50% of the mutation on testing). If they do, then it is likely the variant is a mutation and the cause of the diagnosis. Or second, if a parent has a 50:50 distribution of the mutation, then it could either be a mutation of variable penetrance (the reporting laboratory should have read the literature for you and included this in your report), but if there is no support for this, the variant cannot be interpreted. If this has been previously reported as of variable penetrance then it is very likely to be a mutation and the diagnosis. *Recurrence risk for inheriting the mutation is 50%, but for the phenotype is <50%. For either situation, refer to clinical genetics to discuss recurrence risk and arrangement of prenatal testing, if appropriate;* or

3. previously unreported missense mutation, whether found in a parent or not, cannot be interpreted as pathogenic or not (and the detailed analysis of this will be in your mutation report). *Recurrence risk unclear, and there is no prenatal testing available.*

Rare causes of dominant severe intellectual disability

A growing number of these conditions have been defined, where a 'loss of function' mutation causes severe learning difficulties/developmental impairment (severe/profound intellectual disability/developmental delay in the older literature) and an otherwise either poorly defined or undefinable phenotype (e.g. *DDX3X, CASK, KANSL1, ARID1B, SATB2, SYNGAP1, ANKRD11, SCN1A, DYRK1A, STXBP1, MED13L*).

Interpretation of such mutations depends on their genetic context:

1. If a de novo mutation, the mutation is likely to be the cause of the clinical problem. The recurrence risk is <5%. *Refer to clinical genetics for evaluation of need for prenatal diagnosis.*

2. If previously described and mosaic in a parent, it is likely to be the diagnosis. *Refer to clinical genetics for discussion of the need for prenatal diagnosis, as a positive result cannot be interpreted as meaning an affected child.*

3. If present in a parent, it is most likely to be a harmless variant; keep looking for a diagnosis. *Recurrence risk unknown and prenatal diagnosis not available (as there is no genetic test to offer).*

Tuberous sclerosis (TS) is often diagnosed in a child with infantile spasms. Finding a TSC1 or TSC2 mutation confirms the diagnosis but gives no guide to the severity and extent of the TS phenotype (noting that TSC2 cases as a group are more severely affected than TSC1). Once a child is found to have a mutation then it is more expedient to test the parents for the mutation than to screen them for all the clinical features of TS, as in 1/3 of families a parent will also have the heterozygous mutation. Of de novo cases (2/3 of families) at least 10% are mosaics, making detection of their mutation more difficult, but with the advantage that parents will not need testing and there is no recurrence risk. *Recurrence risk 50% if the non-mosaic parent carries a TSC mutation. If the parent is mosaic then the recurrence risk is unknown, but safest to assume it is up to 50% and offer prenatal diagnosis.*

Autosomal dominant disorders with anticipation

Myotonic dystrophy (1 and 2): clinically this may be distinct, or at least a very likely diagnosis. Congenital myotonic dystrophy is distinct from the other forms, presenting at birth with hypotonia and weakness, with effects on cognition and partial recovery of some aspects in later childhood. This is caused by extremely large triplet repeat expansions and is almost exclusively inherited from affected mothers. For all forms of myotonic dystrophy, if there is a pathogenic mutation then you have your diagnosis, but you now need to consider parental testing and see which is a carrier/minimally affected and refer to an adult neurology or clinical genetics colleague to determine who else is a carrier or affected, and who needs neurology follow-up. *Recurrence risk 50% for inheriting the disorder but more complex in predicting the severity of the phenotype. Referal to clinical genetics as prenatal diagnosis can be complex.*

Myotonic dystrophy type 2 (very rare in children) is caused by mutation in the *CNBP* gene and there is no anticipation. *The recurrence risk for the disease is 50%, however, there is no correlation between disease features and the mutation. Prenatal diagnosis is available but consider referral to clinical genetics to discuss the options with the family.*

Autosomal recessive diseases

SMA is clinically classified by age at onset and the rate of progression and the combined mutations correlate with the phenotype. The mutation pathogenesis is complex in SMA. It is a combination of the lack of functioning *SMN1* genes and the number of copies of *SMN2* genes. *SMN2* have a small amount of residual ability to make a SMN protein, and individuals can have 0 to 6 *SMN2* genes. So, the number of *SMN2* genes can modulate the effect of loss of activity of the two *SMN1* genes in SMA. The most severe form of SMA is when a child inherits no functional *SMN1* genes and one or two *SMN2* genes (0 copies of SMN2 is thought to be lethal). Mutation testing is complex and should only be undertaken by experienced centres. *The recurrence risk in a family is usually 25% for the same SMA phenotype. However, and unusually for a recessive condition, there is a new mutation rate of about 2% for SMN1 mutations. Thus, parental testing is obligatory, and if the child has one (of their two) SMN1 mutation that is de novo, then only one parent is a carrier and the family's recurrence risk is negligible. If other parents in the same family are tested for SMA, be aware that the phenotype can be more or less severe than in the index family. Referral to clinical genetics is usually indicated.*

X-linked recessive diseases

Duchenne and Becker muscular dystrophy are caused by mutations in the extremely large gene DMD. Two thirds of mutations are exon deletions or duplications, and one third are nucleotide changes (half of which are nonsense mutations). Traditionally, this was a very time-consuming gene to test, but modern methodologies use a single test to detect all mutation types; however, this only works in males (who have only one X chromosome).

There is a broad correlation between mutation position and type and the severity of the phenotype. If a deletion or duplication affects the middle section of the protein (a long column of spectrin repeats) and is in frame (i.e. the number of bases removed or added is divisible by 3), then a milder/Becker phenotype is to be expected. The detection of mutations in carrier females is possible, but only completely so when the mutation of the male index case is known. In confirmed cases of DMD/Becker muscular dystrophy, carrier testing of the mother is recommended, not only for counselling for family planning, but also because 10% to 15% of carriers are symptomatic and they are recommended cardiac assessments

If the mother of an affected male is a carrier, the recurrence risk is 50% in further males, and 50% that female offspring will be carriers. If the mother is not a carrier the recurrence risk is up to 20%, because of the proven empirical risk of germline mosaicism in the mother.

X-linked dominant diseases

Rett syndrome is caused by heterozygous mutations in the *MECP2* gene (on the X chromosome), and can be missense, or nonsense mutations or deletions. In 99% of classic cases the mutation is de novo, and not present in the mother. Mosaicism in a carrier mother or an affected child is very rarely detected (but see below). The *MECP2* gene is very polymorphic, with far more missense changes than usually expected. Despite this, it is usually possible to categorize mutations as being pathogenic (as they have been previously reported or altering amino acids that have been observed in the mutations seen in previous affected cases) or as benign (because they exist at a significant prevalence in population databases). Most males inheriting a *MECP2* mutation die in utero, but those few that are born have severe neonatal encephalopathy and manic-depressive psychosis, pyramidal signs, Parkinsonian, and macro-orchidism (PPM-X syndrome). *The recurrence risk should be negligible, but because of empirical risks prenatal diagnosis is usually offered. If the mother is affected, then the recurrence risk for an affected female is 50%. For the parents of an affected male there is a recurrence risk for both affected males and affected females, which is hard to quantify, but prenatal diagnosis should be contemplated.*

Mitochondrial genome diseases

Mutations in the circular DNA each mitochondrion carries are being increasingly recognized, and the phenotype can vary both in features and severity between and within families. The diagnosis should be considered often, but testing is complex and can require multiple tissues and types of testing. Homoplasmy means that all mitochondria carry a mutation/change in their genomes, while heteroplasmy means that only a proportion do, but the proportion can vary from cell to cell and tissue to tissue. For this reason, it can be difficult to predict the mitochondrial phenotype of a mitochondrial mutation. Mutations can be missense, nonsense, deletions, and rearrangements. Mitochondrial testing, phenotyping, and genetic counselling for recurrence risk and prenatal diagnosis are specialist (see Chinnery, 1993).

REFERENCES

Chinnery PF (1993) Mitochondrial Disorders Overview. In: Adam MP, Ardinger HH, Pagon RA, et al. eds. *GeneReviews*. Seattle (WA): University of Washington.

Richards S, Aziz N, Bale S et al. (2015) Standards and guidelines for the interpretation of sequence variants: a joint consensus recommendation of the American College of Medical Genetics and Genomics and the Association for Molecular Pathology. *Genet Med* 17: 405–424.

Resources

GeneReviews is a large and growing resource of articles on genetic diseases, all of which are freely downloadable at https://www.ncbi.nlm.nih.gov/books/NBK1116/

Two free 'browsers' allow visualization of the human genome at any position, gene, or chromosome location, along with a host of embedded analytical and annotation software: Human Genome Browser at http://genome.ucsc.edu/; and Decipher at https://decipher.sanger.ac.uk/

UNIQUE is a UK parent's organization that provides support and information particularly focussed on chromosome anomalies, but increasingly including single genes that cause intellectual disability phenotypes https://www.rarechromo.org/

Genetic Home Reference is an online comprehensive source of information for affected families https://ghr.nlm.nih.gov/

CHAPTER 12

Drug treatments: drugs, vitamins, and minerals

Imti Choonara and Peter Baxter

Key messages

Neonatal drugs

- Use drug doses adjusted for age-specific metabolism (e.g. reduced doses in infants born preterm).
- Administer drugs less frequently (for drugs that are renally excreted).
- Avoid highly protein-bound drugs.

Medication errors

- Tenfold errors occur more frequently in neonates and infants.
- Errors involving aminoglycosides and morphine are particularly dangerous.
- Errors with intravenous drugs are more likely to result in harm.

Anti-infective drugs

- Ceftriaxone is contraindicated in neonates.

General principles

- Avoid polypharmacy.
- Avoid intramuscular administration of medicines.
- Be aware that all medicines have side effects.
- Use the lowest effective dose of a medicine for the shortest duration.

> ## Common errors
>
> - Using drug treatments without a clear diagnosis.
> - Using drug treatments for which there is no justification.
> - Using oral preparations of phenytoin in infants under the age of 6 months.
>
> ## When to worry
>
> - Unexplained adverse clinical change associated with addition of a drug.

INTRODUCTION

Medicines are extremely useful in the treatment of diseases. It is important, however, to recognize that medicines can also be harmful, especially if used inappropriately. It is important to try to use as few medicines as possible and ideally to use the medicine in the lowest dosage that is effective and for the shortest duration of time. This will hopefully reduce the risk of drug toxicity while ensuring that the child receives appropriate treatment.

IS THE TREATMENT EVIDENCE-BASED?

Medicines are licensed by regulatory agencies if they are shown to be more effective than placebo. Unfortunately, medicines may be licensed even if they are less effective than existing treatment. Therefore, one always needs to critically evaluate licensed medicines. An additional problem is that many medicines are not licensed for use in young children because clinical trials have not been performed. This does not automatically mean we should not use any medicine that is not licensed, but that we should always try and evaluate the existing evidence to see whether the medicine is likely to be of benefit or not. The most supportive evidence for efficacy of a medicine is a clinical trial and this is ideally performed as a randomized clinical trial. Clinical trials, however, are not that effective in detecting uncommon side effects. One needs to recognize that new medicines may be associated with side effects that have not been detected in a small randomized clinical trial.

DRUG METABOLISM

Drugs are excreted either by metabolism in the liver or through the kidneys. Drug metabolism is usually decreased in the neonatal period and renal function is also impaired, especially in the affected infant born preterm. The most important metabolic pathway for the elimination of drugs in the liver is the CYP3A4 pathway. The activity of this pathway is reduced at birth, but then increases during the first year of life. Midazolam is an example of a medicine that is eliminated by this pathway, so it is important that one uses lower doses of midazolam in the first year of life and especially in neonates.

Another major metabolic pathway in the liver is the CYP1A2 pathway, which again is reduced at birth and then gradually increases during infancy. The CYP3A4 and CYP1A2 pathways both involve oxidation.

Other pathways include conjugation into a glucuronide or a sulphate. Morphine undergoes conjugation to both morphine 3-glucuronide and morphine 6-glucuronide. The latter is an important metabolite as it has considerable analgesic activity.

Glucuronidation of morphine is decreased in the neonatal period and then increases in activity during the first year of life. As the metabolism of morphine is decreased in the neonatal period, one needs to use lower doses of morphine. Paracetamol undergoes metabolism by both glucuronidation and sulphation. Glucuronidation of paracetamol is reduced in neonates and infants, but sulphation is increased. The overall metabolism of paracetamol is reduced in the neonatal period but from the age of 1 month onwards it is similar to that in older children because of the increased sulphation. Paracetamol is the exception in that for all the other drugs mentioned in this section, drug metabolism is decreased in the first year of life.

Many drugs, such as aminoglycosides and cephalosporins are eliminated by renal excretion. Renal function is impaired in the first few days of life, especially in the neonate born preterm. The dosing interval for these drugs is, therefore, increased in affected neonates born preterm. After the neonatal period renal function is usually normal.

DRUG TOXICITY

The effect of reduced drug metabolism in the neonatal period is illustrated by the grey baby syndrome that was reported in association with chloramphenicol. When chloramphenicol was first used in infants, individuals were unaware that drug metabolism in the early stages of life was reduced. Unfortunately, several infants developed catastrophic cardiovascular collapse and died because they had received too high a dose of chloramphenicol.

Sulphonamides were noted to result in an increased mortality in neonates. This was due to the displacement of bilirubin from albumin and the subsequent development of kernicterus. It is essential, therefore, that one does not use a medicine that is highly protein-bound in affected neonates.

There are cases of drug toxicity that have affected infants where the mechanism is not fully understood. An example is the use of sodium valproate in children under the age of 3 years, especially if the child is on more than one medicine. These children are at greater risk of liver toxicity. This is thought to be due to the activation of different metabolic pathways in young children. These different metabolic pathways can also be enhanced in children with developmental delay or by the use of polypharmacy.

We know that one in 10 children in hospital will experience an adverse drug reaction. One in eight of these adverse drug reactions will be severe and 2% of children admitted to hospital will be admitted directly as a result of an adverse drug reaction. We cannot prevent adverse drug reactions entirely, but we can do our best to reduce the incidence.

MEDICATION ERRORS AND ROUTE OF ADMINISTRATION

Medication errors occur in adults and children. The most frequent type of medication error in children is the wrong dose of the medicine being given. A particular problem in infants is tenfold errors whereby the decimal point is placed incorrectly. Tenfold errors occur more frequently in neonates and infants as one can administer 10 times the dose of a drug from a single ampoule. The clinical impact of a medication error is greater with certain medications, in particular morphine, phenytoin, and aminoglycosides. Medication errors associated with intravenous formulations are more likely to result in significant harm. One needs, therefore, to be especially careful with intravenous medicines.

Medicines are usually given orally. This is the preferred route for children who are able to take medicines orally and who are not critically ill. Intravenous administration of medicines should be reserved for children with severe acute infections or if they are critically ill (i.e. in status epilepticus). Intramuscular medicines are not routinely recommended in neonates, infants, or young children. Oral medicines should be given as a suspension/liquid to infants in the first year of life as they are unable to take tablets. Unfortunately, many medicines are not available in a suitable format for infants and extemporaneous preparations are frequently required. Microtablets may be more acceptable to young children, but are not routinely available for most medicines. In children who cannot take an oral medication, for example, due to vomiting, the rectal route can be used. For some preparations, such as paraldehyde mixed with oil, this is the route of choice.

ESSENTIAL DRUG LISTS

In order to ensure children receive the medicines that are essential, the World Health Organization (WHO) has recently developed an Essential List of Medicines for Children. This is available on the WHO website (www.who.int/medicines/publications/essentialmedicines/en/). One needs to question the routine use of medicines that are not on the WHO Essential List of Medicines for Children.

Antiepileptic drugs

In the neonatal period, intravenous phenobarbital has been shown to be clinically effective and is the first-line drug of choice. Outside the neonatal period, buccal midazolam has been shown to be more effective than rectal diazepam for acute seizures. If intravenous medication is required, then lorazepam is the drug of choice and midazolam, with appropriate dose reduction in the neonatal period, is a good alternative. A particular problem in the first year of life is West syndrome (previously called infantile spasms), for which oral corticosteroids (prednisolone) and vigabatrin are the preferred treatments. In children with West syndrome due to tuberous sclerosis, vigabatrin is the first line of treatment. First line treatment of Dravet syndrome, which also starts in infancy, includes stiripentol or topiramate.

Infants requiring oral medication for epilepsy should ideally be given carbamazepine in preference to sodium valproate, which is more likely to be associated with hepato-toxicity in children under the age of 3 years. Levetiracetam is also increasingly used.

Hepatotoxicity is rare, and exactly how rare is not precisely known, but unfortunately is usually fatal and, therefore, valproate should only be used if carbamazepine or pheno-barbital has been ineffective. Exceptions to this rule apply to certain specific epilepsy syndromes with certain types of epileptic seizure becoming more severe when car-bamazepine, phenytoin, or lamotrigine are added to treatment (see Chapter 20).

Nevertheless, valproic acid should *not be used routinely* in infants with developmental delay or in those receiving more than one anticonvulsant, as hepatotoxicity is signific-antly increased in this group of infants.

Anti-infective drugs

In the neonatal period, intravenous benzylpenicillin and gentamicin are the usual first-line choice of antibiotics. Ceftriaxone is contraindicated in neonates for two reasons. First, it is highly protein-bound and may displace bilirubin and second it has been associated with death in several neonates and infants who have also received calcium supplements. Cefotaxime is the cephalosporin of choice in the neonatal period. The first-line choice of intravenous antibiotic for meningitis in infants will depend upon local resistance. Benzylpenicillin remains the drug of choice for meningococcus and pneumococcus if local strains are penicillin-sensitive. In areas of high resistance, intra-venous cephalosporins, such as cefotaxime or ceftriaxone (except in neonates), can be given. If herpes encephalitis/meningitis is suspected, then high dose aciclovir is recom-mended. For tetanus, intravenous benzylpenicillin is the drug of choice.

Analgesia and antipyretics

A fever is not usually a problem in the neonatal period and antipyretics are not routinely recommended. In the first year of life it is more important to try to determine the cause of the fever than simply to reduce the temperature. If an antipyretic is required, paracetamol is the drug of choice as it is safer than ibuprofen which, as a nonsteroidal anti-inflammatory drug, may cause gastrointestinal symptoms and, rarely, may cause gastrointestinal bleeding. Paracetamol is also the initial drug of choice for mild pain.

If more potent analgesia is required, then one should consider the use of morphine either intravenously or orally.

Sedative agents

For critically ill children or neonates who require sedation, intravenous midazolam is the drug of choice. For infants who are able to tolerate oral or nasogastric medication then chloral hydrate and promethazine are alternatives to midazolam. Sedation should only be used to benefit the infant. It should never be used to make life easier for health professionals.

Antispasmodics

Children with cerebral palsy may have hypertonicity/spasticity of their voluntary muscles. If this is chronic then oral baclofen may be beneficial. Diazepam is also frequently used. Skeletal muscle relaxants are, however, usually of benefit in children only after the first year of life. Baclofen and other muscle relaxants should not routinely be used in infancy, although a carefully assessed trial of their use is reasonable for intractable cases, always remembering the importance of discontinuing treatment unless of clear clinical benefit.

Gastro-oesophageal reflux

Gastro-oesophageal reflux is a physiological event which is self-limiting and is common in infants in the first 6 months of life. Children with chronic neurological problems such as cerebral palsy have an increased risk of severe persistent gastro-oesophageal reflux disease. Not all infants with gastro-oesophageal reflux require medication. If the reflux is causing significant medical problems, such as failure to thrive or excessive vomiting, then one should consider using milk thickeners (e.g. Carobel) or alternatively alginates such as Gaviscon. The efficacy of motility stimulants, such as domperidone and metoclopramide, has not been established in gastro-oesophageal reflux, and are contraindicated by the risk of extrapyramidal unwanted effects in infancy, and should, therefore, not be used. Histamine H2 receptor antagonists, such as ranitidine, again should not routinely be used for gastro-oesophageal reflux. Proton-pump inhibitors, such as omeprazole, should not routinely be used for reflux as they have been shown to be ineffective in infants (Davies et al. 2015).

Diuretics for hydrocephalus

Historically, acetazolamide has been used to try to prevent hydrocephalus. Systematic literature reviews, including Cochrane Reviews, have shown that acetazolamide and furosemide are ineffective in reducing the need for surgical intervention and cause significant harm in increasing the risk of subsequent motor disability and of nephrocalcinosis (Whitelaw, Kennedy, and Brion, 2001). It is best, therefore, to avoid the use of diuretics for post-haemorrhagic hydrocephalus in the neonatal period.

VITAMINS AND MINERALS

Neurological conditions that respond to treatment with vitamins, minerals, or other substances such as amino acids are rare. However, if in doubt it is always worth considering a trial of treatment since a response can be dramatic and can, at times, save a child from further damage. As a general principle, deficiencies occur when there is an inadequate diet, malabsorption, disorders of transport, or with some metabolic disorders. In addition, maternal deficiency can affect newborn infants.

Vitamins and minerals can have possible therapeutic benefits in a wide range of conditions presenting with seizures, encephalopathy, reflex anoxic syncope, extrapyramidal movement disorders, early developmental impairment, weakness/ myopathy, deafness, oculomotor disorders, and retinopathy.

Possible indications and dose ranges are given in Table 12.1. Please refer to later chapters in this volume for more details on the relevant conditions, as well as appropriate doses for specific disorders.

Table 12.1 Possible indications, dose ranges, and some adverse effects of vitamins and minerals

	Specific conditions	Dose range	Route	Adverse effects
Vitamins				
A (retinol)	Vitamin A deficiency Retinitis pigmentosa	Neonate: 5000 IU/day; older child: 5000—10000 IU/day	Oral	Raised intracranial pressure
B1 (thiamine)	Maple syrup urine disease Leigh syndrome Mitochondrial cyto-pathies Pyruvate dehydro-genase deficiency (females) Wernicke encephalo-pathy	Neonate: 5mg/kg/day older child: 50—300mg/day	Oral or IV	Anaphylactic shock may follow injection

Table 12.1 (continued)   Possible indications, dose ranges, and some adverse effects of vitamins and minerals

	Specific conditions	Dose range	Route	Adverse effects
B2 (riboflavin)	Fazio—Londe or Brown—Vialetto—Van Laere syndrome Multiple acyl-CoA dehydrogenase deficiency Mitochondrial cytopathies MTHFR deficiency	50—300mg/day	Oral	
B3 (nicotinamide)	Pellagra Hartnup disease	50—300mg/day	Oral	
B6 (pyridoxine)	Pyridoxine dependency Pyridoxal phosphate dependency (or PNPO deficiency) Hypophosphatasia Epilepsy including West syndrome Homocystinuria Tetanus	Initial: 30—50mg/kg/day; Maintenance: 5—50mg/kg/day; 12—24 hourly	Oral/IV	Immediate: apnoea Long-term: sensory neuropathy
B6 (pyridoxal-5-phosphate)	Pyridoxal phosphate dependency (or PNPO deficiency) Pyridoxine dependency Hypophosphatasia Epilepsy including West syndrome	30—50mg/kg/day; 4—6 hourly	Oral	Immediate: apnoea Long term: sensory neuropathy
B12 (hydroxocobalamin)	B12 deficiency Methylmalonic aciduria	Variable depending on condition being treated	IM	
C (ascorbic acid)	Mitochondrial cytopathies Prolidase deficiency	50-1000mg/daily	Oral	

Table 12.1 (continued)   Possible indications, dose ranges, and some adverse effects of vitamins and minerals

	Specific conditions	Dose range	Route	Adverse effects
D (cholecalciferol)	Rickets (all forms) Hypocalcaemia	400 units/day; rescue therapy 3000-10000 units/day for 2 months	Oral	Nephrocalcinosis, hypercalcaemia
Vitamin E deficiency E (alpha-tocopherol)	Ataxia with vitamin E deficiency Hypobetalipoprotein-aemia	Neonate 10mg/kg/day; older child 100-200mg/kg/day increasing if needed	Oral	
K (phytomena-dione)	Haemorrhagic disease of the newborn Mitochondrial cyto-pathies	1-3mg/day	Oral/IM/IV	Risk of hyperbiliru-binemia in neonates
Biotin	Biotinidase deficiency Leigh syndrome Biotin-responsive encephalopathy Holocarboxylase syn-thetase deficiency	5—30mg/day	Oral	
Folinic acid	Folinic acid-responsive seizures (≈ Pyridoxine depend-ency)	3—5mg/kg/day 12 hourly;	Oral	Immediate: apnoea
	Remethylation defects	5—20mg/day		
Folic acid	Remethylation defects	5—20mg/day	Oral	
Minerals				
Calcium	Hypocalcaemia Rickets		Oral or IV	Nephrocalcinosis
Iron	Iron deficiency		Oral	Hepatopathy

Table 12.1 (continued) Possible indications, dose ranges, and some adverse effects of vitamins and minerals

	Specific conditions	Dose range	Route	Adverse effects
Magnesium gly-cerophosphate	Magnesium defi-ciency	0.6mmol/kg/day (expressed as Mg2+)	Oral	Constipation
Other				
Serine	Serine defi-ciency, e.g. due to 3-phosphoglycerate dehydrogenase defi-ciency	400—650mg /kg/day, 8 hourly	Oral	
Carnitine	Primary or secondary carnitine deficiency Reye syndrome Mitochondrial cyto-pathies	100mg/kg/day initially	Oral or IV	Vomiting/diarrhea, odour
Ubidecarenone (coenzyme Q)	Ubidecarenone defi-ciency	10—300mg/day	Oral	
Idebenone	Mitochondrial cyto-pathy			
Creatine	Creatine-deficiency syndromes	100—2000mg /kg/day	Oral	
Dicloroacetate	Pyruvate dehydro-genase deficiency			Renal tubulopathy, pericardial effusion, neuropathy
Betaine	5,10-MTHFR reductase deficiency; other disorders of folate and cobalamin metabolism	500mg/kg/day, or 2—3g/day in young children and 6—9g/day in older children	Oral	If powder inhaled, severe pneumonia

IM, intramuscularly; IV, intravenously; MTHFR, 5,10-methylenetetrahydrofolate reductase.
Authors' Caveat: Readers should note that recommended doses and routes vary with the information source and with the indication for the vitamin/mineral. Before prescribing, it is therefore advisable to check the dose and route appropriate to the patient in whom treatment is being considered by consulting other on-line references or resources which are listed at the end of this chapter or in chapter 15.

Various vitamin and mineral treatments have also been tried in conditions such as Down syndrome, autism, fragile X syndrome, and Duchenne muscular dystrophy. Formal trials have shown that they are ineffective and should not be used.

Drugs to avoid

It is important that one only uses medicines that have been shown to be effective. This does not mean that we need a large multinational randomized clinical trial before medicines are used in neonates or in infants. It is, however, important to recognize that there needs to be some evidence to justify the use of the medication in an infant.

Doctors throughout the world are very quick to copy colleagues who will start to use a medication with no scientific evidence to justify its use in a particular clinical situation. An example of this is the use of domperidone in infants with mild gastro-oesophageal reflux. Similarly, there does not appear to be any scientific rationale for the use of medicines such as actovegin and citicoline. It is not possible to list all the medicines that are used inappropriately, but each doctor who writes out a prescription for a medication should be able to justify the use of such a medication and this justification needs to be based on articles published in the scientific literature rather than copying the practice of other individuals.

REFERENCES

Davies I, Burman-Roy S, Murphy MS; Guideline Development Group (2015) Gastro-oesophageal reflux disease in children: NICE guidance. *BMJ* 350: g7703.

Whitelaw A, Kennedy C, Brion L (2001) Diuretic therapy for newborn infants with posthemorrhagic ventricular dilatation. *Cochrane Database Syst Rev* 2: CD002270.

Resources

Blau N, Hoffmann GF, Leonard J, Clarke JTR, eds (2006) *Physician's Guide to the Treatment and Follow-up of Metabolic Diseases*. Berlin: Springer-Verlag.

The British National Formulary for Children. Available at https://bnfc.nice.org.uk/

Neurokids Workbook and App (Available on Google Play and the Apple Store).

Scriver CR, Beaidet A, Sly WS, Valle D, Vogelstein B, Childs B, eds (2001) *The Metabolic and Molecular Bases of Inherited Disease*, 8th edn. New York: McGraw-Hill

Valle D, Beaudet AL, Vogelstein B, et al. The Online Metabolic and Molecular Bases of Inherited Disease. Available at https://ommbid.mhmedical.com/book.aspx?bookID=971

World Health Organization. Essential List of Medicines for Children. Available at https://www.who.int/ medicines/publications/essentialmedicines/en/

CHAPTER 13

Nonpharmacological treatment

Ilona Autti-Rämö

Key messages

- Learn the spectrum of normality.
- Give high-risk groups the structured follow-up that they need.
- Teach parents, as a first step, to handle and be in contact with their child.
- Start individually planned interventions when abnormalities persist or increase.
- Establish a quality-control system for the follow-up of at-risk children.

Common errors

- Not involving parents in early intervention.
- Treating a symptom without proper clinical and developmental evaluation.

When to worry

- Regression in development (suspect progressive disease).
- Poor response to visual and/or acoustic stimulation (suspect visual and/or auditory problems).
- Poor social interaction.
- Abnormalities in posture and/or movement that do not respond to adequate handling.

The infant learns more during the first year of life than in any subsequent year. However, the pace of learning is individual. Individual characteristics such as axial tone, genetic predisposition to variants of typical development (e.g. age at first independent steps in crawlers versus bottom shufflers; age at first expressed words with meaning), relationships within the family (including those between the parents and the child) and the challenges which face the child in (or when) learning to take control of his/her body and the environment all have an effect on the developmental trajectories of the individual child. Acute or chronic diseases and physical disabilities, whether hidden or obvious, can lead to developmental trajectories being either delayed or qualitatively different to the normal trajectory with abnormal postures, movements, or social behaviour or, rarely, progressively disordered with stasis then loss of previously acquired developmental skills. Early developmental concerns do not necessarily mean long-term difficulties, but more severe early developmental impairments tend to mean that there will be long-term disabilities. Identification and early intervention will decrease longer-term disability.

PROTOCOL FOR FOLLOW-UP

It is not possible to predict the developmental outcome of infants born with a risk factor for later developmental difficulties without follow-up. It is important that there is a structured protocol for follow-up and that parents are aware of why and how their child is being followed and what kind of interventions may be instituted. If any abnormality is observed, the parents should first be given advice on how to handle and interact with their child in daily life. Often this active contact (tactile, visual, and auditory) and daily 'training' shows, within a matter of a few weeks, how the infant can benefit from such handling and interaction. If the developmental trajectory does not normalize, individual treatment may need to be started. The intensity, content, and length of individual treatment are based on the severity and complexity of the developmental disorder. Usually it is best to start with only one therapist (usually the physiotherapist) and other members of the multiprofessional team (e.g. occupational therapist for visual and play activities, speech therapist for oromotor and feeding functions, psychologist for social interaction and psychological support) are consulted. It is important that the bonding between parents and the child is not disturbed and that the parents are supported in their growth as parents. Their care is the best for their child and the use of their capacity should be encouraged and supported. Pre- or postnatal maternal distress can also have an adverse effect on cognitive, behavioural, and psychomotor development, and so the well-being of the mother needs to be confirmed.

WHAT TO DO WHEN DEVELOPMENT IS ATYPICAL

When there are obvious abnormalities in development — either a pattern of failure to reach developmental milestones or abnormality in posture, movement, or performance of any specific task — one must decide on the treatment strategy. For a strategy to be effective and transformed into therapeutic actions, it must have goals that are SMART (i.e. Specific, Measurable, Achievable, Relevant, and Time-bound). Skilled therapists are important for identifying realistic goals and the optimal ways to challenge the child. The most important part of early intervention, however, is confirmation that the parents have learned what they were encouraged to learn and have changed their day-to-day handling of their child accordingly. It is most important to understand that the infant cannot be helped with individual therapies in isolation; development is not just training but finding ways in which the child can best use his/her abilities. How the child performs in the clinic (capacity) can differ greatly from how the child performs in his/her daily surroundings. Thus, it is often important to make home visits to see how the environment can best be adjusted to facilitate the child's functional abilities.

Delay in early motor development may be due to hypotonia and in these cases the development often normalizes with age. Axial tone affects the way the child needs to be treated and handled.

Delay in motor development may be abnormal or may be an idiosyncratic variation of typical development, e.g. 'dissociated motor development' in which fine motor development proceeds normally but early gross motor development is delayed, or 'bottom shuffling' in which the child does not crawl but is mobile in the sitting position by pushing with the feet. Age of independent walking is delayed in both these movement variations, but most of these children perform normally by preschool age. Indications for individual therapies need to be decided on a case-by-case basis. Counselling and guidance on specific activities to be undertaken at home are often all that is required. These developmental variations are often familial; for example, one of the parents may have had the same pattern of motor development.

Hypotonia is often associated with inactivity and poor muscle strength and the child needs, in all situations, to learn to adopt a wider base for support.

Hypertonia can lead to atypical motor development and posture or movement patterns. The more severe the hypertonia, the more difficult it is for the child to move smoothly and to balance. Hypertonia (e.g. in the neck extensors and shoulder girdle), co-occurring with hypotonia as a compensation for lack of control can be overcome with specific handling techniques. These infants need follow-up and parental coaching, but only rarely intensive treatment.

Asymmetry of posture or movement is sometimes a red-flag feature of an evolving hemiplegic (unilateral) type of cerebral palsy and the asymmetric patterns become more evident as the child initiates active movement.

Delay in overall development may be due to difficulties in vision, hearing, social skills, or cognition. Vision — especially the ability to accommodate — needs to be checked in all cases of delayed development and an ophthalmological assessment should be undertaken if there is any kind of suspicion of delayed or impaired vision. The toys used should have strong contrasts in colour (black/white is best) and the figures and shapes must be easy to perceive. Hearing impairment also affects overall development and hearing should be checked with age-appropriate means. A disorder of social development can be due to neuropsychiatric disorders, impaired attachment, maternal depression, or cognitive delay. All these aetiologies need to be considered to identify the best treatment strategy. Cognitive delay nearly always also causes delay of motor development as this is led by curiosity and the intrinsic need to learn to use one's body and search the environment. Children with delayed cognitive development need much repetition in order to remember causal relationships and learn to use their body in a meaningful way.

Clearly abnormal development (motor and/or cognitive) can be the result of several disorders – described in other chapters of this book – and the level of functional disability can vary from minor to severe. A definite abnormality in an infant is, however, for the parents always a severe disability and it is important that the parents are supported in their parenthood so that the child is always accepted as he or she is.

Individual therapies, technical aids, and orthoses should be planned according to individual needs by a multiprofessional team. Rehabilitation is not about 'fixing' the child but giving him/her the possibility to find his/her potential and learn how to use it in various contexts. It is important to help the parents to understand that their child is unique and special, not something to be ashamed or sad about.

Diagnosis-specific early interventions optimize infant motor and cognitive plasticity, prevent secondary complications, and enhance caregiver well-being. Diagnosis requires a set of diagnostic criteria that are based on the World Health Organization (WHO) International Classification of Diseases, 11th Revision (ICD-11, see Chapter 1). Continuing to embrace outdated, discredited classification systems and diagnostic labels not included in the WHO ICD (e.g. 'the syndrome of intracranial hypertension') leads to confusion, failure to recognize treatable conditions, and an additional iatrogenic burden on the families of infants thus labelled (Mustafayev et al. 2020).

EVIDENCE-BASED THERAPIES

Research on general and disorder-specific early interventions and rehabilitation is continually increasing (Hadders-Algra et al. 2017, Novak and Morgan, 2019) but it is important to bear in mind that a rehabilitation programme may not always be transferrable or generalizable to other countries with differing healthcare systems, organization, and resources.

The following factors have been identified as key ingredients of effective individual therapies (Ziviani et al. 2010, Cioni et al. 2011, Whittingham et al. 2011, Kingston et al. 2012, Eliasson et al. 2014, Fiori et al. 2015, Chorna et al. 2017, Hadders-Algra et al. 2017, Novak et al. 2017, Novak and Morgan, 2019):

- using a theory- and evidence-based method;

- starting early (e.g. in the neonatal intensive care unit) to optimize infant motor and cognitive plasticity, prevent secondary complications, and enhance caregiver well-being;

- setting realistic and meaningful goals while having a family-centred focus;

- helping the child to actively use his/her potential;

- repetition;

- providing the parents means to adjust their interaction with their child; and

- adjusting the environment according to the child's needs.

The amount of practice is of importance. However, it is not the frequency per unit time or duration over time per se that will be beneficial. The daily training activities should challenge the child with joy and enhance their drive to explore their own possibilities and those of the environment. When a parent-coaching intervention is provided, the parents can be taught to implement child-responsive engagement strategies. There is evidence that parent-mediated and therapist-mediated constraint-induced manual training (i.e. encouraging use of the less dextrous hand by preventing use of the other hand) improves hand use (Eliasson et al. 2014) and the principles of such training can be applied to other types of rehabilitation. The goal of rehabilitation is to help the child to cope with the requirements and challenges of the environment and to adjust the environment according to the capacity of the child.

THE ROLE OF TECHNICAL EQUIPMENT/AIDS

- For infants with hypertonia, a supportive baby seat may be helpful in feeding situations as it helps the child to remain in a flexed and symmetrical position.

- Children with any kind of visual problem find it easier to see toys and pictures that have clear contrasts and are not crowded (a simple pattern of black and white is often best).

- For small children, less is often more; think carefully what kind of technical aids or modifications (e.g. to a spoon) are needed and try to find the one best suited to the child that is also easy for the parents to use every day.

Many parents believe that the various types of technical equipment currently being marketed to enhance the child's development are good for the infant. This is not necessarily so, and it is important to check what kind of technical equipment the parents have bought as they may sometimes intensify abnormal movement patterns. For example,

- bouncing swings and infant walking aids may enhance toe walking, increasing hypertonia and spasticity;

- a child placed for too long in a sitting position will spend a reduced amount of time on the tummy (prone), which is necessary for developing active control of extensors.

NOVEL TREATMENT METHODS REQUIRE EVIDENCE OF SAFETY AND EFFICACY

Having a child with a definite developmental impairment is always a shock for the parents and they want to do everything in their power to help their child to achieve typical development. Early intervention with a local multidisciplinary team working in partnership with the family is always important but some intensive treatment programmes can lead to a stressful life, without joy, and weaken or otherwise damage the relationship between the child and the main carers, with negative consequences in the longer term. It is important to remember that one can help the child to find his/her capacity only through activities that the child is willingly involved in.

Some centres provide very intensive, time-consuming, complex, and often expensive treatment programmes with strict treatment protocols that can also include manipulation and various alternative treatment methods that have no evidence-based theory to build upon. There is, however, no evidence, as yet, that such interventions offer any advantage over standard care.

High-tech equipment sometimes provides benefit; however, it may also simply look 'impressive' but be without benefit and with the risk of causing unwanted effects. The use of hyperbaric oxygen therapy exemplifies the need for caution in the face of the power of high-tech to attract the attention of parents of children with a disability. For a brief period this technology was being marketed for use in neurodevelopmental disorders, but has now been discontinued as no adequate proof of benefit in autism spectrum disorders, cerebral palsy, or any other neurodevelopmental disorder of childhood has been reported (Mitchell and Bennett, 2014; Goldfarb et al. 2016).

There is continuing scientific interest in stem cell transplantation for children with cerebral palsy (Eggenberger et al. 2019) and in infants born preterm at high risk of brain injury (Peng et al. 2020), but the lack of a valid animal model has hampered the scope of clinical trials. Clinical studies have included children, rather than infants, over a wide range of ages and aetiologies and treated them with widely differing stem cell dose regimens. Collectively, these studies have shown that severe adverse medical effects of this treatment are uncommon. A limited number of studies have attempted to assess efficacy and have done so at differing times after treatment and with varied outcome measures. The risk of one or more types of bias (see Chapter 3) has been identified in the reporting of most studies included in systematic reviews (Novak et al. 2016, Eggenberger et al. 2019) and more rigour in patient selection and trial methodology is still needed (Jantzie, Scafidi, and Robinson, 2018). Some systematic reviews report a limited positive effect of stem cell transplantation on gross motor function, but long-term benefit to gross motor function, comparable to those required of orthopaedic or other interventions for cerebral palsy, is not clear. Stem cell transplantation is, however, an area in which further developments seem likely and new data continue to emerge (Gu et al. 2020).

High-quality studies are needed for every new intervention in order to prove their efficacy and safety and submitting to unproven therapies from unvalidated sources is unwise (Dan 2016, Novak et al. 2016). The use of current treatments for indications other than those where the treatment is proven to be beneficial also raises ethical concerns about provision of misleading information and giving false hope. In order to support caregivers in navigating the claims of institutions offering therapeutic methods of unproven effect, clinical practitioners need to update their knowledge as new, high-quality studies, systematic reviews, and meta-analyses become available. High-quality evidence of clinically meaningful benefit, rather than only of statistical difference, is the treasure that you seek and critical reading skills are the tools that you will find the most valuable in that quest.

REFERENCES

Chorna OD, Guzzetta A, Maitre NL (2017) Vision assessments and interventions for infants 0-2 years at high risk for cerebral palsy: a systematic review. *Pediatr Neurol* 76: 3—13.

Cioni G, D'Acunto G, Guzzetta A (2011) Perinatal brain damage in children: neuroplasticity, early intervention, and molecular mechanisms of recovery. *Prog Brain Res* 189: 139—154.

Dan B (2016) Stem cell therapy for cerebral palsy. *Dev Med Child Neurol* 58: 424.

Eliasson AC, Krumlinde L, Gordon A et al. (2014) Guidelines for future research in constraint-induced movement therapy for children with unilateral cerebral palsy: an expert consensus. *Dev Med Child Neurol* 56; 125—137.

Eggenberger S, Boucard C, Schoeberlein A, et al. (2019) Stem cell treatment and cerebral palsy: systemic review and meta-analysis. *World J Stem Cells* 11: 891—903.

Fiori S, Guzzetta A (2015) Plasticity following early-life brain injury: Insights from quantitative MRI. *Semin Perinatol* 39: 141—146.

Goldfarb C, Genore L, Hunt C, et al. (2016) Hyperbaric oxygen therapy for the treatment of children and youth with Autism Spectrum Disorders: an evidence-based systematic review. *Res Autism Spect Disord* 29: 1—7.

Gu J, Huang L, Zhang C, et al. (2020) Therapeutic evidence of umbilical cord derived mesenchymal stem cell transplantation for cerebral palsy: a randomized, controlled trial. *Stem Cell Res Ther* 11: 43

Hadders-Algra M, Boxum AG, Hielkema T, Hamer EG (2017) Effect of early intervention in infants at very high risk of cerebral palsy: a systematic review. *Dev Med Child Neurol* 59: 246–258.

Jantzie LL, Scafidi J, Robinson S (2018) Stem cells and cell-based therapies for cerebral palsy: a call for rigor. *Pediatr Res* 83: 345–355.

Kingston D, Tough S, Whitfield H (2012) Prenatal and postpartum maternal psychological distress and infant development: a systematic review. *Child Psychiatry Hum Dev* 43: 683–714.

Mitchell SJ, Bennett MH (2014) Unestablished indication for hyperbaric oxygen therapy. *Diving Hyperb Med* 44: 228–234.

Mustafayev R, Seyid-Mammadova T, Kennedy C, et al. (2020) Perinatal encephalopathy, the syndrome of intracranial hypertension and associated diagnostic labels in the Commonwealth of Independent States: a systematic review. *Arch Dis Child* Epub ahead of print: doi:10.1136/archdischild-2018-315994

Novak I, Walker K, Hunt RW, et al. (2016) Concise Review: stem cell interventions for people with cerebral palsy: systematic review with meta-analysis. *Stem Cells Transl Med* 5: 1014–1025.

Novak I, Morgan C, Adde L et al. (2017) Early, accurate diagnosis and early intervention in cerebral palsy: advances in diagnosis and treatment. *JAMA Pediatr* 171: 897-907.

Novak I, Morgan C (2019) High-risk follow-up: Early intervention and rehabilitation. *Handb Clin Neurol* 162: 483–510.

Peng X, Song J, Li B, Zhu C, Wang X. (2020) Umbilical cord blood stem cell therapy in premature brain injury: Opportunities and challenges. *J Neuro Res* 98: 815–825.

Whittingham K, Wee D, Boyd R (2011) Systematic review of the efficacy of parenting interventions for children with cerebral palsy. *Child Care, Health Dev* 37: 475–483.

Ziviani J, Feeney R, Rodger S, Watter P (2010) Systematic review of early intervention programmes for children from birth to nine years who have a physical disability. *Aust Occup Ther J* 57: 210–223.

CHAPTER 14

Birth asphyxia and other acute encephalopathies in the newborn infant

Gian Paolo Chiaffoni and Daniele Trevisanuto

Key messages

- Each year, approximately 2.7 million infants die during the neonatal period; a quarter of these deaths result from intrapartum-related causes.
- More than 90% of these deaths occur in low-resource countries.
- Antenatal care and access to equipment and skilled health professionals significantly reduce still births and improve perinatal outcome.
- Effective neonatal resuscitation is a cornerstone of the management of the asphyxiated newborn infant.
- The clinical assessment remains central to all investigations for the first evaluation, day-to-day medical care, and follow-up of the newborn infant with acute encephalopathy.
- Prolonged moderate hypothermia reduces mortality and increases survival with normal outcome in asphyxiated neonates.
- Although perinatal asphyxia represents the main reason for neonatal encephalopathy, other causes must be considered.

Common errors

- Low Apgar scores misunderstood as signs of perinatal brain injury.
- Clinical evaluation not standardized and considered to be difficult.

- Neurophysiological/neuroimaging investigations considered the only means to recognize neonatal brain injury.
- Hyperoxygenation of an asphyxiated term newborn infant misunderstood as a way to protect the brain.
- Multiple drug treatment believed to have a role in 'protecting' the brain against post-asphyxial damage.

When to worry

- When a newborn infant born at term is unable to initiate or sustain autonomous breathing.
- When a newborn infant born at term shows decreased alertness, seizures, and apnoeas.
- When a newborn infant presents seizures and multiple signs of central nervous system depression continuing for several days after birth. Remedial action is needed because persistence beyond the first week is likely to indicate poor outcome.

DEFINITION

Neonatal encephalopathy (NE) is a clinical — not aetiological — syndrome characterized by a combination of findings that include *an altered level of consciousness at the time of the examination*. Clinical features may also include seizures, abnormalities of muscle tone, movements, and reflexes, with or without poor respiratory control, and poor feeding. Although NE may be caused by hypoxic-ischaemic encephalopathy (HIE), it does not necessarily imply HIE. NE is the preferred term to describe a neonate depressed at birth, as the condition may be produced by causes different from HIE, such as metabolic disorders, infections, drug exposure, stroke, and malformations. The definition of NE is very frequently confused with other aetiologies and/or clinical conditions. For this reason, it is very important to understand the exact definition of NE and related terms. Taking into consideration that NE may be often caused by HIE, the clinical, diagnostic, and therapeutic considerations related to HIE in the following discussion are intended for NE as well.

Other frequently used and potentially confusing terms are listed below.

HIE

This term describes encephalopathy as defined above with, in addition, evidence that the mechanism is hypoxic-ischaemic in nature. HIE can be defined as mild, moderate, or severe according to a combination of signs and symptoms

Perinatal hypoxia, anoxia, and hypoxaemia

These terms describe partial or total lack of oxygen supply to the brain or blood.

Ischaemia

Reduction (partial) or cessation (total) of blood flow to an organ, such as the brain, which impairs both oxygen and substrate delivery to the tissue.

Perinatal asphyxia

This is an insult to the fetus or newborn infant due to a lack of respiratory gas exchange causing hypoxia and hypercapnia and may be associated with ischaemia. This problem can involve several organs and be of sufficient magnitude and duration to produce functional and/or biochemical changes (e.g. lactic acidosis). Asphyxia leads to increased acidity (decreased pH) in the blood resulting both from the lack of oxygen, referred to as metabolic acidosis, and from hypercapnia (i.e. the build-up of carbon dioxide), referred to as respiratory acidosis. The base deficit is an index of the balance between the respiratory and metabolic components of acidosis, with a larger metabolic (or smaller respiratory) component leading to a more negative base deficit.

Perinatal asphyxia is defined by the presence of all the following criteria (according to the American Academy of Pediatrics, 1997):

- Umbilical arterial cord pH <7.0 and absolute base excess <-12mmol/L;

- Apgar score 0 to 3 at 5 minutes;

- Seizures; and

- Signs of multiorgan (renal, cardiovascular, pulmonary, gastrointestinal) dysfunction/failure.

More recently, the Task Force on Neonatal Encephalopathy of the American College of Obstetricians and Gynecologists (2014) concluded that a multidimensional assessment process was required to assess the likelihood of an acute peripartum or intrapartum hypoxic-ischaemic event being the cause of NE. Neonatal criteria regarded as consistent with hypoxia-ischaemia being causal included:

- Apgar score of <5 at 5 minutes and 10 minutes;

- Fetal umbilical artery acidemia: fetal umbilical artery pH <7.0, or base deficit >12mmol/L, or both;

- Neuroimaging evidence of acute brain injury seen on brain magnetic resonance imaging (MRI) or magnetic resonance spectroscopy (MRS) consistent with hypoxia-ischemia; and

- Presence of multisystem organ failure consistent with HIE.

Absence of other significant risk factors (abnormal fetal growth, maternal infection, neonatal sepsis, chronic placental lesions).

The Task Force expressed the view that no single strategy to identify HIE is infallible but they clearly would not regard fulfillment of only two of the above criteria as very strong evidence of HIE. The timing of an hypoxic-ischaemic insult is not easy to establish. Table 14.1 provides approximate percentages occurring at different times relative to birth with likely causes.

Table 14.1   The timing of hypoxic-ischaemic insult and related causes

Timing of the insult	Approximate percentage of total	Possible related causes
Antepartum	20	Maternal hypotension with uterine haemorrhage, abdominal trauma, IUGR, multiples
Intrapartum	35	Malpresentation, forceps extraction, abruptio placentae, cord prolapse, maternal pyrexia
Intrapartum ± antepartum	35	Stress during labour and delivery in pre-existing antepartum difficult conditions (maternal diabetes, pre-eclampsia, IUGR)
Postnatal	10	Severe apnoeic spells, congenital heart disease, iatrogenic reasons

IUGR, intrauterine growth retardation. (Modified from Volpe 1995).

Hypoxic-ischaemic brain injury

This describes brain injury due to exposure to hypoxia and/or ischaemia, as evidenced by biochemical, electroencephalography (EEG), neuroimaging (MRI), cranial ultrasound, or pathological (postmortem examination) findings. If none of the above is available, additional information from computed tomography (CT) needs to be considered, as well as the risks of radiation exposure at this age.

Neonatal depression

This is a general term that describes the clinical condition of the infant in the immediate postnatal period (approximately the first hour of life) without implying any specific association with the prenatal condition or postnatal investigations.

INCIDENCE

The incidence of HIE ranges from 1 to 8 per 1000 live births in developed countries and is as high as 26 per 1000 live births in low-income countries. (Kurinczuk, White-Koning, and Badawi, 2010).

Birth asphyxia is the cause of more than 20% of all neonatal deaths worldwide. It is estimated that each year more than 800 000 neonatal deaths result from intrapartum-related causes; of these, almost all (99%) occur in low- and middle-income countries (see www.un.org, www.countdown2030.org/2015/2015-final-report).

Furthermore, the World Health Organization (WHO) *World Health Report* (WHO, 2005) estimated that as many as 1 million survivors of birth asphyxia may develop cerebral palsy, intellectual disability, learning difficulties, and other disabilities each year.

CLINICAL NEUROBEHAVIOURAL ASSESSMENT OF THE NEWBORN INFANT

The clinical assessment remains central to all investigations for the first evaluation, day-to-day medical care, and follow-up of the newborn infant. The clinical neurobehavioural assessment of the newborn infant is aimed at:

- Evaluating gestational age, which may be related to specific clinical conditions;

- Identifying signs of neural damage and planning for short- and long-term management; and

- Making a tentative and preliminary evaluation of the prognosis.

The core questions to be answered are:

- What has happened? Is there a structural lesion?

- Where is it located in the central/peripheral nervous system?

- When did it happen? Is it possible to establish whether it was it pre-, peri-, or postnatal?

- Why and how did it happen?

Assessment of the clinical neurobehavioural status must be considered an ongoing process, which needs to be repeated over time, to be adapted to the age and clinical status of the newborn infant, and to be compared with reference values. The essential components are history, general assessment, neurobehavioural assessment conducted in a standardized way, evaluation of the environment and quality of care, and follow-up.

The *history* aims to establish which specific conditions may be related to NE: health problems within the family (in particular unexplained and/or recurrent infant/child deaths, stillbirths, abortions, genetic and/or neurological diseases, seizures, cerebral palsy, intellectual disability), maternal illnesses, drug treatments, or unhealthy behaviours before and during pregnancy (alcohol, smoking, addiction to drugs and/or illicit substances), fetal, perinatal, and postnatal problems. When investigating for perinatal and postnatal problems, specific attention has to be paid to the following:

- Clinical status of the newborn infant at birth and Apgar score at 1 minute and 5 minutes;

- Need for – and response to – resuscitation (including its method and duration) at birth;

- Clinical status of the newborn infant after birth: alertness, cry, social responsiveness, posture, tone, and movements, reaction to stimulation, patterns of breathing, feeding, and sleeping, consolability, breast/bottle feeding, skin-to-skin contact, and nesting;

- Presence of 'unusual' clinical signs, such as purposeless sucking, unusual movements/postures such as boxing, cycling, fisting, unusual behaviours such as frequent yawning and sneezing; and

- How the newborn infant looks day-by-day to caregivers, i.e. stable, improved, or worsened.

When taking history, parents and nurses are to be trusted as the best sources, as they care for the newborn infant day and night. Therefore, specific recommendations must be made to caregivers to record what they observe when caring for the newborn infant, remembering that any unrecorded observation is a missed one.

The *assessment* of the newborn infant has, whenever possible, to be conducted when he/she is awake, in order to get reliable information on the state of consciousness, behaviour, vision, tone, and movements; the only exceptions are situations where newborn infants are stuporous or in a very poor neurological condition and/or therapeutically sedated. It needs to be conducted in a quiet, warm place and without interruptions; the mother should be encouraged to attend, and she should be reassured and kept informed while the assessment is performed. When assessing a newborn infant for suspected NE or other neural damage, a single evaluation is rarely sufficient and usually needs to be repeated twice daily, or sometimes more frequently, but this must be balanced against the risk of extensive evaluation stressing the infant.

With specific reference to excellent reviews of neurobehavioural assessment (Volpe, 2017; Amiel-Tison and Gosselin, 2009; video at www.hammersmith-neuro-exam.com), the main steps of evaluation are summarized as follows:

- Gestational age: this is estimated through history, morphological, and neurobehavioural criteria (e.g. the Dubowitz and New Ballard standardized examination scores);

- General condition: aimed at assessing patterns and/or abnormalities of breathing, circulation, thermal control, feeding and nutrition, level of alertness, and at recognizing malformations and dysmorphic signs;

- Signs of trauma: if present, specifying whether they are birth-related and/or involving head, trunk, spine, limbs, impaired function, or pain;

- Alertness and sleep: highly informative with regard to neurological status. They are recognizable from the 28th week, normally variable during the day, best evaluated through integrated assessment of eye-opening, breathing, spontaneous movements, and crying pattern.

- Visual and auditory communication: visual fixation and tracking, response to sound and consolability, defined by the response of the crying infant to voice or soothing;

- Posture and tone—best evaluated from 24 hours after birth:

  o The spontaneous posture for a newborn infant born at term delivered with a cephalic presentation is of full flexion of all four limbs;

  o Passive tone: defined as muscle tone at rest; that is, minimal contraction of the resting muscle, best evaluated through posture and range of movement with standard manoeuvres (e.g. forward traction/pull to sit, ventral suspension);

  o Active tone: observed during spontaneous movements, best evaluated through motor performance;

  o Spontaneous movements: assessed as spontaneous and/or in response to stimulation, they are normally smooth, symmetrical, and varied; abnormal movements may be slow and stereotyped, or paroxysmal and purposeless, such as chewing and repetitive tongue-thrusting movements;

- Reflexes: both deep tendon and primitive reflexes may be present, absent, decreased, increased, or asymmetrical. The primitive (or inborn automatic) reflexes are automatic responses that appear during the second half of pregnancy, are present at birth (and gradually disappear by 6 months of age). Abnormal findings are reflexes not elicited at birth (suggesting central nervous system [CNS] depression), or reflexes persisting beyond a specific age limit (suggesting CNS damage); the following are used in routine evaluation:

- o   Moro reflex;

- o   Finger grasp and response to traction;

- o   Automatic walking;

- o   Sucking;

- o   Asymmetric tonic neck reflex;

- Cranial nerves (CN), evaluated through their specific sensory and/or motor functions including response to light, visual behaviour, eyelid elevation (II, III CN), extraocular movements (III, IV, VI CN), facial sensibility, biting (V CN), facial motility and taste (VII CN), hearing and vestibular responses (VIII CN), sucking, swallowing, vocalization, taste, and gag reflex (IX and X CN), head and neck movements (XI CN), movements of the tongue (XII CN);

- Peripheral nerves: look for injuries at the level of the brachial plexus (immobile floppy upper limb), phrenic nerve (dyspnea), facial nerve (facial asymmetry), laryngeal nerve (stridor, dyspnea), median nerve, radial nerve (loss of normal hand posture and movement), lumbosacral plexus, sciatic nerve, peroneal nerve; look also for generalized neuropathy: congenital or chronic sensory or sensorimotor neuropathy, acute polyneuropathy;

- Autonomic function: respiratory, cardiovascular, bowel, and bladder functions; and

- Higher cognitive functions: social responsiveness, behavioural responses to tactile, thermal, painful, visual, and auditory stimulation, specifically investigating for latency, habituation, modulated/stereotyped responses.

Abnormal findings leading to suspicion of neonatal CNS damage occur in the following more common clinical presentations:

- *CNS depression*, seen in NE, trauma, other encephalopathies, drug intoxications: characterized by decreased alertness, tone, movements and reflexes, poor feeding;

- *Hyperalertness/seizures*: seen in mild NE caused by HIE, infection, acute dysmetabolism (hypoglycaemia, hypocalcaemia), drug withdrawal (opioids, cocaine, other psychotropes); seizures are clinically differentiated from tremors as they include abnormal eye movements, unresponsiveness to passive flexion of limbs, possible associated apnoea, bradycardia and cyanosis, abnormal EEG, if available; be aware that neonatal seizures may be subtle, that is, only characterized by abnormal gaze, eyelid blinking, sucking and other oral-lingual movements, swimming, boxing, cycling, although in affected infants born at term subtle seizures are rarely the only type of convulsions;

- *Intracranial hypertension,* seen in acute severe infection, intracranial haemorrhage, intracranial mass: signs may include enlarged head and sutures, full/bulging fontanelles, decreased alertness, forced downgaze (sunsetting), bradycardia, apnoea, vomiting, yawning, hypertonia, extensor posturing, opisthotonus;

- *Generalized muscular hypotonia,* seen in HIE (early stages), intracranial haemorrhage, infection, kernicterus, drug exposure: decreased passive and active tone;

- *Axial (i.e. muscles of neck and torso) extensor hypertonia*: rare and severe, seen in HIE, massive intracranial haemorrhage, infection, hyperekplexia (stiff baby syndrome; see Chapter 24 and Gastaut and Villeneuve, 1967), associated with an exaggerated startle response and apnoea.

Once the diagnosis of NE is suspected, the following clinical considerations may be useful in orienting towards possible timing and aetiologies.

- The infant was typical at birth and atypical thereafter: consider the following perinatal/postnatal causes:

  o Intraventricular haemorrhage;

  o HIE, with caution as asphyxiated infants are never entirely typically developing at birth;

  o Acute/congenital inborn error of metabolism;

  o Infection;

  o Progressive disease;

  o Drug withdrawal.

- The infant was atypical at birth, then improved/worsened thereafter: consider the following causes:

  o HIE;

  o Trauma;

  o Intracranial haemorrhage;

  o Progressive/metabolic disease;

  o Anaemia due to fetal-maternal transfusion.

- The neonate was atypical at birth and stable thereafter: consider the following prenatal causes:

  o Developmental malformations of the CNS;

  o Infections (TORCH; T, toxoplasmosis, O, other; R, rubella; C, cytomega-lovirus; H, herpes simplex virus; see also Chapter 22);

  o Prenatal hypoxic-ischaemic brain injury;

  o Inborn errors of metabolism.

CLINICAL PRESENTATIONS OF HIE WITH/WITHOUT MULTIORGAN FAILURE

The Sarnat and Sarnat 1976 classification is the most widely used instrument to identify the prognostic risk of a term neonate with HIE. This classification is based on clinical and EEG findings and enables patients with HIE to be divided into three groups within the first 24 to 48 hours after birth (see Table 14.2). The stages in Table 14.2 are a continuum, reflecting the spectrum of clinical states of infants over 36 weeks gestational age.

Table 14.2 Sarnat and Sarnat (1976) classification

	Stage 1 (mild)	Stage 2 (moderate)	Stage 3 (severe)
Level of consciousness	Hyperalert, irritable	Lethargic or obtunded	Stuporous, comatose
Neuromuscular control	Uninhibited, overreactive	Diminished spontaneous movement	Diminished or absent spontaneous movement
Muscle tone	Normal	Mild hypotonia	Flaccid
Posture	Mild distal flexion	Strong distal flexion	Intermittent decerebration
Stretch reflexes	Overactive	Overactive, disinhibited	Decreased or absent
Segmental myoclonus	Present or absent	Present	Absent
Complex reflexes	Normal	Suppressed	Absent
Suck	Weak	Weak or absent	Absent

Table 14.2 (continued)   Sarnat and Sarnat (1976) classification

	Stage 1 (mild)	Stage 2 (moderate)	Stage 3 (severe)
Moro	Strong, low threshold	Weak, incomplete; high threshold	Absent
Oculovestibular	Normal	Overactive	Weak or absent
Tonic neck	Slight	Strong	Absent
Autonomic function	Generalized sympathetic	Generalized parasympathetic	Both systems depressed
Pupils	Mydriasis	Miosis	Variable, often unequal, poor light reflex
Respirations	Spontaneous	Spontaneous, occasional apnoea	Periodic, apnoea
Heart rate	Tachycardia	Bradycardia	Variable
Bronchial and salivary secretions	Sparse	Profuse	Variable
Gastrointestinal motility	Normal or decreased	Increased, diarrhea	Variable
Seizures	None	Common, focal, or multifocal	Uncommon (excluding decerebration)
EEG findings	Normal (awake)	Early: low-voltage showing continuous delta and theta Later: periodic pattern (awake); seizures focal or multifocal; 1.0—1.5Hz spike-and-wave	Early: periodic pattern with isoelectric phases Later: totally isoelectric
Duration	<24h	2—14 days	Hours to weeks
Outcome	About 100%	80% normal; abnormal if symptoms more than 5—7 days	About 50% die; remainder with severe sequelae

A simplified clinical classification to identify candidates for therapeutic hypothermia has been proposed by The Florida Neonatal Neurologic Network (http://hopefn3.org; see Table 14.3). Figure 14.1 reports inclusion and exclusion criteria for therapeutic hypothermia.

Table 14.3   Clinical score for candidates to therapeutic hypothermia. Presence of seizures or 3 of 6 of the following

Clinical criteria	Signs of encephalopathy	
	Moderate encephalopathy	Severe encephalopathy
1. Level of consciousness	Lethargic	Stupor/coma
2. Spontaneous activity	Decreased activity	No activity
3. Posture	Distal flexion, complete extension, frog leg posture Decerebrate	
4. Tone	Hypotonia (focal or general), hypertonia (focal or truncal) Flaccid	
5. Primitive reflexes		
Suck	Weak or bite	Absent
Moro	Incomplete	Absent
6. Autonomic system		
Pupils	Constricted	Skew deviation/dilated/non-reactive to light
Heart rate*	Bradycardia	Variable
Respirations	Periodic	Apnoea or intubated

*Heart rate should only be used as an entry criterion if the patient is normothermic at the time of staging.

Perinatal asphyxia may involve several organs other than the brain, to different degrees. Vulnerability, clinical presentation, and recoverability are tabulated in Table 14.4.

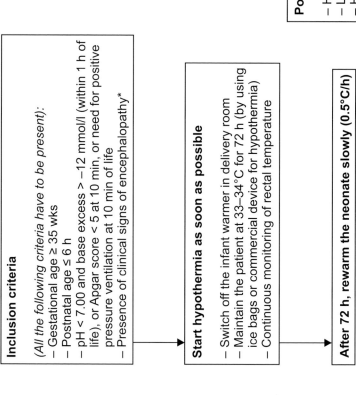

Inclusion criteria

(All the following criteria have to be present):
– Gestational age ≥ 35 wks
– Postnatal age ≤ 6 h
– pH < 7.00 and base excess > –12 mmol/l (within 1 h of life), or Apgar score < 5 at 10 min, or need for positive pressure ventilation at 10 min of life
– Presence of clinical signs of encephalopathy*

Exclusion criteria

– Gestational < 35 wks
– Postnatal age > 6 h
– Major congenital malformations
– Brain haemorrhage

Start hypothermia as soon as possible

– Switch off the infant warmer in delivery room
– Maintain the patient at 33–34°C for 72 h (by using ice bags or commercial device for hypothermia)
– Continuous monitoring of rectal temperature

Potential side effects and solution

– Heart: sinus bradycardia
– Lung: pulmonary hypertension
– Haematology: thrombocytopenia

(Transient increase of 0.5–1.0°C solves the problem in most cases)

After 72 h, rewarm the neonate slowly (0.5°C/h)

*See Table 14.3.

Figure 14.1 Protocol for therapeutic hypothermia

Table 14.4 Multisystem organ injuries

Organ/system	Vulnerability	Clinical presentation	Recoverability
Brain	+ + + +	Apnoea, hypoxia, encephalopathy, coma, seizures	+
Kidneys	+ + +	Acute renal failure	+ + +
Lungs	+ + +	PPHN, ARD, pulmonary haemorrhage	+ + + +
Liver	+ +	Transaminase derangement, Coagulopathy	+ + + +
Heart	+ +	Cardiogenic shock, valvular regurgitation	+ + + +
Blood	+ +	Thrombocytopenia, DIC	+ + + +
Vascular	+ +	Capillary leak, sclerema	+ + + +
Gastrointestinal tract	+ +	Feeding intolerance, necrotizing enterocolitis	+ + + +

PPHN, persistent pulmonary hypertension of the newborn infant; ARD, acute respiratory distress syndrome; DIC, disseminated intravascular coagulation. Vulnerability: +, less likely to occur; + + +, most likely to occur. Recoverability: +, likelihood of complete recovery without impairments is very scarce; + + + +, likelihood of complete recovery without impairments is very likely.

Diagnosis and differential diagnosis of HIE

When assessing a newborn infant with suspected HIE, the differential diagnosis has to be considered including the following conditions, which can mimic neonatal HIE:

- Inborn errors of metabolism, (e.g. nonketotic hyperglycinaemia, disorders of pyruvate metabolism, urea-cycle defects, Zellweger syndrome, and mitochondrial disorders);

- Drug exposure, abstinence syndrome, drug withdrawal;

- Stroke;

- Neuromuscular disorders, including neonatal myopathies;

- Brain tumours;

- Developmental defects;

- Infections.

Many new technologies, when available and reliable, are aimed at documenting early CNS damage and can support the already mentioned central role of clinical assessment in recognizing and evaluating NE.

Laboratory studies in HIE

HIE is a *clinical* diagnosis because the diagnosis is made based on the history, physical and neurological examination with *supporting* biochemical, imaging, and/or EEG investigation. Many of the tests are performed to assess the severity of the brain injury and to monitor the functional status of systemic organs. Laboratory studies should include those listed below (see Table 14.4 and Chapter 10).

- *Arterial blood gas-analysis:* blood gas monitoring is used to assess acid-base status and to avoid hyperoxia and hypoxia as well as hypercapnia and hypocapnia.

- *Serum electrolyte levels:* in severe cases, daily assessment of serum electrolytes is valuable until the infant's status improves. Markedly low serum sodium, potassium, and chloride levels in the presence of reduced urine flow and excessive weight gain may indicate acute tubular damage or syndrome of inappropriate antidiuretic hormone, particularly during the initial 2 to 3 days of life. However, in the absence of excessive weight gain, they may indicate an *appropriate* ADH response to intravascular hypovolaemia (e.g. after haemorrhage or excessive fluid restriction) (Modi, 1998). Failure to treat hypovolaemia will decrease cerebral blood flow and exacerbate HIE. Fluids that maintain intravascular volume and that also will not add free water into the extracellular space are, therefore, often indicated. Conversely, 5% dextrose with 0.18% saline or any solution containing dextrose alone are relatively contraindicated.

- Similar electrolyte changes may be seen during recovery; increased urine flow may indicate ongoing tubular damage and excessive sodium loss relative to water loss.

- *Renal function:* serum urea and creatinine levels and creatinine clearance suffice in most cases.

- *Cardiac and liver enzymes:* these values are an adjunct to assess the degree of hypoxic-ischaemic injury to these other organs. These findings may also provide some insight into injuries to other organs, such as the bowel.

- *Haematological and coagulation system evaluation:* increased nucleated red blood cells, neutropenia or neutrophilia, and thrombocytopenia have been reported.

Coagulopathy includes alteration of prothrombin time, partial thromboplastin time, and fibrinogen levels.

NEUROIMAGING AND NEUROPHYSIOLOGICAL INVESTIGATIONS IN HIE

We can consider three phases of perinatal asphyxia management: antenatal, delivery room, and postnatal management (see Chapters 8 and 9).

PREVENTION OF HIE

Preventing fetal asphyxia through effective obstetric care is greatly preferable to managing an asphyxiated newborn infant. When asphyxia has occurred, the key to effective resuscitation is to restore adequate blood and oxygen supply to vital organs, particularly the brain. This can be achieved through anticipating the need for neonatal resuscitation in the presence of maternal, uteroplacental, and intrapartum risk factors for birth asphyxia, and ensuring updated knowledge and skills in neonatal resuscitation among nurses, midwives, and doctors attending the birth. Once an asphyxiated neonate is born, optimal management must be systematic (see Tables 14.2 and 14.5) and brain-centred.

Table 14.5 The three phases of perinatal asphyxia management: antenatal, delivery room, and postnatal management

Problem	Recommendations
(a) Antenatal phase	
Clinical environment	Clean and warm (26°C) delivery suite; availability of equipment including radiant warmer (37°C), suction system (max. pressure 100mmHg), oxygen (flow rate: 5l/min), self-inflating bag, facial mask, set for neonatal tracheal intubation, medications (epinephrine [adrenaline], volume expanders, sodium bicarbonate)
Fetal heart rate and rhythm abnormalities and/or presence of thick meconium. Scarce fetal movements	Consider emergency caesarean section
(b) Delivery room phase	
Apnoea and/or heart rate <100 beats/min; cyanosis, hypotonia	Neonatal resuscitation including positive pressure ventilation, chest compressions, drugs (see Perlman et al. 2015, Wyllie et al. 2015)

Table 14.5 (continued)   The three phases of perinatal asphyxia management: antenatal, delivery room, and postnatal management

Aspect	Objective	Things to avoid and why
(c) Postnatal management		
Ventilation	To maintain CO_2 in normal ranges (35—45mmHg)	Hypercapnia (causes cerebral vasodilation) Hypocapnia, CO2 <25mmHg (decreases cerebral blood flow and oxygen release from haemoglobin)
Oxygenation	To maintain O_2 in normal range (SaO_2, 85—95% or PaO2 50—75mmHg)	Hyperoxia (increases range free radical damage and decrease cerebral blood flow)
Temperature	To maintain core temperature in normal range (36.5—37.5°C). Consider moderate therapeutic hypothermia (33—34°C for 72h)	Hyperthermia (may increase brain injury)
Blood circulation	To maintain blood pressure (40—60mmHg) and haemoglobin in normal range (consider blood transfusion) Judicious fluid management (40—70ml/kg/day) To consider inotropes based on cardiac function; if good, consider fluids/dopamine; if not good and PPHN, epinephrine and milrinone	Hypotension and anaemia (may decrease cerebral and body perfusion) Fluid overload (may cause cerebral oedema and generalized oedema due to SIADH) Dopamine in case of PPHN increases pulmonary resistances
Metabolic state	To maintain blood glucose levels in normal range (2.2—6.6mmol/l)	Hypoglycaemia (may potentiate excitotoxic amino acid) Hyperglycaemia (may increase oedema, brain lactate)

Table 14.5 (continued) The three phases of perinatal asphyxia management: antenatal, delivery room, and postnatal management

Neurological problems	To control seizures with anticonvulsants (pheno-barbital, phenytoin, lorazepam) and correction of metabolic perturbations (hypoglycaemia, hypocal-caemia, hyponatremia)	
Renal problems	To monitor urine output	Avoid fluid overload
Haematologic problems	Based on coagulation pro-file and platelet count, con-sider fresh frozen plasma and platelet transfusion, respect-ively	
Gastrointestinal problems	Start feeding with caution	Avoid large amount of feed-ing during the acute phase (necrotizing enterocolitis)
Liver function	To evaluate transaminases (alanine transferase, aspartate transferase), clotting (pro-thrombin time, PTT, fibrino-gen), glucose, albumin, biliru-bin, ammonia To monitor levels of drugs metabolized and/or eliminated through the liver	

For reference ranges, see Chapter 10. PPHN, persistent pulmonary hypertension of the newborn infant; SIADH, syndrome of inappropriate antidiuretic hormone; PTT, partial thromboplastin time.

Neuroprotective strategy

Perinatal asphyxia occurs in three phases: primary, secondary energy failure, and ter-tiary phase (Figure 14.2). During secondary energy failure, there are four main mech-anisms determining neuronal cell death: (1) excite-toxic, in which adenosine tri-phosphate (ATP) and glutamate are abundant in the synaptic spaces; (2) accumula-tion of intracellular calcium; (3) formation of free radicals; and (4) production of pro-inflammatory cytokines. The tertiary phase is characterized by many phenom-ena including cell death, remodeling, astrogliosis, and repair. This phase lasts several months (Douglas-Escobar and Weiss, 2015)

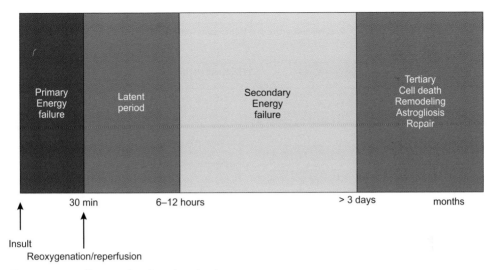

Figure 14.2 Phases of perinatal asphyxia

Experimental studies show that therapeutic hypothermia can be used as a treatment to limit the damage caused by all these processes. A meta-analysis of 11 randomized controlled trials comprising 1505 infants born at term and late preterm with moderate/severe encephalopathy and evidence of intrapartum asphyxia demonstrated the positive effects of moderate hypothermia (33–34°C) for 72 hours on the outcomes listed in Table 14.6. The results of this meta-analysis provide evidence for the benefit of prolonged moderate hypothermia in asphyxiated neonates (Jacobs et al. 2013).

Table 14.6 Effects of therapeutic hypothermia (33–34°C) for 72 hours

	Risk ratio (95% CI)	Number needed to treat (95% CI)
Death or severe disability to 18 months	0.75 (0.68–0.83)	7 (5–10)
Mortality	0.75 (0.64–0.88)	11 (8–25)
Neurodevelopmental disability in survivors	0.77 (0.63–0.94)	8 (5–14)
Cerebral palsy in survivors	0.66 (0.54–0.82)	8 (6–17)

Adapted from Jacobs et al. (2013).

Systemic supportive care

In addition to therapeutic hypothermia, the treatment of patients with HIE is based on a systemic supportive care. The pillars of this approach are summarized in Figure 14.3.

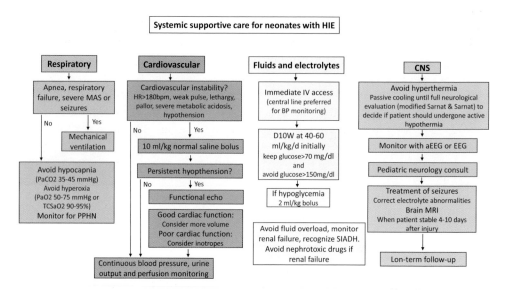

Figure 14.3 Systemic supportive care. aEEG, amplitude-integrated EEG; BP, blood pressure; D10W, dextrose 10% in water; HIE, hypoxic-ischaemic encephalopathy; IV, intravenous; MAS, meconium aspiration syndrome; PPHN, persistent pulmonary hypertension; SIADH, syndrome of inappropriate antidiuretic hormone. (Modified from Douglas–Escobar and Weiss 2015 and http://hopefn3.org.)

Prognosis

A persistently low Apgar score at 10 minutes is associated with death or moderate/severe disability at 18 months and at 6 to 7 years of age (Laptook et al. 2009, Natarajan et al. 2011). However, not all infants with a 10-minute Apgar score of 3 or less had a uniformly poor outcome; 27% and 20% of children with a score of 0 at 10 minutes survived without disability at 2 years (Perlman et al. 2015, Wyllie et al. 2015) or at school age (Natarajan et al. 2011). Persistence of severe encephalopathy on serial neurological examinations, lack of improvement in the abnormal background in the amplitude-integrated EEG and EEG, and MRI evidence of severe injury may be useful to identify infants at highest risk of severe neurological sequelae (Shankaran et al. 2012).

FOLLOW-UP AND OUTCOME AFTER NE

Once the diagnosis of NE has been made and management has been started, one of the major concerns for both family and caregivers is the expected/suspected short- and long-term outcome. This will influence the child's and the family's future life and, if not favourable, will challenge the family's ability to cope with the child's problems and society's ability to meet the child's special needs. The prognosis of NE is highly unpredictable because of different aetiologies, timing of occurrence and diagnosis, management options, and environmental factors.

OUTCOME AFTER NEONATAL HIE

NE caused by cerebral hypoxia-ischaemia due to perinatal asphyxia is an important cause of neonatal mortality and morbidity. The outcome is influenced by the combination of duration and severity of the insult to the brain, gestational age, presence and duration of seizures, associated problems from infection, trauma, and metabolic alterations. The following predictors of mortality and neurological morbidity after perinatal hypoxia-ischaemia have been reported (Levene and de Vries, 2011):

- Extended period (up to 20min) of very low (≤3) Apgar scores;

- Prolonged delay in establishing spontaneous respirations after birth;

- Severity and duration of intrapartum metabolic acidosis (umbilical artery pH 7.00);

- Neonatal neurological examination findings: in particular, unfavorable signs are Sarnat stage 3 and persistently abnormal neurological examination;

- Brain imaging (ultrasound, MRI) findings;

- EEG or amplitude-integrated EEG findings; and

- Visual, brainstem auditory, somatosensory evoked potentials findings.

With specific attention to the neonatal neurological examination, follow-up studies (Sarnat et al. 1976; Finer et al. 1981; Robertson and Finer, 1985; Low et al. 1985; Levene et al. 1986) have shown that mild HIE has a very low risk of death or major neurodevelopmental disability), although a recent systematic review (Conway et al. 2018) has shown that approximately one quarter of infants with mild HIE have an abnormal outcome defined as death, motor, or developmental delay at follow-up to 18 months. Moderate HIE is associated with few deaths and 75% survival without major neurological deficits. Severe HIE has a very poor outcome, with a 50% to 100% mortality rate and severe disability (cerebral palsy, intellectual disability, sensory-neural impairment, epilepsy) in up to 75% of survivors.

Other studies (Thompson et al. 1997; Miller et al. 2004) have correlated outcome to early neurological signs through numerical scoring systems. In summary, the prognosis for children with HIE depends on the severity and duration of the neurological abnormalities, with a significant risk of death after severe HIE and major developmental problems after moderate or severe HIE.

According to the recent review by Volpe (2017), the occurrence of neonatal neurological features provides a reliable indicator of infants at risk of subsequent significant neurological deficits. In particular, the aspects most useful in estimating the prognosis include the severity of the neurological syndrome, the presence of seizures, and the duration of the abnormalities. The severity, when systematically quantitated, was found to correlate directly with the incidence of neurological sequelae: infants who suffered a severe syndrome had the highest rate of mortality and sequelae (Ishikawa et al. 1987; Ellenberg and Nelson, 1988; Caravale, Allemand, and Libenson, 2003; Miller et al. 2004). However, later neurodevelopmental follow-up has also identified some cognitive and motor disabilities in infants that had mild NE (van Khoji et al. 2008; van Handel et al. 2012).

The presence of neonatal seizures was found to increase the risk of neurological sequelae (Sarnat and Sarnat 1976; Ishikawa et al. 1987; Ellenberg and Nelson, 1988; Caravale, Allemand, and Libenson, 2003; Miller et al. 2004), in particular if seizures occur in the first 12 hours and/or are difficult to control.

The duration of neonatal neurological abnormalities is useful in identifying the infant at greatest risk of sequelae. Several studies reported that the majority of infants who showed no abnormalities after about 1 week of life (Sarnat and Sarnat 1976; Caravale, Allemand, and Libenson, 2003) were normal at follow-up, and 10% had only mild abnormalities. Although the disappearance of abnormalities by 1 to 2 weeks is an excellent prognostic sign, the possibility of learning disturbances at school age cannot be conclusively ruled out (Volpe, 2017).

The study by Mercuri et al. (1999) showed that specific clinical patterns can be observed in infants with HIE and these can be related to the pattern of lesion on brain MRI. In particular, as it was reported by other recent studies (Martinez-Biarge et al. 2011; Cheong et al. 2012) while infants with normal MRI or minimal changes tended to show only minor tone abnormalities after the first week of life, infants with more severe lesions, such as basal ganglia lesions show persistent and diffuse neurological abnormalities. Infants with white matter changes but intact basal ganglia show a different clinical pattern with improved sucking reflex and behaviour and less severe tone abnormalities. They also reported that the neurological examination performed after the second week of life is a reliable indicator of outcome in these infants. Other recent studies (Walsh et al. 2017) reported that, although the significance of milder MRI abnormalities for long-term outcome is unclear, there is a strong association between moderate-severe MRI injuries and long-term neurodevelopmental deficits (Rutherford et al. 2010; Martinez-Biarge et al. 2011). Therefore, infants with mild NE deserve greater focus and future investigation, with particular emphasis on the potential benefits of neuroprotective strategies.

Ellis et al. (1999) reported that there are very few studies in low-income countries of outcome in HIE survivors and that only 36% of survivors with any grade of HIE were normal at 1 year. Growing attention is being paid to less severe forms of disability in older children surviving neonatal HIE, such as minor motor impairments, attention-deficit/hyperactivity disorder, significant perceptual-motor or cognitive difficulties, and abnormalities in brain MRI (Barnett et al. 2002; Moster, Lie, and Markestad, 2002; Marlow et al. 2005).

Regular clinical follow-up over time enables prognosis to be estimated appropriately. This follows from evaluating performance according to postnatal age (corrected up to 2 years for gestational age) and normal ranges (see Chapters 5 and 6), recognizing delayed or disrupted developmental trends and taking quality of professional care into account. Any estimate of long-term prognosis made before 8 to 12 months of corrected age has a wide margin of error.

REFERENCES

American Academy of Pediatrics, American College of Obstetrics and Gynecologists (1997) *Guidelines for Perinatal Care*, 4th edn. Washington, DC: AAP and ACOG.

Amiel-Tison C, Gosselin J. (2009) Clinical assessment of the infant nervous system. In: Levene MI, Chervenak FA, *Fetal and Neonatal Neurology and Neurosurgery*, 4th edn. Philadelphia: Churchill Livingstone Elsevier, pp. 128–154.

Barnett A, Mercuri E, Rutherford M, et al. (2002) Neurological and perceptual-motor outcome at 5–6 years of age in children with neonatal encephalopathy: relationship with neonatal brain MRI. *Neuropediatrics* 33: 242–248.

Caravale B, Allemand F, Libenson MH (2003) Factors predictive of seizures and neurologic outcome in perinatal depression. *Pediatr Neurol* 29: 18–25.

Cheong JL, Coleman L, Hunt RW, et al. (2012) Prognostic utility of magnetic resonance imaging in neonatal hypoxic-ischemic encephalopathy: substudy of a randomized trial. *Arch Pediatr Adolesc Med* 7: 634–640.

Conway JM, Walsh BH, Boylan GB, Murray DM (2018) Mild hypoxic ischaemic encephalopathy and long-term neurodevelopmental outcome-A systematic review. *Early Hum Dev* 120: 80–87.

Douglas-Escobar M, Weiss MD (2015) Hypoxic-ischemic encephalopathy: a review for the clinician. *JAMA Pediatr* 169: 397–403.

Ellenberg JH, Nelson KB (1988) Cluster of perinatal events identifying infants at high-risk for death or disability. *J Pediatr* 113: 546–552.

Ellis M, Manandhar N, Shrestha PS, Shrestha L, Manandhar DS, Costello AM. (1999) Outcome at 1 year of neonatal encephalopathy in Kathmandu, Nepal. *Dev Med Child Neurol* 41: 689–695.

Finer NN, Robertson CM, Richards RT, Pinnell LE, Peters KL (1981) Hypoxic-ischaemic encephalopathy in term neonates: perinatal factors and outcome. *J Pediatr* 98: 112–117.

Gastaut H, Villeneuve A (1967) The startle disease or hyperekplexia: pathological surprise reaction. *J Neurol Sci* 5: 523–542.

Ishikawa T, Ogawa Y, Kanayama M, et al. (1987) Long-term prognosis of asphyxiated full-term neonates with CNS complications. *Brain Dev* 948–953.

Jacobs SE, Berg M, Hunt R, Tarnow-Mordi WO, Inder TE, Davis PG (2013) Cooling for newborns with hypoxic ischaemic encephalopathy. *Cochrane Database Syst Rev* (1): CD003311.

Kurinczuk JJ, White-Koning M, Badawi N (2010) Epidemiology of neonatal encephalopathy and hypoxic-ischaemic encephalopathy. *Early Hum Dev* 86: 329–338.

Laptook AR, Shankaran S, Ambalavanan N, et al. (2009) Outcome of term infants using Apgar scores at 10 minutes following hypoxic-ischemic encephalopathy. *Pediatrics* 124: 1619—1626.

Levene MI, Sands C, Grindulis H, Moore JR (1986) Comparison of two methods of predicting outcome in perinatal asphyxia. *Lancet* 1: 67—69.

Levene MI, de Vries LS (2011) Hypoxic-ischaemic encephalopathy. In: Martin RJ, Fanaroff AA, Walsh MC, eds. *Neonatal-Perinatal Medicine: Diseases of the Fetus and Infant*, 9th edn. St Louis: Elsevier Mosby, pp. 952—976.

Low JA, Galbraith RS, Muir DW, Killen HL, Pater EA, Karchmar EJ (1985) The relationship between perinatal hypoxia and newborn encephalopathy. *Am J Obstet Gynecol* 152: 256—260.

Marlow N, Rose AS, Rands CE, Draper ES (2005) Neuropsychological and educational problems at school age associated with neonatal encephalopathy. *Arch Dis Child Fetal Neonatal Ed* 90: F380—387.

Martinez-Biarge M, Diez-Sebastian J, Kapellou O, et al. (2011) Predicting motor outcome and death in term hypoxic-ischemic encephalopathy. *Neurology* 76: 2055—2061.

Mercuri E, Guzzetta A, Haataja L, et al. (1999) Neonatal neurological examination in infants with hypoxic ischaemic encephalopathy: correlation with MRI findings. *Neuropediatrics* 30: 83—89.

Miller SP, Latal B, Clark H, et al. (2004) Clinical signs predict 30-month neurodevelopmental outcome after neonatal encephalopathy.*Am J Obstet Gynecol* 190: 93—99.

Modi N (1998) Hyponatraemia in the newborn. *Arch Dis Child Fetal Neonatal Ed* 78: F81—F84.

Moster D, Lie RT, Markestad T (2002) Joint association of APGAR scores and early neonatal symptoms with minor disabilities at school age. *Arch Dis Child Fetal Neonatal Ed* 86: F16—F20.

Natarajan G, Shankaran S, Laptook AR, et al. (2011) Apgar scores at 10 min and outcomes at 6-7 years following hypoxic-ischaemic encephalopathy. *Arch Dis Child Fetal Neonatal Ed* 98: F473—F479.

Perlman JM, Wyllie J, Kattwinkel J, et al. (2015) Part 7: Neonatal Resuscitation: 2015 International Consensus on Cardiopulmonary Resuscitation and Emergency Cardiovascular Care Science With Treatment Recommendations. *Circulation* 132 (16 Suppl 1): S204—S241.

Robertson C, Finer NN (1985) Term infants with hypoxic-ischaemic encephalopathy: outcome at 3.5 years. *Dev Med Child Neurol* 27: 473—484.

Rutherford M, Ramenghi LA, Edwards AD, et al. (2010) Assessment of brain tissue injury after moderate hypothermia in neonates with hypoxic-ischaemic encephalopathy: a nested sub-study of a randomised controlled trial. *Lancet Neurol* 9: 39—45.

Sarnat HB, Sarnat MS. (1976) Neonatal encephalopathy following fetal distress: a clinical and electroencephalographic study. *Arch Neurol* 33: 696—705.

Shankaran S, Laptook AR, Tyson JE, et al. (2012) Evolution of encephalopathy during whole body hypothermia for neonatal hypoxic-ischemic encephalopathy. *J Pediatr* 160: 567—72.

Thompson CM, Puterman AS, Linley LL, et al. (1997) The value of a scoring system for hypoxic-ischaemic encephalopathy in predicting neuro-developmental outcome. *Acta Paediatr* 86: 757—761.

Van Khoji BJ, van Handel M, Uiterwaal CS, et al. (2008) Corpus callosum size in relation to motor performance in 9- to 10-year-old children with neonatal encephalopathy. *Pediatr Res* 63: 103—108.

Van Handel M, de Sonneville L, de Vries LS, et al. (2012) Specific memory impairment following neonatal encephalopathy in term-born children. *Dev Neuropsychol* 37: 30—50.

Volpe JJ (1995) *Neurology of the newborn*, 3rd ed. Philadelphia: WB Saunders.

Volpe JJ (2017) *Neurology of the Newborn*, 7th edn. Philadelphia: Saunders Elsevier.

Walsh BH, Neil J, Morey J, et al. (2017) The frequency and severity of magnetic resonance imaging abnormalities in infants with mild neonatal encephalopathy. *J Pediatr* 187: 26—33.

WHO (2005) *The World Health Report 2005: Make Every Mother and Child Count*. Geneva: World Health Organization. https://www.who.int/whr/2005/whr2005_en.pdf.

Wyllie J, Bruinenberg J, Roehr CC, Rüdiger M, Trevisanuto D, Urlesberger B (2015) European Resuscitation Council Guidelines for Resuscitation 2015: Section 7. Resuscitation and support of transition of babies at birth. *Resuscitation* 95: 249—263.

Resources

American College of Obstetricians and Gynecologists (2014) Executive summary: Neonatal encephalopathy and neurologic outcome, second edition. Report of the American College of Obstetricians and Gynecologists' Task Force on Neonatal Encephalopathy. *Obstet Gynecol* 123: 896—901.

Ballard JL, Khoury JC, Wedig K, Wang L, Eilers-Walsman BL, Lipp R (1991) New Ballard score, expanded to include extremely premature infants. *J Pediatr* 119: 417—423.

Carlo WA, Goudar SS, Jehan I, et al. (2010) First Breath Study Group. Newborn-care training and perinatal mortality in developing countries. *N Engl J Med* 362: 614—623.

Cowan F, Rutherford M, Groenendaal F, et al. (2003) Origin and timing of brain lesions in term infants with neonatal encephalopathy. *Lancet* 361: 736—742.

Countdown to 2015 for maternal newborn and child survival. A decade tracking progress maternal, newborn, child survival: the 2015 Report. Available at: http://countdown2030.org/reports-and-articles/2015-final-report. Accessed October 1, 2018.

de Vries LS, Toet MC (2006) Amplitude integrated electroencephalography in the full-term newborn. *Clin Perinatol* 33: 619—632.

Edwards AD, Brocklehurst P, Gunn AJ, et al. (2010) Neurological outcomes at 18 months of age after moderate hypothermia for perinatal hypoxic ischaemic encephalopathy: synthesis and meta-analysis of trial data. *BMJ* 340: 1—7.

Ehret DY, Patterson JK, Bose CL (2017) Improving neonatal care: a global perspective. *Clin Perinatol* 44: 567—582.

Murray DM, Bala P, O'Connor CM, et al. (2010) The predictive value of early neurological examination in neonatal ischaemic encephalopathy and neurodevelopmental outcome at 24 months. *Dev Med Child Neurol* 52: e55—e59.

Spitzmiller RE, Phillips T, Meinzen-Derr J, Hoath SB (2007) Amplitude-integrated EEG is useful in predicting neurodevelopmental outcome in full-term infants with hypoxic-ischemic encephalopathy: a meta-analysis. *J Child Neurol* 22: 1069—1078.

The Florida Neonatal Neurologic Network. Available at: http://hopefn3.org.

The millennium development goals report 2015. Available at: https://www.un.org/millenniumgoals/2015_MDG_Report/pdf/MDG 2015 rev (July 1).pdf. Accessed October 1, 2018.

United Nations Children's Fund (2015) Levels and trends in child mortality. Available at: https://unicef.org/publications/files/Child_Mortality_Report_2015_Web_9_Sept_15.pdf. Accessed October 1, 2018.

Wall SN, Lee AC, Carlo W, et al. (2010) Reducing intrapartum-related neonatal deaths in low- and middle-income countries — what works?*Semin Perinatol* 34: 395—407.

CHAPTER 15

Inherited metabolic encephalopathies of infancy

Barbara Plecko

Key messages

- Inherited metabolic encephalopathies can be suspected from the presence of biomarkers of the condition in plasma, urine, or cerebrospinal fluid and then confirmed by Sanger sequencing of the relevant gene(s).
- Cranial imaging may give additional diagnostic clues, if interpreted by experienced neuroradiologists.
- Early diagnosis is crucial to prevent irreversible brain injury because some of these disorders are amenable to specific treatments, such as supplementation of compounds or enzymes, special diets, or drugs that eliminate toxic compounds.
- In patients with chronic encephalopathies with nonspecific clinical presentations, a combination of broad biomarker testing and next generation sequencing is the most efficient way to establish a diagnosis. This will allow genetic counselling and future family planning.

Common errors

- Inborn errors of metabolism are ultra-rare and only exist in textbooks.
- The field of inborn errors can be separated from the field of child neurology.

> ## When to worry
>
> - Every acute encephalopathy of unclear aetiology needs an urgent diagnostic work-up for inborn errors of metabolism, including urgent laboratory analysis to rule out hypoglycemia, disturbances of acid-base balance, and hyperammonaemia.
> - Determination of amino acids and acylcarnitines in plasma as well as organic acids in urine should be performed if there is any clinical suspicion of abnormalities of these compounds, even if routine parameters give normal results.
> - Treatment trials with thiamine and biotin should be considered in patients with suggestive symptoms or compatible radiological findings until results of selective screening analyses are available.

DEFINITION

Metabolic disorders are caused by gene defects that encode metabolic pathway enzymes involved in the synthesis, degradation, or the transport of molecules. Metabolic disorders are rare diseases with an incidence below 1:2000. Most of these inborn errors of metabolism (IEM) cause a metabolite pattern that allows for a quick diagnosis by special analytical techniques. Many IEM are amenable to specific treatment, but timely initiation is crucial to avoid irreversible brain injury. Next generation sequencing (NGS) will enable broader recognition of many IEM. This chapter will focus on IEM presenting in the first year of life.

IEM can be grouped into those with acute onset and those with a chronic, sometimes progressive course of disease. In most cases IEM will affect the central nervous system (CNS), but some affect the peripheral nervous system or muscle. Typical clinical features of IEM with acute presentation include:

- acute encephalopathy,
- seizures,
- muscular hypotonia, and
- movement disorders.

Symptoms and signs in chronic presentations are:

- early developmental impairment,
- muscular hypotonia,
- epilepsy,

- micro- or macrocephaly,

- movement disorders,

- multisystem disease, and

- neurological regression.

The main mechanisms underlying CNS disease are:

- toxicity,

- substrate deficiency,

- imbalance of neurotransmitters, and

- storage disorders.

Many metabolic disorders are amenable to specific treatment, and early diagnosis is crucial to prevent adverse outcome. This has led to the establishment of newborn infant screening programmes in many countries across the world. Disorders included in newborn infant screening programmes are selected by their incidence, availability of reliable testing methods and specific treatment, as well as cost-effectiveness. Every child neurologist should be aware of the list of disorders included in the local national newborn infant screening programme. In light of continuous worldwide migration, it may be appropriate for children born elsewhere to undergo the national neonatal screening programme at a later age.

INTOXICATION TYPE DISORDERS: ACUTE ENCEPHALOPATHY

This group comprises IEM that lead to the accumulation of neurotoxic compounds, due to disturbed degradation of nutritional protein/nitrogen, as in urea cycle defects or organic acidurias. About 70% of patients present in the newborn period, while the remainder will present later in life (e.g. at the time of weaning from breast milk, during puberty, or at the time of common febrile or nonfebrile illnesses). The typical presentation in the neonatal period is a term newborn or infant, that presents with lethargy and poor feeding after a symptom-free interval. Symptoms at first are nonspecific but worsen to somnolence and coma within hours to days, probably accompanied by seizures. Usually the first suspicion is an underlying infection or, in older children, an exogenous intoxication. Abnormal breathing patterns may mislead towards the suspicion of pneumonia. Electroencephalogram will show diffuse slowing and, eventually, some epileptic discharges. Ultrasound and cranial magnetic resonance imaging (MRI) are usually nonspecific or may reveal brain oedema. In some organic acidurias (e.g.

propionic acidaemia or methylmalonic acidaemia), basal ganglia injury can be a radiological hallmark of the disease. An affected infant with encephalopathy needs to have cardiac, hepatic, and renal involvement assessed by laboratory analysis and ultrasound.

The most important step in a child with unclear acute encephalopathy is to perform routinely an extended set of laboratory evaluations, including the following:

- acid base balance,

- blood glucose,

- electrolytes,

- lactate,

- ammonia, and

- ketone bodies in urine.

The constellation of respiratory alkalosis with elevated ammonia (>100µmol/l) is highly suggestive of a urea cycle defect: hyperammonaemia drives central tachypnoea with subsequent low pCO2 levels. Usually, children become symptomatic if ammonia levels rise (>150µmol/l). Be aware that some laboratories will give ammonia levels in µg/dl which is higher than in µmol/l by a factor of 1.7 (NH_3 170µg/l $= 100µmol/l$). Metabolic acidosis with an increased anion gap ($[Na + K] - [NaHCO_3 + Cl] > 22$) should prompt the search for accumulating acid compounds, such as lactate or organic acids. Toxic compounds may inhibit other enzymes (e.g. in gluconeogenesis), so that hypoglycaemia may accompany metabolic decompensation as it is frequently observed in propionic acidaemia. The same inhibitory effect can cause secondary hyperammonaemia, also typically seen in propionic or in methylmalonic acidaemia. In that case, hyperammonaemia will be associated with metabolic acidosis.

Positive ketone bodies in an affected neonate should always alert the clinician to look for IEM, as they are clear indicators of a catabolic state. In contrast, disorders of long-chain fatty acid oxidation, such as very-long-chain or long-chain acyl-CoA dehydrogenase deficiency (VLCAD or LCHAD), show nonketotic or hypoketotic hypoglycaemia, metabolic acidosis, and eventually hyperammonaemia as laboratory hallmarks. These long-chain fatty acid oxidation disorders provoke a combination of energy depletion resulting from lack of acetyl-CoA production, as well as a build-up of toxic long-chain acylcarnitines leading to cardiac, hepatic, and muscle involvement.

Diagnosis of intoxication type disorders warrants urgent quantitative analysis of amino acids and acylcarnitines in plasma as well as orotic and organic acids in urine.

This package of investigations should be done even in the absence of abnormal routine laboratory parameters as metabolic acidosis may be absent in maple syrup urine disease and glutaric aciduria. Finally, the diagnosis has to be confirmed at a molecular level by Sanger sequencing of the respective gene to allow genetic counselling and prenatal diagnosis in forthcoming pregnancies (see Chapter 11).

Emergency treatment for all intoxication type disorders is the immediate discontinuation of protein supply for 24 hours to a maximum of 48 hours, together with a high glucose intake, given as an infusion at a calculated rate, and subsequently also lipids in order to provide a high caloric intake. Lipids must not be given intravenously in case of suspected fatty acid oxidation disorders. In severely affected infants this disorder requires insertion of a central venous line to provide 100 to 120cal/per kilogram of body weight per day. Careful continuous administration of low-dose insulin (e.g. 0.01IE/kg/h) may be needed to avoid hyperglycaemia, especially in the presence of metabolic acidosis.

Correction of metabolic acidosis is required only if pH levels drop below 7.1. In the case of hyperammonaemia, special drugs (e.g. sodium benzoate, phenylbutyrate, L-carbamylglutamate, or L-arginine) may be administered to lower ammonia levels rapidly. Supplementary L-carnitine (100–200mg/kg/d IV) is given to avoid secondary deficiency because many accumulating compounds are excreted as acylcarnitine products. In suspected long-chain fatty acid oxidation disorders, however, no L-carnitine should be given because long-chain fatty acid acylcarnitines have a toxic effect.

Children in a metabolic coma should be referred immediately to a metabolic centre experienced in haemodialysis or haemofiltration to prevent irreversible brain injury. Long-term treatment for urea cycle defects and organic acidurias is by a protein restricted diet, eventually supplemented by special amino acid mixtures and nitrogen scavengers. Long-term treatment of long-chain fatty acid oxidation defects is by fat restriction and supply of medium-chain fatty acids.

ENERGY DEFICIENCY

In neonates and infants, the brain consumes about 70% of total body energy. Thus, energy deficiency conditions at that age frequently manifest with seizures or acute encephalopathy. The final energy producing fuel for all of our cells is adenosine triphosphate (ATP), which is derived from the breakdown of glucose, fat, and proteins and is produced by oxidative phosphorylation within the respiratory chain. In the fed state, glucose is the main energy source, while beyond enteral glucose absorption, ATP production depends on the breakdown of liver glycogen, followed by fatty acid oxidation and gluconeogenesis. IEM in any of these pathways will cause recurrent hypoglycaemia that can start within hours after birth. Moreover, glucose metabolism is regulated by hormones such as insulin, cortisol, and growth hormone. In neonates and infants, the most frequent manifestation of hypoglycaemia is a symptomatic seizure. Prolonged profound hypoglycaemia may lead to MRI changes with signal alterations, which are pronounced in the occipital region on T2-weighted images. These changes may be reversible but may also be associated with irreversible brain injury and secondary epilepsy.

In the diagnostic work-up of recurrent hypoglycaemia, the history questioning the interval to the last meal, the physical examination, as well as the amount of glucose needed to achieve normoglycaemia may give important clues to diagnosis. A large-for-dates infant with an unpredictable occurrence of hypoglycaemia and an increased glucose demand will most probably have a mother with diabetes or suffer from congenital hyperinsulinism, while an infant with stunted growth, enlarged liver, and the need for frequent feeding to avoid preprandial hypoglycaemia will most probably suffer from glycogen storage disease type 1. Medium-chain acyl-CoA dehydrogenase deficiency, the most prevalent defect in fatty acid oxidation, with an incidence of 1:10 000, typically presents with hypoketotic or nonketotic hypoglycaemia in a previously unaffected infant that had reduced nutritional intake at the time of a febrile infection or gastroenteritis. In disorders where hypoglycaemia is accompanied by the accumulation of toxic compounds (e.g. in the case of long-chain fatty acid oxidation defects), hypoglycaemia may be accompanied by involvement of other organs, such as hepatopathy or cardiomyopathy with, sometimes, fatal arrhythmia. A child with hypoglycaemia, vomiting, and hepatopathy following the introduction of fruits and vegetables will most likely suffer from hereditary fructose intolerance.

Again, the extended list of routine laboratory evaluations may give important clues to diagnosis and warrants analysis — at best — of a 'critical' blood sample drawn at the time of hypoglycaemia. It is best, if services have a package of tubes ready to be added to routine measurement of transaminases and blood count etc., for the following laboratory analyses:

- blood glucose (if no critical sample available, do preprandial, no extra fasting),

- blood gases,

- uric acid,

- lactate,

- cholesterol, triglycerides,

- urinary ketones,

- free fatty acids — if available,

- blood ketone bodies-acetoacetate and hydroxybutyrate — if available,

- acylcarnitines,

- amino acids in plasma,

- organic acids in urine, and

- insulin, cortisol, human growth hormone (most valid at times of hypoglycaemia).

Immediate correction of hypoglycaemia is of utmost importance and, thereafter, controlled maintenance of glucose homeostasis by frequent feeding or parenteral supply. Long-term treatment depends on the underlying defect and is beyond the scope of this chapter.

As ATP production is the final common pathway of all energy fuels, defects in the mitochondrial respiratory chain also manifest as energy deficiency. The most severe form is that of primary lactic acidosis with metabolic acidosis due to massive lactate accumulation (>6mmol/l). Children may experience bouts of lethargy or present with Leigh syndrome with hypotonia, dystonia, eye movement disorders, swallowing difficulties, and seizures. Metabolic analyses are identical to intoxication type disorders to exclude secondary lactic acidosis along other with IEM. When measuring lactate, blood should be drawn without a tourniquet as this may cause an artificial increase of peripheral lactate. Further diagnostic work-up for mitochondrial disease has switched from biochemical analysis in muscle biopsies to primary molecular testing. As the number of known mitochondrial genes exceeds 250, genetic testing needs to be performed by NGS techniques.

IEM WITH CHRONIC PRESENTATIONS

Chronic presentations of IEM may be assigned to the following groups:

- hypotonia,

- metabolic epilepsies (see Chapter 16),

- early developmental impairment/intellectual disability with or without epilepsy,

- movement disorders,

- multisystem disease with or without dysmorphism,

- neurodegeneration (predominantly of white or of grey matter).

Discussions on IEM with chronic presentation are often structured according to the affected cell organelle (e.g. mitochondriopathies, peroxisomal disorders, lysosomal storage disease). This approach is very important when it comes to metabolic screening tests but is less helpful for the clinician faced with a disease of unclear aetiology. Table 15.1 lists metabolic screening tests and diseases according to affected cell organelles. The diagnostic work up by a symptoms-related approach is discussed in this chapter.

Table 15.1 Biomarkers for selective screening of organelle diseases manifesting in the first year of life

Diseases	Cell organelle	Urine	Plasma	CSF
CDG syndromes	Endoplasmatic reticulum or Golgi apparatus	—	Transferrin pattern for N-glycosylation ApoCIII electrophoresis for some O-glycosylation defects	—
Leigh syndrome	Mitochondria	—	Lactate	Lactate
Mitochondrial depletion syndromes	Mitochondria	—	Lactate eventually glycine	Lactate
MPS	Lysosomes	Proteoglycans	—	—
Mucolipidosis II Sialidosis	Lysosomes	Oligosaccharides	—	—
Niemann-Pick type A	Lysosomes	—	—	—
Gaucher disease	Lysosomes	—	—	—
GM1 gangliosidosis	Lysosomes	Oligosaccharides	—	—
GM2 gangliosidosis	Lysosomes	—	—	—
PBD (Zellweger syndrome)	Peroxisomes	—	Very-long-chain fatty acids, pristanic acid, phytanic acid, pipecolic acid	—

CSF, cerebrospinal fluid; CDG, carbohydrate deficiency glycoprotein; MPS, mucopolysaccharidosis; PBD, peroxisome biogenesis disorders.

MUSCULAR HYPOTONIA

Muscular hypotonia, if profound, can be evident from birth, or cause delayed acquisition of motor milestones. In neonates and infants, it may be difficult to differentiate central from peripheral hypotonia, unless the presence of seizures, for example, clearly favours CNS disease. Complete absence of deep tendon reflexes is more likely to occur with peripheral disorders, but the ratio of central to peripheral aetiology in general is 4:1. Treatable IEM should be considered first and measurement of total carnitine and acylcarnitines is mandatory to detect carnitine transporter defects or fatty acid oxidation defects. Analysis of acylcarnitines and lactate in plasma and organic acids in urine will allow a quick diagnosis of treatable entities and could also reveal other (probably untreatable) IEM. Hypotonia can also be a sign of neurotransmitter defects with dystonia only emerging at a later age. Aromatic acid decarboxylase deficiency (AADC) is the most severe defect in neurotransmitter synthesis with reduced formation of dopamine as well as serotonin. In addition to massive hypotonia, these patients will present with bradykinesia, episodes of tonic upward gaze (oculogyric crisis), and also autonomic dysfunction with low body temperature and blood pressure instability. While supplementation of L-Dopa and serotonin agonists have limited effects, studies on intracerebral AADC-gene therapy with stereotactic injections are very promising.

It has to be mentioned that glycogen storage disease may also present with prominent muscular hypotonia, therefore, child neurologists should always check for organ enlargement as part of their physical examination. In a child manifesting with muscular hypotonia and feeding difficulties during early infancy we would consider Pompe disease in the differential diagnosis. Patients typically have mild to moderate elevation of serum creatine kinase (CK). Patients with infantile Pompe disease manifesting at less than 6 months of age will have a hypertrophic cardiomyopathy with typically enlarged QRS complexes on electrocardiogram while onset at more than 6 months of age leads to involvement of skeletal muscle, but not of cardiac muscle. Early initiation of enzyme replacement therapy can be beneficial, but may need combined immunosuppression against induced antibody formation.

An infant with hypotonia may also suffer from a mitochondrial or a peroxisomal disease with pure neurological symptoms or multisystem disease. Pyruvate dehydrogenase deficiency (PDH) and Leigh syndrome are the most prevalent disorders and can be delineated by radiological findings with marked overlap. X-linked PDH deficiency is more prevalent in males and may show additional corpus callosum hypoplasia or agenesis, while Leigh syndrome has no sex preponderance and leads to typical bilateral basal ganglia and brainstem involvement. PDH can be treated by thiamine supplementation (100–300mg/d) and a ketogenic diet. Most patients with Leigh syndrome are not amenable to specific treatment, but a subgroup has been identified harbouring a gene defect in thiamine transporter SLC19A3 who may benefit from early high dose thiamine (200mg/d p.o.) and biotin (10mg/kg/d p.o.) supplementation.

Very-long-chain fatty acids (VLCFA) in plasma are the key metabolite to test for peroxisomal disorders, but the metabolite pattern may vary depending on single enzyme defects or peroxisomal biogenesis defects in which all biochemical functions are affected. Rarely, additional testing of pristanic and phytanic acid in plasma and determination of VLCFA in fibroblasts may be needed. While Zellweger syndrome, due to a peroxisomal biogenesis disorder, is recognizable by dysmorphic signs and multi-organ involvement, single enzyme defects, such as peroxisomal Acyl-CoA-oxidase deficiency, can manifest with isolated, profound hypotonia.

In every child with early developmental impairment (EDI) or intellectual disability, organ systems have to be checked thoroughly. For example, a male with hypotonia, brittle hypopigmented hair, and skin laxity could have Menkes disease due to mutations in the X-linked *ATP7A* gene and determination of copper and ceruloplasmin in serum will be helpful to establish a diagnosis. A male with congenital cataracts and muscular hypotonia may have Lowe syndrome and should be checked for aminoaciduria.

INTELLECTUAL DISABILITY WITH OR WITHOUT MICROCEPHALY

While intellectual disability is a frequently encountered problem, only 3% of its underlying aetiology is caused by IEM. Nevertheless, metabolic disorders deserve a one-time diagnostic test in order not to miss treatable conditions. Conditions with epilepsy as the main presenting symptom are covered in Chapters 16 and 20. Phenylketonuria can still be named as a paradigm for preventable cognitive impairment caused by IEM. More recently discovered entities with specific treatment options are defects in serine biosynthesis, that may also lead to congenital or secondary microcephaly and epilepsy. Supplementation with L-serine, 200 to 600mg/kg/day, and evt. L-glycine will improve cognitive outcome and seizure activity. Intellectual disability and microcephaly, usually associated with seizures, are also a hallmark of glucose transporter deficiency, and warrant simultaneous determination of cerebrospinal fluid (CSF) and blood glucose or genetic testing of the glucose transporter deficiency type 1 (GLUT1) gene, including multiplex ligation-dependent probe amplification (MLPA) analysis to cover for deletions. In GLUT1 deficiency, early initiation of a ketogenic diet leads to marked clinical improvement. Microcephaly, EDI and intellectual disability can also be a sign of defects in homocysteine metabolism, as cobalamin C- or methylenetetrahydrofolate reductase (MTHFR) deficiency. As a result of the increasing popularity of vegan diets, nutritional vitamin B12 deficiency is becoming more common than IEM, affecting vitamin B12 metabolism. Serum concentrations of vitamin B12 should be determined in every infant with elevated homocysteine levels, especially when breastfed.

Defects in creatine metabolism may present with primary EDI and intellectual disability, autistic features, expressive speech defects, and epilepsy. Two defects of autosomal recessive inheritance, guanidinoacetate methyltransferase deficiency, and L-arginine: glycine amidinotransferase (GAMT and AGAT), affect creatine synthesis, while the most prevalent defect is an X-linked defect of creatine transport. Magnetic resonance spectroscopy (MRS) may reveal decreased creatine levels in grey matter in all three disorders. Oral supplementation of creatine (300–400mg/kg/d) is beneficial in AGAT and GAMT deficiency, but unfortunately the X-linked creatine transporter defect is not amenable to treatment, at least in males.

Diagnostic tests in a child with suspected intellectual disability should comprise analysis of plasma amino acids, acylcarnitines, plasma homocysteine, urinary organic acids, purine, and pyrimidines in urine, guanidinoacetate in urine, or plasma as well as a urinary creatine/creatinine ratio. As some patients with mucopolysaccharidosis have very subtle or sometimes no signs pointing towards a storage disorder, measurement of urinary glycosaminoglycans is also recommended. Diagnosis of serine deficiency as well as of GLUT1 deficiency warrants simultaneous sampling of blood followed by a spinal tap in the unfed state with determination of the blood to CSF glucose ratio and amino acids.

MULTISYSTEM DISEASE WITH OR WITHOUT DYSMORPHIC SIGNS

Many IEM manifest as multisystem disorders. The most prevalent group of mitochondriopathies has an estimated incidence of 1:10 000 and can present with 'any symptom in any organ at any age'. Manifestations of mitochondriopathies are more prevalent in organs with high energy demand, such as the brain, the retina, the kidney, and the heart. Nystagmus with neonatal liver failure may also eventually be seen by the child neurologist for consultation and is indicative of a distinct mitochondrial depletion syndrome due to defects in DGUOK. Lactate is the most important biomarker to test for mitochondriopathies but is not necessarily elevated and should be determined in CSF whenever possible. Elevated CNS/CSF lactate can also be detected by MRS, but is nonspecific and can also be elevated in non-mitochondrial disorders (e.g. Krabbe disease). The genetic background of mitochondriopathies is complex, as some disorders are caused by mutations or deletions of mitochondrial DNA (mtDNA) inherited from mothers only, while the majority are caused by nuclear genes encoding respiratory chain enzymes, assembly factors for the formation of the different complexes, import of cofactors, or replication of mtDNA. Disorders affecting mtDNA can lead to recognizable syndromic manifestations, such as maternally inherited Leigh syndrome, or entities manifesting later in life, such as Kearns–Sayre syndrome and mitochondrial encephalomyopathy, lactic acidosis, and stroke-like episodes (MELAS) syndrome. Treatment options in mitochondriopathies are emerging, as some patients benefit from cofactor therapy with selected vitamins such as thiamine or riboflavin, coenzyme Q10, or a 1:1 modified Atkins diet.

Carbohydrate deficiency glycoprotein (CDG) syndromes are another continuously growing group of IEM with multisystem involvement. Glycosylation defects may affect N- or O-glycosylation with more than 100 genes known to date. Patients with N-glycosylation defects present with muscular hypotonia, strabismus, and feeding difficulties from an early age. Additional manifestations are manifold, including hepatopathy, coagulation defects, hormonal disturbances, and skin as well as skeletal anomalies. The most prevalent type is CDG1a, due to phosphomannomutase (PMM2) deficiency. Patients have typical gluteal fat pads and inverted nipples as subtle, but highly suggestive signs. Cardiac MRI (cMRI) may show cerebellar hypoplasia/atrophy. The pattern of transferrin isoforms in plasma by high-performance liquid chromatographic or electrophoresis serves as a screening test for N-glycosylation defects and allows distinction of two groups (type I or type II pattern), which guides further molecular work-up. Treatment is purely symptomatic, aside from SLC35A2 CDG syndrome that presents with EDI, epilepsy, facial dysmorphism, and skeletal involvement and may respond to oral galactose. Patients with O-glycosylation defects can present with muscular hypotonia, arthrogryposis, seizures, eventual eye involvement, and complex brain malformation such as cobblestone lissencephaly or hindbrain malformation. This group of O-glycosylation disorders comprises congenital muscular dystrophies with serum CK elevation, which may easily be missed in the complex clinical presentation. The most severe forms are Walker-Warburg syndrome and muscle eye brain disease. Isoelectro focusing of serum apolipoprotein C-III serves as a screening test, but is only able to detect a minority of these patients, while the rest are identified by NGS techniques. Recently, combined N- and O-glycosylation defects have been described with cutis laxa and hypotonia as dominant clinical features.

Gaucher syndrome type II is the most severe form of glucocerebrosidase deficiency with onset within the first few months of life. Children show visceromegaly, strabismus, dysphagia, and spasticity and have to be diagnosed by enzymatic analysis.

Zellweger syndrome (ZS) is a well-known metabolic disorder that often allows diagnosis at a glance. Newborn infants present with massive hypotonia, broad forehead, and ptosis. Cataracts and hepatorenal cysts can be found and cMRI reveals perisylvian polymicrogyria leading to therapy resistant epilepsy. Stippling of the patella is another suggestive sign and easily proven on X-ray. ZS is the most severe form of peroxisomal biogenesis defects and leads to the absence of all peroxisomal enzymes with elevation of VLCFA, but also pristanic, phytanic, and pipecolic acid in plasma. Patients with peroxisomal bifunctional protein deficiency are clinically undistinguishable from classic ZS, but VLCFA in plasma may be normal, while pristanic acid is elevated. Diagnosis may need additional biochemical testing in fibroblasts. Treatment is purely symptomatic and the life span is markedly reduced.

Smith–Lemli–Opitz (SLO) syndrome is caused by a defect in cholesterol synthesis. Patients present with typical facial features including ptosis, tented mouth, anteverted nares, microcephaly, syndactyly of toes, and hypospadia. Patients may have brain malformation affecting the corpus callosum, cerebellum, or frontal regions of hemispheres or have simple holoprosencephaly. Plasma cholesterol is markedly decreased, while 7- and 8-dehydrocholesterol in urine is markedly increased. Treatment with cholesterol (50–100mg/kg/) and simvastatin (0.5–1mg/kg/d) can be beneficial in less severely affected cases.

Some lysosomal storage disorders may manifest in the neonatal period or even as hydrops fetalis. In mucolipidosis, patients show coarse facial features and skeletal involvement, while patients with mucopolysaccharidosis type I (MPS I) present with hernia, macrocephaly, frequent upper respiratory tract infections, and, eventually, spinal deformities, before signs of CNS involvement become more obvious.

IEM WITH NEURODEGENERATION

This group is characterized by a short span of typical early development, followed by neurological regression, usually initiated by a period of slowed developmental progress and plateauing. MRI pattern recognition is an important clue to diagnosis.

Disorders mainly affecting grey matter manifest with cognitive decline, seizures, and often affect the retina.

Early infantile neuronal ceroid lipofuscinosis (NCL) manifests with secondary micro-cephaly and seizures as well as retinitis pigmentosa, which may be easily missed in the beginning. Electroretinogram is superior to fundoscopy in detecting retinitis pig-mentosa. Infants with GM2 gangliosidosis present at the age of 4 to 8 months with macrocephaly, developmental plateauing, and typical acoustic myoclonus with lack of habituation upon repetition. Cherry red spot may be present from age 4 months and precede obvious visual impairment. Both NCL and GM2 gangliosidosis can be con-firmed only by enzyme analysis.

Canavan disease presents with psychomotor regression from the age of 3 to 4 months, followed by progressive visual impairment, epilepsy, and macrocephaly. Diagnosis is suspected by organic acid analysis or MRS with elevated N-acetylaspartate in grey mat-ter.

Disorders affecting white matter lead to spasticity, while cognition is initially preserved and seizures only occur in the later course of the disease. Krabbe disease and mitochon-drial disorders are included in the list as IEM causing early onset leukodystrophies, while some entities, such as vanishing white matter, are pure genetic disorders and not considered as metabolic diseases.

Some disorders, such as Pelizaeus–Merzbacher disease, affect the formation of myelin and follow-up MRI is required to distinguish delayed myelination from primary hypo-myelination. In white matter disorders, the MRI is usually markedly abnormal. The pattern of leukodystrophic changes, if interpreted by experienced neuroradiologists or clinicians, may allow recognition of the underlying disease, as is the case in Krabbe disease or in Canavan disease.

In grey matter disorders, MRI changes can be very subtle in the initial phase and altered signal intensity of white matter may be present. The later stages of grey matter dis-orders are typically accompanied by marked brain atrophy, which is nonspecific. A cherry red spot is a hallmark of lysosomal storage disorders such as GM2 gangliosidosis,

Niemann-Pick, and Farber disease and fundoscopy is mandatory in every infant with developmental decline.

RESOURCES

Agana M, Frueh J, Kamboj M, Patel DR, Kanungo S (2018) Common metabolic disorder (inborn errors of metabolism) concerns in primary care practice. *Ann Transl Med* 6(24): 469. Open access at http://atm.amegroups.com/article/view/23102/html

eVM — Vademecum Metabolicum. An excellent free App for iOS (also available for Android): https://apps.apple.com/us/app/evm-vademecum-metabolicum/id1123172322

Gene reviews. Open access at https://www.ncbi.nlm.nih.gov/books/NBK1116/advanced/

van Rijt WJ, Koolhaas GD, Bekhof J, et al. (2016) Inborn errors of metabolism that cause sudden infant death: a systematic review with implications for population neonatal screening programmes. *Neonatology* 109(4): 297—302. Open access at https://www.karger.com/Article/FullText/443874

CHAPTER 16

Neonatal seizures

Barbara Plecko

Key messages

- Electroencephalogram is mandatory to diagnose neonatal seizures.
- Neonates with recurrent seizures need to be admitted to an intensive care unit.
- Exclusion of hypoglycaemia, electrolyte imbalance, infectious work-up, and cranial imaging are mandatory first line investigations.
- About 10% to 20% of neonates with recurrent seizures of unclear aetiology need extended second-line investigations to identify metabolic or genetic causes of their epilepsy, some of which are amenable to specific treatment.

Common errors

- Subtle seizures are often unrecognized.
- Physiological episodic phenomena may be over diagnosed as seizures.

When to worry

- Seizures are resistant to therapy.
- History of siblings with neonatal seizures and poor prognosis.

DEFINITIONS

The newborn period is defined as the first 4 weeks of life and comprises the time of birth, postpartum adaptation, and first weeks of infantile development. The estimated incidence of neonatal, clinically recognized seizures is around 2% in infants born at term and around 5% to 13% in neonates with a birthweight <1500g. According to the clinical setting, one can distinguish three scenarios:

- Clinical seizures diagnosed by observation only;

- Electroclinical seizures documented by observation and ictal electroencephalogram (EEG) patterns; and

- Electrographic seizures with an ictal EEG pattern with a duration >10 seconds but no clinical correlate.

It is common for neonatal seizures to be very subtle and for nonconvulsive seizures to remain largely unrecognized by pure clinical observation. On the other hand, there is also a tendency to overestimate physiological episodic phenomena as being of epileptogenic nature.

Therefore, the clinical diagnosis of neonatal seizures is unreliable and EEG investigations are mandatory in every newborn infant with unclear, episodic phenomena. If the newborn infant shows signs of neurological impairment in between seizures, the diagnosis of epileptic encephalopathy is made.

A newborn infant with recurrent seizures should be admitted to a neonatal intensive care unit for continuous monitoring of vital signs (i.e. heart rate, respiratory rate/apnoeas, oxygen saturation, blood pressure).

CLINICAL APPROACH

Recognition of neonatal seizures can be difficult and needs a high degree of suspicion whenever episodic or repetitive patterns are observed clinically. Neonatal seizures are usually focal, brief, and subtle with motor automatism and eye blinking or eye opening. As the newborn infant's brain is largely unmyelinated and synapses are still immature, generalized seizures are not seen in this young patient group. Involvement of all four extremities at that age rather represents bilateral epileptic discharges with some degree of synchrony. While clonic seizures are easily recognized clinically and electrographically, myoclonic, tonic, or subtle seizures (as listed in Table 16.1) may need repeated EEG recordings to prove their epileptogenic nature.

In infants born at term, subtle seizures are by far the most common seizure type (Table 16.1). In infants born preterm the prevalence of seizure types differ, about 50% are clonic, 33% tonic, 26% are subtle, and 10% are myoclonic. Autonomic signs (increase/decrease in heart rate, blood pressure, etc.) along with seizures are more frequent in infants born preterm (37%) than in infants born at term (6%).

Combinations of episodic symptoms are more likely than single symptoms to represent seizure events. On the other hand, some nonepileptic episodic phenomena may be distinguished from seizures by clinical criteria. Jitteriness is distinguished from clonic seizures by preceding triggering stimuli, interruption by changes in position, and lack of abnormal eye movements. Sleep myoclonus is distinguished from seizures by its occurrence only during rapid eye movement sleep phase I, the non-stereotyped clonic jerks mainly affecting the upper limbs, but also the legs and face, with normal muscle tone in between the myoclonus.

Table 16.1 Different seizure patterns according to clinical recognition and the consistency of typical ictal electrographic patterns

Semiology	Ictal EEG correlate	Aetiology
Clonic (25–30%) (focal, segment-ary, or bilateral)	+++ repetitive spikes	Various, frequent in stroke
Myoclonic (15–20%) erratic, frag-mentary, or more generalized	— to +++	Various, frequent in meta-bolic disorders
Tonic (5%) (resembling decerebrate rigidity)	— to +++ rhythmic Delta activity	Most often structural brain anomalies
Subtle seizures 50–70% (nystag-mus, tonic eye deviation, blinking, limb posturing, pedalling move-ments, repetitive sucking/chew-ing, recurrent apnoea, vasomotor change)	— to ++ flattening of EEG (more than one EEG tra-cing may be needed to show epileptic discharges)	Various, frequent in HIE

Numbers in brackets are estimates of respective frequencies in neonates born at term (Pitt and Pressler, 2005). ++, frequent feature; —, absent; +++, prominent feature. EEG, electroencephalogram; HIE, hypoxic-ischaemic encephalopathy.

NEONATAL SEIZURE SYNDROMES

According to the International League Against Epilepsy (ILAE), there are three epilepsy syndromes that manifest within the first 4 weeks of life.

Benign familial neonatal seizures (BFNS) have their onset between day 2 and day 15 of life with very frequent focal tonic and bilateral clonic seizures. Neurological status is normal and seizures remit spontaneously. EEG shows frontal spikes propagating to temporal zones. Family history is positive and in keeping with autosomal domi-nant inheritance. The prognosis is favourable in most cases. BFNS are caused by muta-tions in either of two genes (*KCNQ2* or *KCNQ3*), both of which encode voltage-gated potassium channel subunits.

Early myoclonic encephalopathy (EME) seizures consist of fragmentary myoclonic jerks. EEG shows a burst-suppression pattern. The aetiology is variable and includes cortical dysgenesis and also metabolic disorders, such as pyridoxine-dependent epilepsy (PDE) and nonketotic hyperglycinaemia.

Early infantile encephalopathy with epilepsy (EIEE) is also called Ohtahara syndrome. Patients have tonic spasms and bilateral seizures, indistinguishable from West syndrome. EEG shows a burst suppression pattern and from age 4 to 6 months may develop into typical hypsarrhythmia and West syndrome. The causal background is heterogeneous (brain malformations, Aicardi syndrome, dentate-olivary dysplasia) and prognosis is usually poor.

EEG

Video EEG over 40 to 60 minutes including a sleep phase, is standard for investigating seizures in the neonate. Because of the small head size, the number of electrodes is reduced to nine: four on each side in temporoparietal row and one as Cz. Experience and knowledge of normal EEG patterns in neonates born at term and preterm is required, as pathological paroxysmal features are not easily recognized in this young age group.

In the neonatal period discharges are frequently focal with decreasing prevalence from temporal to occipital and to central and frontal in term as well as infants born preterm. Usually there is abnormal background activity in interictal periods. Infants born at term produce sharp waves, spikes, and sharp and slow waves at the onset of seizures, while rhythmic delta activity is the most common ictal pattern in infants born preterm. In both groups, ictal patterns may vary in frequency, morphology, duration, or propagation during a single event or from one seizure to another. Seizures tend to be longer (around 10min) in term than in neonates born preterm (2−3min). There is no correlation of EEG patterns, onset of seizures, or frequency to the underlying aetiology. Status epilepticus (SE) is diagnosed in newborn infants if there is over 50% spike wave activity in a 30-minute EEG tracing and is more frequent in infants born at term. Severely abnormal background activity usually indicates poor prognosis, unless attributable to drugs (e.g. phenobarbitone, morphine, surfactant, etc.).

CORRELATION OF EEG AND CLINICAL SEIZURES

It is a common problem that clonic seizures are often clinically recognized, while subtle seizures easily escape clinical detection (Malone et al. 2009, Murray et al. 2008). When matching EEG data to clinical video observation, only 27% of seizure events were diagnosed correctly. As neonates have spikes and waves as physiological EEG patterns, rhythmic activity over 10 seconds plus clinical symptoms have to be present to diagnose an electroclinical seizure. Therefore, ictal EEG recording is of utmost importance. Conventional EEG (cEEG) is able to detect about 90% of seizure events correctly, as most seizures propagate to the surface in neonates. In certain circumstances cEEG may show ictal events without clinical seizures. These so called 'electrographic-only' events are mostly seen after the administration of antiepileptic drugs (electroclinical uncoupling) or with very high seizure activity (e.g. SE). It is likely that these purely electrographic seizures impact long-term prognosis and should be treated with anticonvulsants.

Amplitude-integrated EEG (aEEG) is an established method for long-term monitoring of neonates at risk or under treatment for repeated seizures. Single channel aEEG (Figure 16.1) will pick up about 25%, while two channel aEEG will pick up about 50% of seizures. This gross limitation is due to restriction of seizure detection to the central zone and to the fact that low amplitude spike wave discharges escape detection by aEEG.

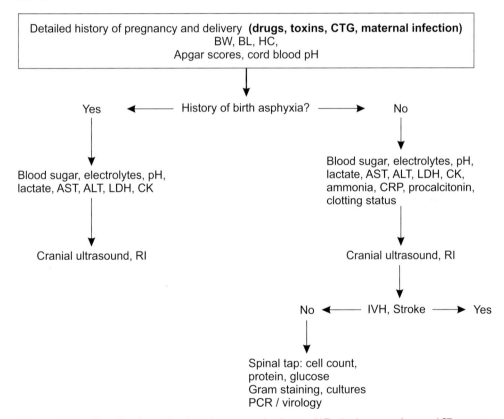

Figure 16.1   First-line investigations in neonatal seizures ALT, alanine transferase; AST, aspartate transferase; BL, birth length; BW, birthweight; CK, creatine kinase; CRP, C-reactive protein; CTG, cardiotocography; HC, head circumference; IVH, intraventricular haemorrhage; LDH, lactate dehydrogenase; PCR, polymerase chain reaction; RI, resistance index.

COMMON AETIOLOGIES OF NEONATAL SEIZURES

Neonatal seizures are rarely idiopathic and therefore need a standardized first and second line diagnostic work-up (Figures 16.1 and 16.2).

The most common causes of neonatal seizures are:

- birth asphyxia,

- intracranial haemorrhage (if born preterm) or ischaemic stroke (if born at term), and

- central nervous system (CNS) infection.

As seizures have the potential to induce apoptosis they represent an independent and often additional threat to the developing brain. When seizures are observed in a newborn infant, easily treatable causes have to be considered first. Immediate assessment of blood sugar and electrolytes will help to detect underlying hypoglycaemia, hypo- or hypernatremia, hypocalcaemia, or hypomagnesemia. Imbalance of glucose or electrolytes are usually part of a more complex derangement, such as preterm birth, infection, anoxia, or intracranial haemorrhage, and should not be considered as isolated conditions unless proven otherwise.

For the following section it is recommended that locally established normal laboratory values be considered, taking into account whether the infant is born at term or preterm, as well as strict dependency on postnatal age in days (Rennie, 2012).

Hypoglycaemia is frequently seen in infants born preterm and is associated with seizures in about 50% of cases. Correction and maintenance of normal blood glucose levels is mandatory in every newborn infant.

Hyponatraemia may occur in association with intracranial haemorrhage or CNS infections, most likely due to inappropriate secretion of antidiuretic hormone (ADH). It may also occur with excessive fluid restriction or fluid replacement lacking electrolytes (e.g. pure 5% or 10% dextrose) or as a result of appropriate ADH secretion in response to loss of intravascular volume (e.g. into a large cephalhaematoma) or dehydration.

Hypernatremia may be caused by excessive administration of sodium bicarbonate to buffer acidosis or by dehydration.

Hypocalcaemia is largely prevented by adequate calcium and phosphorous supply in the parenteral or enteral nutrition. While early hypocalcaemia within the first days of life is difficult to treat, later occurrence around day 7 has a favourable response.

Hypomagnesemia can present with focal or multifocal convulsions along with restlessness as an isolated finding in the occasional patient and responds well to intravenous or oral correction.

BIRTH ASPHYXIA

Around 50% to 75% of neonatal seizures are caused by birth asphyxia and about 64% of asphyxiated neonates will experience seizures. Asphyxiated neonates usually start seizing before day 2, when acute cell death and damage by secondary cytotoxins has reached its maximum impact. Head cooling or whole body cooling has clearly reduced seizure burden and the overall prognosis of asphyxiated infants born at term. Seizure semiology is variable and ictal EEG is necessary to assess the epileptic character of the clinical manifestations and to detect subtle seizures or even non-convulsive SE. Interictal background activity at age 1 week is a helpful prognostic marker for outcome in children who experienced perinatal asphyxia. Seizures in asphyxiated neonates are often accompanied by other signs, such as apathy, hypo- or hypertonia, absence of Moro reflex, and bulbar signs, indicating hypoxic-ischaemic encephalopathy (HIE).

Caution should be exercised when ascribing seizures to hypoxia/asphyxia as this may prevent patients from receiving a correct diagnosis of an eventually treatable condition such as meningitis or genetic conditions such as PDE. To attribute seizures to an anoxic event a careful history of peripartum risk factors has to be taken (i.e. dips on cardiotocography, meconium staining, abruption of placenta, cord prolapse, slow or fixed fetal heart rate, prolonged labour, Apgar scores, cord blood pH). Usually, but not always, asphyxiated neonates suffer from involvement of organs other than the CNS (e.g. transient renal failure or cardiac insufficiency). High plasma lactate is a sign of anaerobic glycolysis.

High blood concentrations of lactate dehydrogenase and creatinine kinase may reflect tissue damage and, though nonspecific, serve as laboratory indicators of birth asphyxia. Cranial imaging by ultrasound, computed tomography (CT), or magnetic resonance imaging (MRI) may reveal blurring of the posterior part of the internal capsule or diffuse brain oedema and a high resistance index, indicating poor cerebral perfusion. Cranial ultrasound, as a bedside method, allows serial investigation with minor burden for the patient, while for CT and MRI, the burden of transport and sedation has to be weighed against the higher diagnostic yield of these imaging techniques. Neonatal MRI may be done in a 'feed and wrap' setting without sedation or anaesthesia. Whenever possible CT should be avoided because of the associated irradiation of the newborn infant's brain.

STROKE

Around 15% to 30% of neonatal seizures are due to ischaemic infarction, with or without sinus venous thrombosis or intracranial haemorrhage, the latter especially in infants born preterm. These events usually occur between day 1 and 5 of life. Seizures are usually focal, clonic, unilateral, and more stereotyped and rarely lead to SE. The ictal EEG may show spikes in the Rolandic region and the interictal EEG is asymmetric with unilateral or focal continuous or discontinuous abnormal patterns. In contrast to asphyxiated neonates, patients with haemorrhage or ischaemic stroke do not show signs of encephalopathy. Focal neurological deficits, if they are to appear, often do not become evident before 3 to 4 months corrected age. Nevertheless, intraventricular haemorrhage associated with repeated convulsions in an infant born preterm indicates a rather poor prognosis. Cranial ultrasound is a suitable method to detect most intra-cerebral haemorrhages and infarctions, with less sensitivity for events of the posterior fossa or pathology close to cortical areas or in the subdural and subarachnoid spaces.

CNS INFECTIONS

Besides asphyxia and stroke as the two major causes of neonatal seizures, meningitis or encephalitis have to be considered. Intracranial infections account for 3% to 20% of neonatal seizures in different reported series (Shellhaas, Glass, and Chang, 2018). CNS infections usually occur during the first week of life, especially after day 2 or 3. Meningitis may be part of systemic septicaemia, as in E. coli sepsis of the newborn infant, but may occur as an isolated meningitis, especially with Citrobacter or Proteus mirabilis. Viral infections in the newborn infant are mainly caused by Toxoplasma gondii, rubella, herpes simplex I and II, cytomegalovirus, or coxsackie B. In the absence of a suggestive history of birth asphyxia and after having obtained normal imaging on cranial ultrasound, every newborn infant with unexplained seizures should undergo a lumbar puncture (Figure 16.1).

RARE AETIOLOGIES OF NEONATAL SEIZURES

In neonates with repeated seizures but a normal birth history and normal first-line investigations, rare aetiologies have to be considered, especially if seizures are therapy-resistant. In this situation, second-line investigations have to be performed (Figure 16.2), taking into consideration:

- metabolic-genetic disorders,

- other chromosomal/genetic disorders, and

- cerebral dysgenesis.

Metabolic disorders are genetically determined inborn errors of metabolism that usually have a biomarker in urine, plasma, or cerebrospinal fluid (CSF). As some metabolic conditions manifesting with neonatal epilepsy are amenable to treatment, they have to be considered in every newborn infant with therapy-resistant seizures of unknown aetiology (Dulac et al. 2014). Only early detection will enable optimal outcome. The following entities have been selected either because they have treatment options available or because they are relatively common.

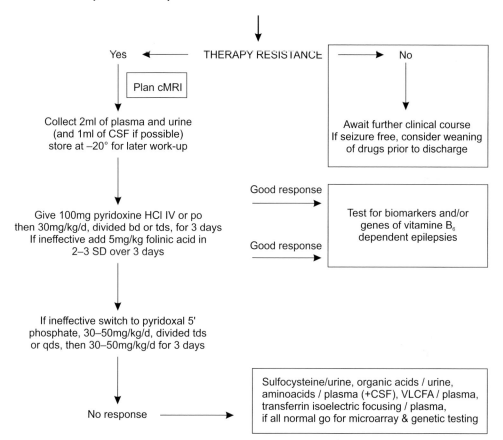

Figure 16.2 Second-line investigations and cofactor trials in neonatal seizures. cMRI, cranial magnetic resonance imaging; CSF, cerebrospinal fluid; HCl, hydrochloride; IV, intravenous; po, *per os*; SD, single dosages; VLCFA, very-long-chain fatty acids.

Vitamin B$_6$ (pyridoxine)-dependent epilepsies (PDE)

PDE is one of the more common vitamin responsive encephalopathies. We now know of four metabolic-genetic-defects that can manifest with neonatal seizures and have a positive response to vitamin B$_6$ (Table 16.2).

Table 16.2 Biomarkers for vitamin B_6-dependent epilepsies with neonatal onset

Disorder	Urine	Plasma	CSF	Gene
PNPO def.	(vanillactate)	pyridoxamine	pyridoxamine	PNPO
CH		Alk Phosph, Ca, Ph, PLP		ALPL
Antiquitin def.	AASA, P6C (PA)	AASA, (PA)	AASA, PA	ALDH7A1
PLPBP def.	–	–	–	PLPBP

CSF, cerebrospinal fluid; PNPO, pyridox(am)ine 5'-phosphate oxidase deficiency; def., deficiency; CH, congenital hypophosphatasia; Alk phosph, alkaline phosphatase; Ca, calcium; Ph, phosphate; PLP, pyridoxal 5'-phosphate; AASA, alpha-aminoadipic semialdehyde; PA, pipecolic acid; PLPBP, pyridoxal 5'-phosphate-binding protein.

Vitamin B_6 is an important cofactor in neurotransmitter and amino acid metabolism. The underlying genetic defects cause either reduced formation, or inactivation, or reduced cellular uptake or impaired intracellular homeostasis of pyridoxal 5'-phosphate (PLP, the active form of vitamin B_6) and can be differentiated by specific biomarkers (Table 16.2). Pyridoxine hydrochloride is the most common available vitamin B_6 compound for oral or intravenous administration, while PLP is available as a chemical compound for oral administration only in most countries outside of Asia. It is important to have a protocol in place for a standardized trial of vitamin B_6 (Figure 16.2). The first administration of vitamin B_6 can lead to apnoea and comatose state, thus resuscitation equipment should be at hand. If patients have a favourable response to vitamin B_6, diagnosis should be confirmed by genetic testing and treatment should not be withdrawn because of the risk of seizure recurrence within days to weeks. All four disorders described below will need lifelong treatment with supra-physiological doses of vitamin B_6, while common anticonvulsants may be tapered and discontinued.

Antiquitin deficiency

The majority of PDE cases are caused by an autosomal recessive defect of antiquitin, an enzyme involved in the lysine degradation pathway, causing endogenous inactivation of PLP by accumulating compounds. The incidence is 1:64 000. About 30% of patients have a history of complicated delivery, leading the clinician to misattribute seizures as being symptomatic of HIE. Abdominal distension and vomiting, as well as hypoglycaemia and lactic acidosis have been reported. Therapy-resistance, systemic signs, sleeplessness, and erratic myoclonus resembling drug-withdrawal should alert the clinician to test for pyridoxine dependency. Patients with antiquitin deficiency need lifelong pyridoxine therapy with the usual maximal daily dose being 200 to 300mg, divided into two to three doses. Dosages above 500mg/day may lead to sensory or even motor neuropathy, which in most cases is reversible. Despite early specific treatment, about 70% of patients have intellectual disability of varying degree. Add-on of a lysine-restricted diet or high dose arginine supplementation to improve developmental outcome are under investigation.

Pyridoxal phosphate-dependent epilepsy

This autosomal recessive disorder is caused by pyridox(am)ine 5′-phosphate oxidase (PNPO) deficiency and impaired formation of PLP. It has been differentiated from PDE in that seizures are resistant to pyridoxine but do respond to the administration of PLP. About 70 patients have been reported so far with therapy-resistant, neonatal, mainly myoclonic seizures often accompanied by burst suppression pattern on EEG. Preterm birth and fetal distress are common. Oral (or intravenous) administration of PLP at 30 to 50mg/kg/day, divided into three to four doses, leads to cessation or clear reduction of seizures and improvement of EEG activity. It has become apparent that about half of the patients with PNPO deficiency have residual enzyme activity and show pyridoxine-responsiveness. With early treatment, outcome can be more favourable than previously assumed. As PLP may be hepatotoxic, the powder should be dissolved immediately before administration, the lowest effective dose used, and transaminases and liver function checked regularly.

Congenital hypophosphatasia

Patients with congenital hypophosphatasia (CH) suffer from poor bone mineralization due to an autosomal recessive defect of tissue-nonspecific alkaline phosphatase (TNSALP). TNSALP also regulates the cellular uptake of PLP, thus the severe form of the disease may present with neonatal pyridoxine-responsive seizures before skeletal problems become apparent. Alkaline phosphatase levels in serum are markedly reduced. Aside from pyridoxine-responsive seizures, patients with CH may suffer from a lethal brainstem degeneration. A recently licensed enzyme replacement therapy is not expected to treat CNS manifestations of the disease, as it does not cross the blood–brain barrier.

Pyridoxal 5′-phosphate-binding protein deficiency

Pyridoxal 5′-phosphate-binding protein (PLPBP) (previously published as PROSC) deficiency is a recently discovered defect causing vitamin B_6 dependent epilepsy due to impaired intracellular PLP homeostasis. The clinical presentation is indistinguishable from antiquitin and PNPO deficiency but about 40% of published cases have congenital or acquired microcephaly. In contrast to the above mentioned entities, PLPBP deficiency has no specific biomarker. Patients may respond to pyridoxine or PLP.

Biotinidase deficiency

This disorder affects the recycling of biotin (vitamin H), an essential cofactor of many carboxylases in glucose, protein, and lipid metabolism. As it is easily treatable, biotinidase deficiency is included in the neonatal screening programmes of many countries. Seizures have been recognized as the presenting symptom in 38% of 78 patients and are accompanied by other symptoms such as muscular hypotonia or breathing problems. Seizures are mainly myoclonic and resistant to anticonvulsant therapy in about 50% of cases. Analysis of urinary organic acids by gas chromatography will reveal elevated lactate, 3-OH iso-valeric acid, methylcitrate, and methylcrononyl-glycine, but as these metabolic findings vary, measurement of biotinidase in serum is used to establish the diagnosis. Oral treatment with biotin, 5 to 10mg/day leads to complete resolution of symptoms if started early.

Molybdenum cofactor and isolated sulphite oxidase deficiency

Patients with molybdenum cofactor deficiency (MoCD) as well as with isolated sulphate oxidase deficiency (iSOD) present with feeding difficulties and neonatal tonic—clonic seizures with a high tendency towards SE. MRI shows toxic brain oedema followed by extensive cystic white matter changes and global brain atrophy. Molybdenum (Mo) acts as a cofactor of three different enzymes involved in cysteine degradation. It has been shown that the neurological phenotype is due to impairment at the step of sulphite oxidation. Synthesis of Mo cofactor is encoded by three different genes (*MOCS1*, *MOCS2*, and *GEPH*). Elevated sulphocysteine serves as a reliable diagnostic biomarker for MoCD as well as of iSOD, while a bedside sulphite dipstick test in urine may give false positive as well as false negative results. In MoCD, low urinary uric acid and homocysteine in plasma, as well as elevated xanthine and hypoxanthine in urine can be found. The diagnosis is confirmed by molecular testing. Two thirds of patients with MoCD have mutations in *MOCS1* and lack molybdenum cofactor precursor Z. These patients with MoCD type A can be treated by daily intravenous infusions of purified cyclic pyranopterin monophosphate (cPMP). The window of opportunity is short as irreversible brain injury may occur within days to weeks after onset.

Nonketotic hyperglycinaemia

Nonketotic hyperglycinaemia (NKH) is one of the more frequent metabolic epilepsies but is unfortunately untreatable as it affects a nonessential amino acid. The autosomal recessive defect leading to NKH is located in one of the four subunits of the glycine cleavage system. Patients with NKH usually present a few days after birth with severe epileptic encephalopathy, profound hypotonia, chronic hiccups, and myoclonic jerks accompanied by prolonged apnoea. In the surviving patients the initial burst suppression pattern evolves into hypsarrhythmia and infantile spasms by around 3 months of age. Elevated plasma and CSF glycine as well as an increased CSF:plasma ratio >0.08 in the classic and >0.04 in atypical forms, are diagnostic of NKH. Diagnosis needs to be confirmed by molecular analysis and eventually by enzyme assay in lymphoblasts. A protein-restricted diet, administration of sodium benzoate for alternate glycine elimination, and dextromethorphan, an NMDA receptor antagonist, have been tried without convincing results in typical NKH cases; however, they seem to be promising in atypical cases if implemented early. Beyond these listed entities where neonatal seizures are the hallmark of a metabolic-genetic disease, seizures can be part of the clinical spectrum in other treatable or untreatable metabolic disorders such as urea cycle defects, propionic- or methylmalonic acidaemia, peroxisomal disorders, or congenital disorders of glycosylation syndromes. These disorders have to be considered, if the extended routine laboratory investigation reveals hyperammonaemia or metabolic acidosis. Measurement of ammonia needs rapid processing and cooling to avoid false elevation caused by storage at room temperature.

Chromosomal anomalies with neonatal seizures

Chromosomal lesions leading to epilepsy can be divided into three major subgroups: duplication syndromes, where additional genetic material is present; deletions, where a segment of genetic material is lost; and disruption, where only one or a few genes are affected. If dysmorphic features are present along with epilepsy, the likelihood of chromosomal anomalies is about 50%. Some of those chromosomal disorders are associated with brain malformation.

Disorders of cerebral dysgenesis

Several disorders of cerebral dysgenesis can manifest with neonatal seizures with a broad spectrum ranging from focal cortical dysplasia to more generalized syndromes such as lissencephaly or double cortex. MRI is superior to CT in detecting areas of cortical dysplasia and should be the investigation of choice in this selection of patients. As subcortical U-fibres are largely unmyelinated until the end of the second year of life, discrimination of cortical dysplasia may change with age and repeated MRI may be necessary in 6 to 9 month intervals if no other explanation has been identified. Complex brain malformation is often caused by chromosomal or monogenetic defects and parents need genetic counselling for further family planning. Table 16.3 lists some chromosomal abnormalities associated with brain malformation. These anomalies can be detected by chromosomal microarray analysis.

Table 16.3 Chromosomal anomalies associated with cortical malformations

Condition	Chromosomal anomaly
Lissencephaly	Mille—Dieker syndrome (del17p13.3)
Polymicrogyria	1p36 deletion
	Monosomy 1q44
	Duplication 11q12—11q13
	Monosomy 3p
	Trisomy 5p
	Partial monosomy 18p
	Partial monosomy 21q
	22q deletion
	Duplication 3q
Double cortex	Trisomy 9p
Heterotopia	Deletion 4q
	Ring 17
	Trisomy 13
	Trisomy 19
	69XXX

A growing number of genes are being identified that regulate neuronal migration and cortical structures. Mutations in these genes (e.g. *TUBA1A*, *LIS1*, *ARX*, etc.) can occur de novo or, rarely, be present as gonadal mosaicism and cause severe congenital brain malformations that are only detected by Sanger sequencing of single genes, gene panel analysis, or next generation sequencing (NGS).

MONOGENIC EPILEPTIC ENCEPHALOPATHIES

The past decade has unravelled a rapidly growing list of monogenic disorders with neonatal onset of epileptic encephalopathies without gross structural defects that are caused by mutations in various genes encoding ion channels (e.g. KCNQ2, SCN2A, SCN8A), synaptic vesicle trafficking (e.g. STXBP1) or regulatory proteins (e.g. CDKL5). Recognition by epileptic phenotype or EEG patterns is hardly possible and diagnostic work-up warrants application of larger gene panels or NGS. Inheritance can be auto-somal recessive or sporadic; genetic counselling is based on the identification of the respective gene mutation in the index patient.

TREATMENT OF NEONATAL SEIZURES

Every newborn infant, born at term or preterm, that suffers from recurrent seizures should be admitted to a neonatal intensive care unit for monitoring of vital signs.

The drug most commonly used in the treatment of neonatal seizures is phenobarbitone (Phb), even though studies on its effect were disappointing and animal studies have shown apoptosis in the presence of very high concentrations. In many countries it is still used as a first-line drug and a loading dose of 40mg/kg will lead to cessation of seizures in about 50% of patients with neonatal seizures. Maintenance dosage should keep phenobarbitone plasma levels around 25mcg/ml Electroclinical uncoupling is frequent and aEEG or daily EEG studies should be performed to detect electrographic-only events. There is no guideline supporting the use of phenobarbitone for the pre-vention of seizures in high-risk neonates. Phenytoin will stop neonatal seizures in around 45% of patients. The usual loading dose is 15 to 20mg/kg with a maximum speed of 1mg/kg/min and ECG monitoring to monitor for cardiac arrhythmia. Because of its non-linear pharmacokinetics and variable protein binding in affected neonates, phenytoin is more difficult to handle and its impact on cerebellar growth is a potential serious side effect.

A 2004 Cochrane review reported poor efficacy of combination therapy of phenobar-bitone plus phenytoin (Booth and Evans, 2004). This unsatisfactory situation has led to the use of benzodiazepines, especially clonazepam or midazolam, as second-line drugs in many European countries (Vento et al. 2010). Clonazepam at a dosage of 0.1mg/kg has been effective in newborn patients unresponsive to phenobarbitone. Midazolam with an initial bolus of 0.15mg/kg followed by dosages up to 0.1mg/kg/h by continu-ous infusion was highly effective in a non-randomized study. Continuous administra-tion of benzodiazepines can lead to apathy, poor feeding, and apnoea and may aggrav-ate sleep myoclonus.

There are recent reports on the successful use of off-label, newer antiepileptic drugs, such as levetiracetam (10mg/kg on day 1, 20mg/kg on day 2, and 30mg/kg on day 3) or topiramate (1mg/kg with stepwise increase to 4mg/kg/day), in neonates with refractory seizures, but no formal studies have been performed. Neonates with repetitive tonic, asymmetric seizures may have KCNQ2 mutations and benefit from carbamazepine. Valproate is not recommended for the treatment of neonatal seizures because of poten-tial hepatotoxicity.

About 48% of infants born preterm but only 30% of infants born at term with neonatal seizures will develop epilepsy in later life. No antiepileptic therapy has yet been shown to be effective in the prevention of later-onset epilepsy. This has led to the more recent practice of discussing the weaning and discontinuation of anticonvulsant therapy before discharge from hospital in patients who are seizure-free and have a normal EEG record.

In the presence of therapy-resistant neonatal seizures it is strongly recommended to consider treatable inborn errors of metabolism and to give a standardized vitamin trial with pyridoxine and/or PLP and eventually folinic acid as soon as one, or a maximum of two, conventional drugs have failed. To prevent irreversible brain injury in children with potentially treatable disorders such as PDE, this trial has to be undertaken early during the course of disease, as proposed in Figure 16.2.

REFERENCES

Booth D, Evans DJ. (2004) Anticonvulsants for neonates with seizures. *Cochrane Database Syst Rev* (4): CD004218.

Dulac O, Plecko B, Gattaulina S, Wolf NI (2014) Occasional seizures, epilepsy, and inborn errors of metabolism. *Lancet Neurol* 213: 727—739.

Malone A, Ryan CA, Fitzgerald A, Burgoyne L, Connolly S, Boylan GB. (2009) Interobserver agreement in neonatal seizure identification. *Epilepsia* 50: 2097—2101.

Murray DM, Boylan GB, Ali I, Ryan CA, Murphy BP, Connolly S. (2008) Defining the gap between electrographic seizure burden, clinical expression and staff recognition of neonatal seizures. *Arch Dis Child Fetal Neonatal Ed* 93: F187—91.

Pitt M, Pressler R (2005) Neurophysiological testing in the newborn infant. *Early Hum Dev* 81: 939—946.

Rennie JM (2012) *Rennie and Robertson's Textbook of Neonatology*, 5th edn. London; Churchill Livingston.

Shellhaas RA, Glass HC, Chang T (2018) Neonatal Seizures In: Swaiman KF, Aswhal S, Ferriero DM, et al. eds *Swaiman's Pediatric Neurology* 6th edn, p 130 (Table).

Vento M, de Vries LS, Alberola A, et al. (2010) Approach to seizures in the neonatal period: a European perspective. *Acta Paediatr* 99: 497—501.

Resources

Mathis D, Beese K, Rüegg C, Plecko B, Hersberger M (2020) LC-MS/MS Method for the Differential Diagnosis of Treatable Early Onset Inherited Metabolic Epilepsies. *J Inherit Metab Dis* https://doi.org/10.1002/jimd.12244[Epub ahead of print]

Ramantani G, Schmitt B, Plecko B, et al. (2019) Neonatal seizures. Are we there yet?*Neuropediatrics* 50: 280—93.

Wheless J, Willimore J, Brumback RA, eds (2009) *Advanced Therapy in Epilepsy*. New York: McGraw Hill.

Wilson MP, Plecko B, Mills PH, Clayton P (2019) Disorders affecting vitamin B6 metabolism. *J Inherit Metab Dis* 42: 629—646.

CHAPTER 17

Acute encephalopathy and traumatic brain injury

Tiina Talvik, Fenella Kirkham, Tuuli Metsvaht, and Inga Talvik

---

Key messages

Acute encephalopathy

- Altered level of consciousness is the essential clinical feature of acute encephalopathy.
- In infants, look for disturbed behaviour, poor feeding, irritability, and high-pitched cry.
- Recognize extraocular palsies, facial weakness, hemiparesis, and seizures.
- Recognize decorticate or decerebrate (extensor) posturing, loss of pupillary reflexes.
- Always measure blood glucose and ammonia.
- Treat for bacterial meningitis, Herpes simplex encephalitis; consider anti-tuberculous therapy.
- Emergency computed tomography or magnetic resonance imaging is essential.
- Provide supportive intensive care, whatever the cause.
- Seek specialist help when you suspect an inherited metabolic or genetic syndrome.

Traumatic and inflicted traumatic brain injury

- Distinguish inflicted head injury from accidental traumatic head injury.
- Inflicted injury requires multidisciplinary management.

Common errors

Acute encephalopathy

- Missing meningitis/encephalitis is a very common error — beware!
- Withholding antimicrobial treatment if infection is a possibility: if in doubt, treat.
- Performing lumbar puncture without neuroimaging when Glasgow Coma Scale <9 or brainstem signs.

Traumatic and inflicted traumatic brain injury

- Misinterpreting history given by caregivers.
- Failing to diagnose fractures caused by previous abuse.
- Failing to identify retinal haemorrhages.

When to worry

- Lethargy, coma, progressive decrease in level of consciousness.
- Restlessness in an infant with depressed level of consciousness.
- Hypotension; bradycardia with hypertension.
- Persistent seizures or status epilepticus not controlled with medication.
- Persistent vomiting, recurrent apnoeas, forced downgaze (sunsetting).
- Emergence of focal neurological symptoms or extensor posturing.
- Acute hemiplegia.
- Acute focal or generalized seizures.
- Acute acquired encephalopathy/injury without reasonable explanation.
- Inconsistent history from caregivers following trauma.

DEFINITION

Acute encephalopathy refers to a state of rapid deterioration of brain functions, almost always presenting as an alteration in the state of conscious level, which may or may not be accompanied by focal neurological signs.

CAUSES

There are many possible causes of acute encephalopathy, the two most frequently encountered being traumatic brain injury (TBI) and infection. A recent study of 130 children from four resource-limited settings in Africa identified 45% of cases as TBI and 55% as infective encephalopathy. In this chapter, traumatic, metabolic, toxic, and cerebrovascular causes are considered. Infection and postinfective causes are considered in Chapter 19; non-infectious causes that may mimic infection are considered in this chapter. It is important to note, however, that cases of acute infective encephalopathy with rapid deterioration, and even death, may occur without fever (e.g. there have been recent reports of this due to shigellosis and salmonellosis with only mild diarrhoea). Neoplastic and systemic conditions are also possible causes, but will not be considered in this chapter.

The initial differential diagnosis of acute encephalopathy is usually based on the presence or absence of fever and neuroimaging findings (Figure 17.1). However, remember that in infancy, sepsis may present with temperature instability rather than fever.

GENERAL PRINCIPLES OF MANAGEMENT

The key to rational assessment of the clinical state of the infant is systematic examination, with repeated recording of level of consciousness, pupillary responses, pulse, respiratory rate, and blood pressure. The simple AVPU scale (awake; responds to verbal stimulus; responds to pain; completely unresponsive) may be used in the emergency department but on admission to the paediatric department, assessment of consciousness should be based on observable behavioural responses to stimulation: eye opening, verbal response, and motor response that in combination make up the Glasgow Coma Scale (GCS). In infants the scoring is modified to be age-appropriate (Table 17.1). A total score is obtained by summing the scores on the eye opening, verbal, and motor subscales, but the three clinical observations that constitute the subscale scores are more informative than the total score.

CLINICAL ASSESSMENT OF A CHILD WITH ACUTE ENCEPHALOPATHY

History of the present illness and previous medical and family history, medication/access to medication in the household that may have been accidentally ingested, and history of illness in contacts are all potentially relevant. In the youngest children, the symptoms and signs may be subtle, such as poor feeding or poor social cognition, and easily missed by caregivers.

On examination, assess level of consciousness using the GCS. Assess airway, breathing, and circulation. Measure the blood pressure. In addition, look for a rash (purpuric in meningococcal infection or bleeding disorders, variable in viral infection); signs of inflicted injury or neglect; cardiac murmurs; signs of lower respiratory tract infection (tuberculosis, mycoplasma, pneumococcus); hepatosplenomegaly; any other diagnostic clues on general examination. Measure the occipitofrontal head circumference (OFC) with a disposable paper measuring tape and plot on the centile chart that is

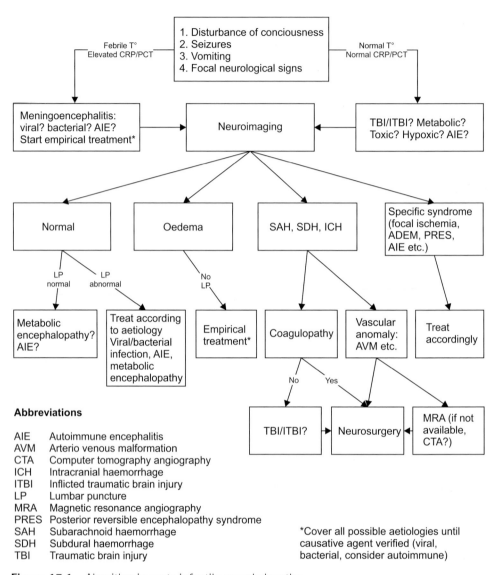

Figure 17.1   Algorithm in acute infantile encephalopathy

appropriate for age and sex: macro- or microcephaly are potentially relevant. Note any separation of the cranial sutures, which may signify intracranial hypertension. Fullness and firmness of the anterior fontanelle, examined, if possible, with the infant supported in a sitting position, can be a useful additional sign. The fontanelle may be sunken in several acute intracranial events.

Table 17.1 Glasgow Coma Scale modified for infants

Eye opening	Spontaneous	4
	To verbal stimuli	3
	To pain only	2
	No response	1
Verbal response	Coos and babbles	5
	Irritable cries	4
	Cries to pain	3
	Moans to pain	2
	No response	1
No response	Moves spontaneously and purposefully	6
	Withdraws to touch	5
	Withdraws in response to pain	4
	Pathological flexion in response to pain	3
	Extension in response to pain	2
	No response	1

Raised intracranial pressure (ICP) may accompany both traumatic and non-traumatic acute encephalopathies. Low cerebral perfusion pressure (CPP; i.e. arterial blood pressure minus ICP) leads to cerebral ischaemia and has consistently been shown to be an important determinant of outcome following TBI and non-TBI in children. Individualized autoregulation-guided CPP management in patients with severe TBI may be of benefit (Donnelly et al. 2017). Cerebral ischaemia itself causes cerebral oedema, which compounds the rise in ICP from other causes (e.g. trauma, metabolic derangement). A progressive, uncontrolled increase in ICP ultimately causes death by brainstem compression.

Persistent unexplained vomiting, loss of upgaze, or forced downgaze (sunsetting) may indicate increasing pressure on the tegmentum caused, for example, by hydrocephalus. If the infant is awake but drowsy, try to assess eye movements. Depressed level of consciousness may be associated with focal neurological signs or with abnormal posturing to noxious stimulation. This may be decorticate (flexion of the upper limbs and extension of the lower limbs, also referred to as pathological flexion) or decerebrate with extension of all four limbs. The emergence of such signs and/or abnormal respiratory patterns may indicate life-threatening deterioration.

Laboratory and radiological assessment of a child with acute encephalopathy

Remember the value of simple laboratory tests: white cell count (and increase in immature cells or 'shift to the left') may be seen in infection or prolonged seizure; acute-phase proteins such as C-reactive protein; cell count in the cerebrospinal fluid (CSF); CSF protein; paired plasma and CSF glucose (you cannot interpret one without the other); lumbar CSF pressure measured with a manometer or, more easily in an infant, with a tape measure held next to a vertically orientated, sterile, thin-bore flexible plastic tube (e.g. intravenous [IV] giving set), attached via a three way tap to the lumbar puncture needle.

Tests for non-infective causes of meningitis/meningo-encephalitis should include consideration of antibody-mediated illness (autoimmune encephalitis, see Chapter 19) and haemophagocytic lympho-histiocytosis (HLH). In practice, investigation for a possible infective cause (see Chapter 19) may also be required.

Ultrasound is good for defining the size of the cerebral ventricles, but less informative in describing extra cerebral and subdural spaces or abnormalities of the cerebral parenchyma. Therefore, computed tomography (CT) or magnetic resonance imaging (MRI) are needed to confirm ultrasound findings. MRI is the method of choice in children; CT has better availability and is often possible to perform without sedation, therefore, CT is used in acute settings for the rapid detection of intracranial blood and oedema. However, the risks of a high radiation dose must be kept in mind when evaluating young children. If the CT is normal, cranial MRI is mandatory in cases of acute encephalopathy, except when there is known trauma that is likely to explain the clinical condition of the child.

Clinical management of a child with acute encephalopathy

The GCS score (Table 17.1) and vital signs should be systematically monitored over time. If seizures are a feature, does the infant return to his or her usual self between seizures? Identify seizure type, duration, any localizing features, conscious level, and responsiveness between seizures. If the GCS is <8 or there is a decreasing level of consciousness, admit the patient to the intensive care unit and manage airway. Restore normal circulating blood volume and manage seizures and CPP.

A child with encephalopathy needs empirical treatment at presentation, often several days before a definitive diagnosis is available. When an infective cause is suspected, an antimicrobial and aciclovir as an antiviral should be commenced. Recommended antimicrobial regimens include ampicillin and an aminoglycoside such as gentamicin. However, resistance of *Escherichia coli* to ampicillin has been reported. Cefotaxime is often added, although resistance to this antibiotic has also been reported.

If there is acute hydrocephalus, consider investigation and treatment for tuberculous meningitis in addition. Better outcome is associated with the starting of appropriate therapy before the conscious level deteriorates (see Chapter 19).

Status epilepticus is less likely to be refractory to medical therapy if treated early with appropriate medication (Table 17.2) (see also Chapter 20).

Table 17.2 2 Anticonvulsants used for seizures with acute encephalopathy

Drug	Route of administration	Paediatric dose adminis- tration
Drugs used as first line treatment of status epilepticus		
Diazepam Rectal	IV bolus	0.25—0.5mg/kg 0.5—0.75mg/kg*
Lorazepam	IV bolus	0.1mg/kg
Midazolam	Buccal, nasal IV	0.15—0.3mg/kg* 0.1mg/kg
Drugs in established status epilepticus or acute encephalopathy with seizures		
Phenytoin	IV infusion	20mg/kg at 1mg/kg/min
Phenobarbital	IV bolus	15—20mg/kg
Levetiracetam**	IV over 5 mins	40mg/kg

IV, intravenous. * May be repeated. ** Lyttle et al. (2019).

Management of intracranial hypertension

Consideration of surgical placement of an ICP monitor is desirable but not possible in some clinical settings. Management aims to optimize CPP and reduce ICP. Methods include positioning (head straight, trunk and head at 30° to horizontal); temperature regulation to avoid fever (and, in post-hypoxic brain injury, controlled normo- or mild hypothermia to 33—34 °C; see also discussion of hypothermia in Chapter 14; note that therapeutic hypothermia is not useful and may even be harmful in TBI); sedation with or without muscle relaxation; external ventricular drainage of CSF; operative decompression; osmotherapy with hypertonic saline or, for acute short-term management of an emergency, mannitol.

Hyperventilation is no longer recommended as the resulting vasoconstriction can worsen cerebral ischaemia. PCO2 target should be set around 35mmHg, but lower values may be accepted for short period(s) of time, e.g. to gain time until surgery can be performed. Early consultation with neurosurgical colleagues is important for early discussion of ICP monitoring and/or surgical removal of space occupying causes of ICP (e.g. extradural haematoma, large tumour or drainage if hydrocephalus is present) and/or surgical decompression. There is possible benefit of decompressive craniectomy (DC) in traumatic and nontraumatic coma for both survival rates and long-term outcome of survivors. Similarly, DC may result in improved outcome in children with elevated ICP regardless of underlying cause and even with unilateral or bilaterally dilated pupils present as a result of brain herniation. It may also be used as rescue therapy when maximal conservative measures for reduction of ICP have failed. However, as the operation is associated with complications, careful individual assessment of each situation is necessary. Boluses of glycerol or mannitol achieve transient reduction in ICP; there is, however, a risk of a significant 'rebound' (i.e. subsequent rise in ICP). The role of this treatment is, therefore, confined to severe acute deterioration due to raised ICP, to buy time to institute other measures to reduce ICP. Hypertonic saline has achieved faster and greater reduction in ICP and is associated with the most favourable effect on the cerebral circulation. In non-traumatic acute encephalopathy, hypertonic saline is associated with lower mortality when compared to mannitol or normal saline. The benefit is sustained for longer when given as a continuous infusion.

SPECIFIC NONINFECTIOUS ACUTE ENCEPHALOPATHIES THAT MAY MIMIC INFECTION

Infection and postinfective causes are considered in Chapter 19.

Haemopha-gocytic lympho-histiocytosis (HLH) may cause meningoencephalitis and significant neurological sequelae. The term HLH encompasses the recessively inherited primary form, familial HLH (or FHL) — mostly affecting young children — and secondary HLH — predominantly associated with infections or malignancies. Common features are fever, pancytopaenia, hypertriglyceridaemia, hypofibrinogenaemia, and hepatosplenomegaly. The majority have a pronounced inflammatory response with high blood concentrations of cytokines and ferritin in association with deficient lymphocyte cytotoxic activity. Importantly, they also develop meningoencephalitis that may be severe. About 66% will have neurological symptoms — with seizures, meningism, and irritability being the three most common — and/or abnormal CSF findings at the time of diagnosis. CT and MRI findings of HLH are ring-enhancing parenchymal lesions (at times calcified), which are nonspecific and mimic abscesses. In the immunosuppressed child increased diffusion at the centre on diffusion-weighted imaging may help differentiate these lesions from an abscess, which has restricted diffusion at the centre. Prompt treatment (etoposide and marrow transplantation) of active HLH at onset or relapse may reduce neurological sequelae, and this is important to consider in undiagnosed encephalopathy.

In long-term survivors, neurological sequelae – usually neurodevelopmental impairment and epilepsy – are reported in approximately 15% of cases. Late sequelae affect approximately 25% of those with abnormal CSF at onset and are about three times as common as in those with normal CSF. Approximately 75% of children aged less than 12 months at the time of diagnosis have abnormal CSF without any neurological symptoms.

Aicardi–Goutières syndrome is a rare, genetically determined disorder with a phenotype classically characterized by episodic acute irritability with or without fever. It is associated with elevated levels of interferon in the CSF and often with an increased CSF white cell count. Chilblains and other skin manifestations may be seen (see also Chapter 19, Differential diagnosis and Chapter 23, Other investigations).

Acute necrotizing encephalopathy (ANE) is predominantly a disease of infants and young children. It is characterized by fever, acute encephalopathy, seizures, and rapid progression to coma within days of onset of a viral illness; more frequently influenza A, but also influenza B, parainfluenza, human herpesvirus 6, and others.

T2-weighted cranial MRI classically shows multiple symmetrical lesions affecting primarily the thalami but also the upper brainstem tegmentum, periventricular white matter, putamina and cerebellum (Figure 17.4 e1). A genetic form of the disease, ANE1, is recognized with mutations in the gene Ran Binding Protein 2 (*RANBP2*; OMIM 601181). The thermolabile polymorphism in the Carnitine Palmitoyltransferase 2 (*CPT2*) gene is also associated with this condition and other acute encephalopathies.

Acute disseminated encephalomyelitis (ADEM) is a monophasic inflammatory multifocal demyelinating disorder of the CNS, usually appearing after an infection and by definition including a degree of encephalopathy (i.e. alteration/depression of conscious level). It is a rare disorder and very unlikely to present in the first year of life. There may also be focal neurological signs. MRI typically shows multifocal large areas of demyelination in white matter but grey matter involvement (e.g. lesions in thalamus and basal ganglia; Figure 17.4 d1) also occurs. Diagnosis is based on the combination of clinical and radiological features and exclusion of diseases that mimic ADEM. Treatment is with intravenous methylprednisolone 30mg/kg, up to a maximum dose of 1g/day, for 3 to 5 days (level of evidence, class III). Higher doses have been used in severe forms of steroid-resistant post-infectious encephalomyelitis. This is usually followed by oral steroid (prednisone 1mg/kg/d) tapered over 4 to 6 weeks, but might be unnecessary if symptoms improve. Monitor for hyperglycaemia, hypokalaemia, high blood pressure, and mood disorders. Outcome is usually favourable, with good functional recovery and mortality rates less than 5%. Recently, ADEM has been found to be associated with myelin oligodendrocyte (MOG) antibodies in over 50% of children under 11 years old.

These children have a higher rate of relapse, or develop other demyelinating disorders (Hacohen and Branwell, 2019).

Posterior reversible leukoencephalopathy syndrome (PRES) is a condition also recognized on the basis of encephalopathy with the classic clinical signs such as seizures, visual disturbances, headache, impaired consciousness, associated with high signal change (vasogenic oedema) on MRI, involving the white matter in parieto-occipital areas (with frequent involvement of the frontal lobe; Figure 17.4 c2, c3). Both hemispheres are usually affected, albeit often asymmetrically. Risk factors include hypertension, hypotension, treatment with tacrolimus, cyclosporin, cyclophosphamide, methotrexate, and some of the newer immunosuppressive and antineoplastic agents. It is very rare in the first year of life. PRES is most often associated with leukaemia/lymphoma (up to 72% of cases) complicating the course of 2.1% to 4.5% of children with acute lymphoblastic leukaemia, and less often associated with solid tumour or non-malignant diseases (HLH/thalassemia major/sickle cell disease [SCD]/Fanconi anaemia/congenital dyskeratosis/megakaryocytic thrombocytopenia).

Mild encephalitis/encephalopathy with reversible splenial lesion (MERS) has been described in the context of viral and bacterial infections in children. The common neurological symptoms include seizure, behavioural changes, altered consciousness, and motor deterioration. The lesions may be in the splenium or other parts of the corpus callosum and show hyperintensity on T2-weighted and fluid-attenuated inversion recovery (FLAIR) sequences with corresponding reduced diffusion (Figure 17.4 c1).

Vaccinations and acute encephalopathy

Recent reviews of cases of long-term neurological impairment with onset of acute epileptic encephalopathy immediately following diphtheria-tetanus-pertussis (DTP) vaccination have found that the majority of these had a *SCN1A* gene deletion. They were, in fact, cases of Dravet syndrome (see Chapter 20) and their neurological outcome was no different from those with the same gene deletion, but in whom the onset of seizures was unrelated to vaccination. There are isolated reports of aseptic meningitis, without any known long-term sequelae, following measles, mumps, and rubella (MMR) vaccination. The risk is less than 1 in 534 000 vaccinations. Research in the 1990s suggesting a link between vaccination and autism has now been discredited and the publications retracted. The resulting debate on this issue led to a large amount of high-quality epidemiological research that has provided reassurance that there is no such link. There is no evidence of increased risk of encephalopathy after DTP/Haemophilus influenzae B (Hib) or MenC vaccines 15 to 35 days after MMR vaccine.

Migraine

Migraine may present as encephalopathy, with or without hemiplegia, but it is a diagnosis of exclusion. There is usually a parent with migraine. Electroencephalography may be asymmetrically slow and diffusion-weighted MRI may show focal abnormality (Figure 17.4 a3).

TBI AND INFLICTED TBI

Definitions

TBI results from external force being absorbed by cranial and intracranial structures. It may be closed or penetrating. It is a major cause of death and disability worldwide, especially in infancy and childhood. TBI is characterized by extra or subdural haemor-rhages, often accompanied by cerebral contusion.

TBI including inflicted TBI

Causes in infancy include falls, or being a passenger in a road traffic accident, but the focus should always be on safeguarding and whether the infant is the victim of deliber-ate inflicted TBI (ITBI). ITBI may be caused by direct impact or shaking, often accom-panied by areas of hypoxia-ischaemia. Pathological data indicate that ITBI is probably a better term than the previously used 'shaken-baby syndrome' as it does not suggest that there is only a single mechanism by which brain injury is caused. The level of viol-ence used is recognized by others as excessive, dangerous, and likely to harm the child.

Caregivers at risk of abusive behaviour generally have unrealistic expectations of their children and may exhibit a role reversal whereby the caregivers expect their needs to be met by the child. Professionals should be aware that a crying infant is at higher risk of ITBI, especially when parents are complaining of excessive crying and are in a social position that could put pressure on the family situation. The actual duration of crying at a given moment seems to be less relevant than the parents' perception of the crying over the long term.

Epidemiology of TBI

The incidence of TBI in childhood is high and higher if measured prospectively rather than retrospectively (Table 17.3). TBI is an increasing cause of death in resource-poor countries and is the underlying cause in almost half of acute encephalopathies.

Clinical approach

Take a careful and exact history. Look for consistency in accounts given by the dif-ferent people involved. Does their version of events stay constant? Assess the injury: open, closed, or penetrating? Focal or diffuse? Associated soft-tissue trauma; damage

Table 17.3 Incidence of traumatic brain injury by region

Location	What is measured	Rate	
South West England and Wales, UK	SDH under 1 year of age	21 per 100 000	Jayawant et al. (1998)
Scotland, UK	SDH under 1 year of age (retrospective)	11.2 per 100 000	Barlow, Milne, and Minns (1998)
Scotland, UK	SDH under 1 year of age (prospective)	24.6 per 100 000	Barlow and Minns (2000)
North Carolina, USA	Hospital surveillance (prospective)	29.7 per 100 000	Keenan et al. (2003)
Canada	Hospital surveillance (retrospective)	40 cases/year	King et al. (2003)
Germany	Estimation	100—200 per year	Matschke et al. (2009)
Switzerland	Nationwide	14 per 100 000 live births	Fanconi and Lips (2010)
New Zealand		14.7—19.6 per 100 000	Kelly and Farrant (2008)
Estonia	Retrospective	13.5 per 100 000	Talvik et al. (2006)
Estonia	Prospective	40.5 per 100 000	Talvik et al. (2006)

SDH, subdural haemorrhage.

to internal organs? Focal neurological signs? Are subtle seizures contributing to apparent depression of consciousness? ITBI is often seen in association with bruising, a torn frenulum, retinal haemorrhages, and fractures of long bones or ribs.

Investigation of TBI

- Blood clotting screen.

- Ophthalmoscopy (retinal haemorrhage in ITBI).

- Cranial CT scanning. CT to verify the possibility of intracranial haemorrhage (see Table 17.4) and brain oedema remains the first choice in all trauma patients with a GCS <15 or in a high risk category, including children (Shavit et al. 2019). Among 13 000 children with negative CT, no patient required operation later. If CT and clinical findings (in suspected ITBI also skeletal survey and retina) are normal no further investigations are needed.

- MRI. MRI of the head is needed within 2 to 5 days if CT is abnormal or if initial CT is normal but clinical evaluation is/remains abnormal or the patient presents in the subacute stage. In case of suspected ITBI and spinal cord injury (e.g. flaccid quadriplegia), MRI of the whole spine may be required urgently. MRI must include T2*-weighted imaging or susceptibility-weighted imaging (SWI) sequences and diffusion-weighted imaging (DWI) that are sensitive to small haemorrhages. MRI is more sensitive than CT for evaluation of diffuse axonal injury with small haemorrhages, brain oedema, and infarctions. Note that between 5 to 10 days MRI and DWI findings may 'pseudo-normalize' and after 14 to 21 days longer-term changes, such as atrophy and encephalomalacia, may develop. Repeat the MRI despite normalized/normalizing clinical signs, if initial CT or MRI scans show abnormalities.

- Other imaging points

    o Spinal cord injury without radiographic abnormalities (SIWORA) is often seen in paediatric trauma patients. A large head compared to body size applies great forces to the neck in case of shaking or severe trauma.

    o Cranial ultrasound in young infants (screening), but should be followed by CT or MRI in suspected ITBI as subdurals are not excluded.

    o Skull X-ray is not recommended in TBI as it is unreliable in predicting the presence and degree of brain injury. In 15% to 30% of cases, skull fracture is associated with intracranial injury. Almost 50% of intracranial injuries occur without fracture and 21% of fractures detected with CT are missed by X-ray.

    o Skeletal survey in traffic trauma or suspected ITBI, including repeat chest X-ray at 7 days for rib fractures that are not apparent on initial X-ray; in 30% to 40% of children with inflicted injuries, signs of previous inflicted injury are present: e.g. old fractures, chronic subdural haemorrhage.

    o Ultrasound and/or CT of abdomen.

Management

Assess the level of consciousness with the GCS (Table 17.1). If GCS score is <8 or there is a deteriorating conscious level, admit to the intensive care unit and manage the airway. Restore normal circulating blood volume and manage seizures and CPP. In possible ITBI, involve the interdisciplinary safeguarding team, which will include not only relevant nursing and medical members of the hospital team but also a family doctor that knows the family, and other agencies that will keep the child safe at home. This will vary by country but may include a social worker and a police officer with specialist safeguarding training and experience.

Table 17.4   Causes of intracranial haemorrhage in infancy

Cause	Clinical or imaging feature	Possible other features	Comment/ management
Inflicted	SDH, ICH	External signs of abuse, inconsistent history, discrepancy between history and injury severity	Abdominal trauma, skeletal survey CT, MRI, surgery if necessary
Trauma	SDH, EDH, ICH	External signs of trauma	CT, surgery if necessary
Haemorrhage	SDH, ICH, SAH	Signs of bleeding outside the CNS (e.g. nosebleed) and/or bruising, CNS parenchymal haemorrhage; bruises	Coagulation profile
Stroke including AVM/VST	SDH, ICH, SAH	Focal neurological signs	MRI, MRA
Infection	SDH	Fever; differentiate focal infection from meningitis (see Chapter 19)	Enhancement with contrast, lumbar puncture if not contraindicated
Metabolic disorder	SDH, ICH	Previous developmental impairment or arrest	MRI, metabolic screening

AVM, arteriovenous malformation; CNS, central nervous system; CT, computed tomography; EDH, extradural haemorrhage; ICH, intracranial haemorrhage; MRA, magnetic resonance angiography; MRI, magnetic resonance imaging; SAH, subarachnoid haemorrhage; SDH, subdural haemorrhage; VST, venous sinus thrombosis.

Outcome of TBI and inflicted brain injury

The majority of children with ITBI have poor outcomes. About 20% die and only 20% survive without impairment. The remainder have impairments in their motor and cognitive abilities, language, vision, and behaviour. These impairments affect future educational and social attainment. The reasons for the poor outcomes in infants and children who sustain ITBI are not known but are probably attributable to associated ischaemia and hypoxia.

ACUTE METABOLIC ENCEPHALOPATHIES

The clinical presentation in children with a metabolic encephalopathy is nonspecific. In neonates it usually occurs after a symptom-free period following delivery. Poor feeding, vomiting, central hypotonia with limb hypertonia, abnormal movements followed by seizures and coma may occur (see Chapter 15). In older infants, it may be associated with periods of metabolic stress (e.g. fasting, intercurrent infection). Inborn errors of metabolism should always be considered in children — and especially infants — with unexplained changes in their conscious level, alongside CNS infections (bacterial or viral), haemorrhage, hypoxia and/or ischaemia, or suspected poisoning.

Management

Supportive management is as for any child with an encephalopathy. Specific therapy depends upon the underlying disorder and the biochemical abnormalities. The three main biochemical disturbances associated with an encephalopathy due to inherited errors of metabolism are hypoglycaemia, hyperammonaemia, and metabolic acidosis. Therefore, the important investigations are ammonia, glucose, pH, serum lactate, and organic acids (see also Chapter 15 for a fuller discussion).

The most common causes of severe hyperammonaemic encephalopathy in children are enzyme deficiencies of the urea cycle (Figure 17.2), which functions to convert highly toxic ammonia arising from the catabolism of amino acids to non-toxic urea. Hyperammonaemia may also occur in children with organic acidaemias and, less commonly, in fat oxidation disorders. The outcome for children with hyperammonaemic encephalopathy is generally poor. However, permanent CNS damage can be limited by a rapid reduction in blood ammonia.

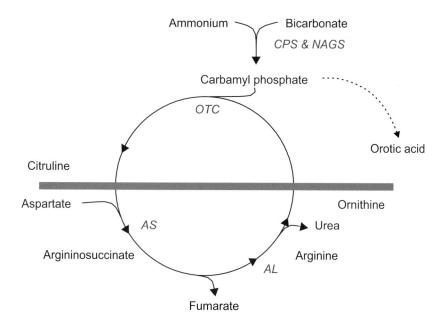

Figure 17.2 The urea cycle. AL, argininosuccinate lyase; AS, argininosuccinate synthetase; CPS, carbamoyl phosphate synthetase; NAGS, N-acetylglutamate synthase; OTC, ornithine transcarbamylase.

Although hypoglycaemia is a common nonspecific feature of many affected infants, it may arise as a result of the following disorders:

- fat oxidation (most common),

- glycogen metabolism,

- gluconeogenesis,

- glucose transport,

- galactose and fructose conversion to glucose, or

- ketone metabolism.

Blood sugar must be measured in the laboratory as well as on BM stix or Dextrostix in any child with an encephalopathy with the following essential investigations:

- true blood glucose,

- lactate,

- free fatty acids, 3-hydroxybutyrate, acyl carnitines,

- insulin, urinary cortisol,

- organic acids,

- later: growth hormone.

Figure 17.3 shows the principles of glucose metabolism. Once identified the principles of management are

- glycogen storage disorders: maintain glucose with nocturnal enteral feeding;

- fatty oxidation defects: regular feeding, give carnitine supplements;

- gluconeogenesis defects: avoid fasting (tolerance increases with age);

- growth hormone/cortisol: replace as appropriate;

- organic acids/amino acids: may be vitamin-responsive, protein restriction;

- galactosaemia/fructosaemia (HFI): avoid galactose/fructose respectively;

- insulin excess: central venous line, glucose — at least 10% but sometimes requires higher concentrations; continuous enteral feeding with a glucose polymer, soma-tostatin, ± diazoxide.

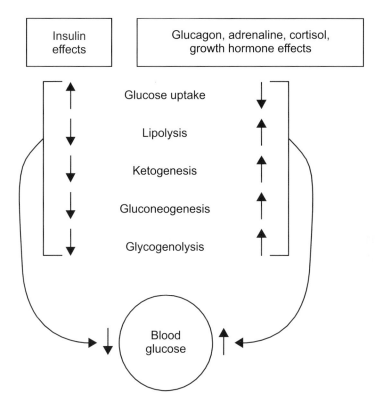

Figure 17.3 The principles of glucose metabolism

Metabolic acidosis is very common in affected infants and children and is most often caused by sepsis, poor tissue perfusion, and/or hypoxia. Severe metabolic acidosis is most often associated with the *organic acidaemias* (mainly propionic and methyl-malonic acidaemia) and *disorders of ketone body utilization*. The absence of acidosis does not exclude these disorders. In contrast to secondary causes of metabolic acidosis, sodium bicarbonate is usually a necessary part of therapy.

Some inborn errors of metabolism present with an acute encephalopathy without prominent biochemical abnormalities of blood glucose, ammonia, or acid/base balance and should still be considered in a child with an unexplained encephalopathy, even if initial biochemical investigations are normal. These include, for example, *pyridoxine-dependent seizures, maple syrup urine disease, sulphite oxidase deficiency*, and *glutaric aciduria type 1* (see Chapter 15). Identification and counselling for any underlying inherited error of metabolism will require the advice of a clinical geneticist.

ACUTE TOXIC ENCEPHALOPATHIES

The most common cause of acute toxic encephalopathy is sepsis, but remember that the crawling infant may be able to access drugs or poisons in the home. Deliberate poisoning will rarely occur.

Figure 17.4 Imaging for diagnosis and differential diagnosis of encephalopathy. T2-weighted magnetic resonance imaging (MRI) unless stated. Viewed from below, i.e. left side is seen as right side of image. Column a: (1) widespread focal cortical involvement (arrow) in Herpes simplex encephalitis in a neonate; (2) oedema/infarction (arrow) in sagittal venous sinus thrombosis secondary to iron deficiency anaemia; (3) parieto-occipital focal oedema consistent with reversible ischaemia (arrow; see also Figure 18.2b) in an unconscious child with unilateral slowing and a family history of hemiplegic migraine.

Column b: focal lesions (1) focus of high signal density in the left frontal white matter (arrow) in a child with anti-N-methyl-D-aspartate receptor antibody encephalitis who recovered after steroids, plasma exchange, and cyclophosphamide; (2) right-sided high signal on T1-weighted imaging (arrow) in a child presenting with hemichorea and a raised antistreptolysin O titre, who recovered after 2 weeks of penicillin and prednisolone; (3) recent large infarct (arrow) in a child presenting with confusion and a reduced conscious level; small strokes rarely cause coma.

Column c: posterior involvement (1) abnormality of splenium bilaterally (arrows) on DWI in a child who recovered rapidly from acute coma; (2) posterior abnormality bilaterally (arrows) consistent with posterior reversible encephalopathy syndrome in an immunosuppressed male with juvenile chronic arthritis and hypertension in whom (3) bilateral border zone ischaemia was demonstrated on DWI (arrows) the day after a period of hypotension.

Column d: thalamic abnormality (1) bilateral thalamic involvement (arrows) in acute disseminated encephalomyelitis after acute otitis media; (2) bilateral thalamic ischaemia (arrows) in a child with (3) venous sinus thrombosis (arrow) and severe iron deficiency anaemia (haemoglobin 4g/dL) who recovered fully after anticoagulation.

Column e: widespread symmetrical abnormality. Fluid-attenuated inversion recovery MRI showing (1) bilateral symmetrical basal ganglia, thalamic, white matter (arrows) and (2) bilateral cerebellar involvement (arrows) in acute necrotizing encephalopathy in a child with acute sepsis for which the differential diagnosis includes (3) Leigh syndrome with bilateral symmetrical basal ganglia involvement (arrows) on computed tomography.

Column f: Cerebellar involvement in (1) cerebellitis with descent of the cerebellar tonsils (arrows) in the context of rising titres to Epstein—Barr virus (2) unilateral infarction (arrow) in a child with (3) basilar occlusion (arrow) which was thrombolysed 11 hours after presentation with good outcome.

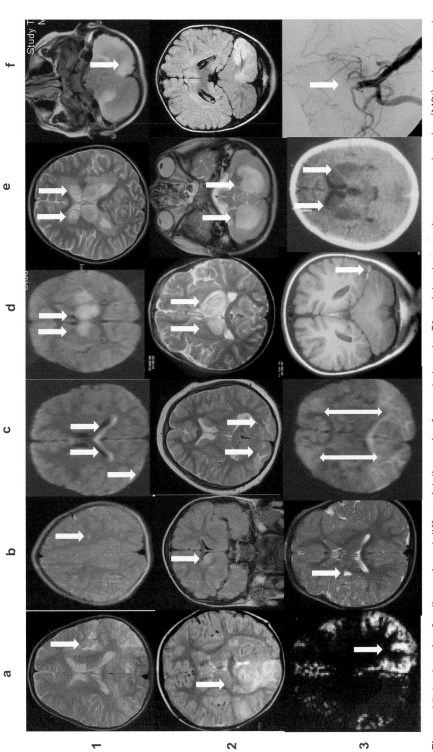

Figure 17.4 Imaging for diagnosis and differential diagnosis of encephalopathy. T2-weighted magnetic resonance imaging (MRI) unless stated. Viewed from below, i.e. left side is seen as right side of image.

REFERENCES

Barlow KM, Milne S, Minns RA (1998) A retrospective epidemiological analysis of non-accidental head injury in children in Scotland over the last 15 years. *Scot Med J* 43: 112—114.

Barlow KM, Minns RA (2000) Annual incidence of shaken impact syndrome in young children. *Lancet* 356: 1571—1572.

Donnelly J, Czosnyka M, Adams H, et al. (2017) Individualizing thresholds of cerebral perfusion pressure using estimated limits of autoregulation. *Crit Care Med* 45: 1464—1471.

Fanconi M, Lips U (2010) Shaken baby syndrome in Switzerland: results of a prospective follow-up study, 2002- 2007. *Eur J Paediatr* 169: 1023—1028.

Hacohen Y, Banwell B (2019) Treatment approaches for MOG-Ab-associated demyelination in child. *Curr Treat Options Neurol* 21: 2.

Jayawant SS, Rawlinson A, Gibbon F, et al. (1998) Subdural hemorrhages in infants: population based study. *BMJ* 317: 1558—1561.

Keenan HT, Runyan DK, Marshall SW, Nocera MA, Merten DF, Sinal SH (2003) A population-based study of inflicted traumatic brain injury in young children. *JAMA* 290: 621—626.

Kelly P, Farrant B (2008) Shaken baby syndrome in New Zealand, 2000-2002. *J Paediatr Child Health* 44: 99—107.

King WJ, MacKay M, Sirnick A; Canadian Shaken Baby Study Group (2003) Shaken baby syndrome in Canada: clinical characteristics and outcomes of hospital cases. *Can Med Assoc J* 168: 155—159.

Lyttle MD, Rainford NEA, Gamble C et al. (2019) Levetiracetam versus phenytoin for second-line treatment of paediatric convulsive status epilepticus (EcLiPSE): a multicentre, open-label, randomised trial. *Lancet* 393: 2125-2134. https://doi.org/10.1016/S0140-6736(19)30724-X

Matschke J, Voss J, Obi N, et al. (2009) Nonaccidental head injury is the most common cause of subdural bleeding in infants<1 year of age. *Pediatrics* 124: 1587—1594.

Shavit I, Rimon A, Waisman Y, et al. (2019) Paediatric Research in Emergency Departments International Collaborative (PREDICT). Performance of two head-injury decision rules evaluated on an external cohort of 18,913 children. *J Surg Res* 245: 426—433.

Talvik I, Metsvaht T, Leito K, et al. (2006) Inflicted traumatic brain injury (ITBI) or shaken baby syndrome (SBS) in Estonia. *Acta Paediatr* 95: 799—804.

Resources

Alnemari AM, Krafcik BM, Mansour TR, Gaudin D (2017) A comparison of pharmacologic thera-peutic agents used for the reduction of intracranial pressure after traumatic brain injury. *World Neurosurg* 106: 509—528.

Banerjee JS, Heyman M, Palomäki M, et al. (2018) Posterior reversible encephalopathy syndrome: risk factors and impact on the outcome in children with acute lymphoblastic leukemia treated with Nordic protocols. *J Pediatr Hematol Oncol* 40: e13—18.

Barthelemy EJ, Melis M, Gordon E, et al. (2016) Decompressive craniectomy for Severe Traumatic Brain Injury: A Systematic Review. *World Neurosurg* 88: 411—420.

Fink EL, von Saint Andre-von Arnim A, Kumar R, et al. (2018) Traumatic brain injury and infectious encephalopathy in children from four resource-limited settings in Africa. *Pediatr Crit Care Med* 19: 649—657.

Paediatric Accident and Emergency Research Group. The management of a child (aged 0-18 years) with a decreased conscious level. An evidence-based guideline for health professionals based in the hospital setting. RCPCH and BAEM 2008 https://www.nottingham.ac.uk/paediatric-guideline/home2.htm

Pinto PS, Meoded A, Poretti A, et al. (2012) The unique features of traumatic brain injury in children: review of the characteristic of the pediatric skull and brain, mechanisms of trauma, patters of injury, complications, and their imaging findings — part 2. *J Neuroimaging* 22: e1—17.

Shein SL, Ferguson NM, Kochanek PM, et al. (2016) Effectiveness of pharmacological therapies for intracranial hypertension in children with severe traumatic brain injury — results from an automated data collection system time-synched to drug administration. *Pediatr Crit Care Med* 17: 236—245.

Talvik I, Alexander R, Talvik T (2008) Shaken baby syndrome and baby's cry. *Acta Paediatr* 97: 782—785.

van der Meer C, van Lindert E, Petru R (2012) Late decompressive craniectomy as rescue treatment for refractory high intracranial pressure in children and adults. *Acta Neurochir Suppl.* 114: 305—10.

Welch TP, Wallendorf MJ, Kharasch ED, et al. (2016) Fentanyl and midazolam are ineffective in reducing episodic intracranial hypertension in severe pediatric traumatic brain injury. *Crit Care Med* 44: 809—818.

Young AMH, Kolias AG, Hutchinson PJ (2017) Decompressive craniectomy for traumatic intracranial hypertension: application in children. *Childs Nerv Syst* 33: 1745—1750.

Zama D, Gasperini P, Berger M, et al. (2018) A survey on hematology-oncology pediatric AIEOP centers: the challenge of posterior reversible encephalopathy syndrome. *Eur J Haematol* 100: 75—82.

CHAPTER 18

Stroke

*Fenella Kirkham, Rael Laugesaar, Tiina Talvik, Tuuli Metsvaht,
and Inga Talvik*

Key messages

- Seizures, as well as hemiparesis, are a common presentation of stroke.
- Neuroimaging, including the venous sinuses, should be performed as early as possible.
- Intracerebral haemorrhage may require urgent neurosurgery.
- In children without prior cardiac disease, exclude shunting at cardiac or pulmonary level.
- In arterial ischemic stroke consider aspirin (5mg/kg acutely, 1–3mg/kg for at least a year) to reduce recurrence risk.
- In extracranial artery dissection and cardioembolic stroke some centres anticoagulate although aspirin is equivalent.
- In cerebral venous sinus thrombosis consider anticoagulation
- Surgical decompression for unconscious children with closed fontanelle and brain swelling following stroke may occasionally be life-saving.

Common errors

- Delay in recognizing that a child has had a stroke.
- Misdiagnosing Todd paresis after focal seizure as stroke or vice-versa.
- Delay in recognizing depressed conscious level and risk of raised intracranial pressure.
- Difficulty in distinguishing between hemiplegic migraine and stroke.

- Mistaking parieto-occipital infarction due to venous sinus thrombosis as arterial stroke.
- Mistaking haemorrhagic infarction due to sinovenous thrombosis as haemorrhagic stroke.
- Reducing instead of supporting blood pressure when cerebral perfusion pressure is low.

When to worry

- Any age: lethargy, decrease in level of consciousness, seizures, vomiting, focal weakness, recent trauma or infection (any viral or bacterial head and neck).
- Neonate: seizures, cardiorespiratory instability, posturing, limb weakness.
- Postneonatal infants: acute focal weakness with or without seizures and/or disturbed consciousness (focal weakness emerging may be presumed perinatal stroke).
- Hypotension especially if there has previously been hypertension.

TYPES OF STROKE

Stroke is one of the most common causes of death and disability in childhood, and presentation is particularly common in the first year of life. Haemorrhagic stroke (HS) (Figure 18.1 a), arterial ischaemic stroke (AIS) (Figure 18.1 b–f), and cerebral venous sinus (sinovenous) thrombosis (CVST) (Figure 18.1 g, h) are increasingly recognized causes of focal signs and encephalopathy (see Chapter 17) in childhood, leading to lifelong morbidity and mortality. Intraventricular haemorrhage is a disorder of infants born preterm, but also seen, rarely, in infants born at term, in which there is bleeding from immature germinal matrix vessels in the subependymal layer, lateral to the lateral ventricles. Germinal matrix haemorrhage may be complicated by compressive obstruction of the medullary veins causing periventricular venous haemorrhagic infarction, which is not conventionally classified as 'stroke' in infants, and in this volume is considered with other infantile causes of hydrocephalus (see Chapter 23).

Diagnosis of stroke is frequently delayed and is often not considered in the differential diagnosis. There have been controversies about the optimal timing for investigation and emergency management strategies, but a consensus is now emerging. The next section of this chapter suggests an evidence-based pathway for investigation and management. More details can be found in the UK Royal College of Paediatrics and Child Health, American Heart Association Stroke Council, American Society of Hematology and American College of Chest Physicians guidelines (see Resources).

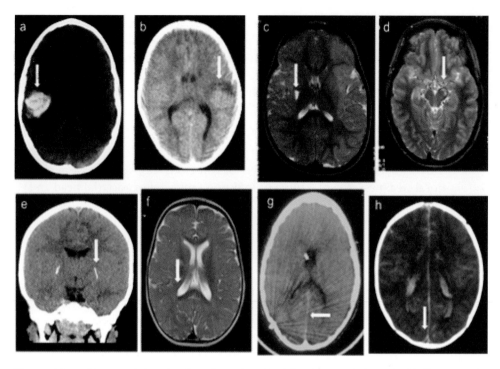

Figure 18.1 Emergency imaging in unilateral stroke. (a) computed tomography (CT) scan showing acute intracerebral haemorrhage with surrounding focal oedema in a child presenting in coma after a focal seizure; (b) CT scan showing infarction in a child with a hemiparesis after minor trauma; (c) magnetic resonance imaging (MRI) showing a small infarct in a child with arteriopathy of the middle cerebral artery after chickenpox; (d) abnormal collateral arteries seen as filling defects on MRI in moyamoya disease; (e) coronal CT showing curvilinear high density foci consistent with mineralization of the lenticulostriate arteries; (f) MRI showing acute infarction in a 6-month-old child with sickle cell disease with a normal MRA but a patent foramen ovale on bubble echocariography; (g) CT scan showing straight sinus venous thrombosis in a young child with acute seizures and reduced conscious level in the context of HbSC disease and shunted hydrocephalus from infancy who was not anticoagulated and died a brain death; (h) venous thrombosis in the sagittal sinus associated with intraventricular haemorrhage: empty delta sign on contrast CT scan.

Epidemiology of stroke

The population prevalence of perinatal AIS is 20 per 100 000 live births (Lee et al. 2005) and for perinatal HS is 6.2 per 100 000 live births (Armstrong-Wells et al. 2009). The incidence of childhood stroke (from 30d—18y) in Estonia was 2.73/100 000 person-years; 1.61/100 000 for AIS, 0.87/100 000 for HS, and 0.25/10 000 for CVST (Laugesaar et al. 2010). This is in line with data from the South of England for AIS (1.60 per 100 000 per year, highest in children aged <1 year (4.14 per 100 000 per year) (Mallick et al. 2014). For Canada the data for AIS (1.72/100 000/year; neonates 10.2/100 000 live births) were also similar (DeVeber et al. 2017), while the incidence of CVST was

0.67 cases per 100 000 children per year, with 67% under the age of 3 years (DeVeber et al. 2001). Neuroimaging will increase diagnostic yield in acutely affected children, for example those in intensive care.

Clinical clues to diagnosis

Neonatal stroke may present as cardiorespiratory instability, seizures, abnormal posturing, or limb weakness. Clinical assessment is often hampered by the fact that the infant is ventilated.

Presumed perinatal stroke typically presents with asymmetry in tone and/or motor function around age 6 to 10 months with relative preservation of cognitive function.

AIS in postneonatal infants typically presents as focal weakness with or without seizures and/or disturbed consciousness. Take a history for underlying conditions and recent trauma or infections, including chicken pox, within the previous year. Note any recent, apparently minor, infections causing upper respiratory tract symptoms or general malaise as well as more serious bacterial infections such as bacterial and tuberculous meningitis. Family history of stroke or neurocutaneous syndromes is important.

In *CVST* (Figure 17.4 a2, d2, d3; Figure 18.1 g, h) in neonates and infants, clinical symptoms are frequently nonspecific and may be subtle but may include seizures, depressed level of consciousness, vomiting, and headache. Typically, there is a comorbid illness, such as head and neck infection, with other prominent risk factors, including dehydration.

HS typically presents with acute loss of consciousness, sometimes with seizures or focal signs (see above).

Clinical examination should note the pattern of motor impairment and features of vasculitis or hypertension; also include a careful heart examination and a search for neurocutaneous stigmata, including the café-au-lait spots of neurofibromatosis, as well as linear sebaceous naevus and incontinentia pigmenti.

Differential diagnosis

There is a wide differential diagnosis for stroke in infancy (Table 18.1, Figure 18.2). When there is an acute stroke protocol, other conditions mimicking stroke, including migraine (Figure 17.4a3, Figure 18.2b) and epilepsy as well as posterior reversible encephalopathy syndrome (PRES) (Figure 18.2a), may be more common and it is important to exclude them before treatment is considered (DeLaroche et al. 2018). Cerebral abscess (Figure 18.2 c) should be considered, especially when cyanotic heart disease and/or endocarditis is present (infarcts, haemorrhages, and mycotic aneurysms may be seen). Although metabolic stroke is rare, hypoglycaemia (Figure 18.2d), MELAS

(Figure 18.2e) and OCT deficiency (Figure 18.2f) are relatively easy to exclude with blood tests for glucose, lactate, and ammonia in the acute phase.

In infancy, separation of prior stroke and stroke of recent onset is particularly difficult, as presumed perinatal stroke may present apparently acutely to the family, even if there was a history of seizures in the neonatal period. Imaging in these cases typically shows focal porencephaly or encephalomalacia secondary to intrauterine or perinatal stroke in an arterial distribution, e.g. middle or anterior cerebral artery territory, or unilateral periventricular white matter hyperintensities with or without ventriculomegaly related to antenatal periventricular venous infarction (Kirton et al. 2008; Kirton et al. 2010). Other causes of hemiplegia presenting in the first year of life include neuronal migration disorders and schizencephaly (Kirkham et al. 2018).

Table 18.1 Aetiology, differential diagnosis, investigation, and management in the child with suspected stroke

Aetiology	Clinical/laboratory/ neuroradiological features	Specific treatments to be considered
Space-occupying mass	Focal signs, seizures, deteriorating level of consciousness	Surgical opinion
Spontaneous intracerebral haemorrhage (Fig 18.1 a, h)	Sudden onset, obvious on plain CT, may be secondary to CVST so CTV/MRV, distinction between aneurysm and AVM may require MR and conventional arteriography	Surgical opinion? decompression, exclude haemorrhagic diatheses, polycystic kidneys, and other genetic causes of AVM or aneurysm
Ischaemic stroke, anterior circulation (Fig 17.4 b3; 18.1 b–f) e.g. or posterior circulation e.g. cerebellar (Fig 17.4 f2,3) or brainstem	Preceding transient ischaemic attacks in some cases, at <24h may be subtle changes on CT but MRI often required	Consider thrombolysis at <4.5h for anterior or<12h for posterior circulation stroke if haemorrhage excluded Consider thrombectomy in case of basilar artery thrombosis Surgical opinion? decompression or drainage (Fig 18.3).
Tumour	Preceding headache and other symptoms and signs, CT with or without MRI	Surgical opinion
Cerebral abscess	Fever, obvious on contrast CT	Antibiotics including cover for anaerobes

Table 18.1 (continued) Aetiology, differential diagnosis, investigation, and management in the child with suspected stroke

Aetiology	Features	Treatments
CVST (Fig 17.4 a2, d2,3; 18.1 g,h)	Focal signs, seizures, deteriorating level of consciousness, haemorrhage or ischaemia, or normal CT; needs CTV or MRV	Anticoagulation, exclude prothrombotic disorders especially prothrombin 20210 and factor V Leiden mutation
Accidental head injury	History of head injury	Surgical opinion
Extradural or intracerebral hematoma	Obvious on plain CT	Consider anticoagulation; may be suitable for interventional neuroradiology
Extracranial dissection	Fat-saturated T1 MRI of neck shows blood in vessel wall	Anticoagulation contraindicated; may be suitable for interventional neuroradiology if haemorrhage in view of recurrence risk
Intracranial dissection	Double lumen may be demonstrated on MR arteriography or conventional arteriography	Surgical opinion? decompression
Diffuse brain oedema	Exclude CSVT on CTV or MRV	
Non-accidental injury	Retinal haemorrhages on fundoscopy, bruises, fractures	Child protection
Subdural or intracerebral haemorrhage/effusion Intracerebral haemorrhage		Neurosurgery opinion Surgical opinion
Hemispheric ischaemia, diffuse brain oedema	Exclude secondary CVST	Surgical opinion? decompression Consider anticoagulation or thrombectomy for CSVT
Acute disseminated encephalomyelitis (ADEM)	Demyelination on MRI, may have had infection	Corticosteroids?, intravenous immunoglobulin

Table 18.1 (continued) Aetiology, differential diagnosis, investigation, and management in the child with suspected stroke

Aetiology	Features	Treatments
Congenital heart disease	Exclude CVST, dissection, moyamoya, aneurysm, embolus	Discuss with cardiologists
Sickle cell disease	Exclude CVST, dissection, moyamoya, aneurysm, embolus	Exchange transfusion, very slowly Appropriate management of stroke syndrome
Other anaemias including iron deficiency	Exclude CVST, PRES (Fig 17.4 2,3; 18.2 a), focal cerebral arteriopathy of childhood, dissection, moyamoya, aneurysm, embolus through PFO	Appropriate management of anaemia and stroke syndrome; transfusion not usually needed but should be very slow if undertaken
Haemolytic-uraemic syndrome	Anaemia, jaundice, Burr cells on blood film, AIS, CVST, or PRES	Dialysis; appropriate management of anaemia and stroke syndrome
Nephrotic syndrome	Typically CVST	Anticoagulate? acutely and in relapse
Inflammatory bowel disease	CVST, PRES, focal cerebral arteriopathy of childhood	CVST? anticoagulate acutely and in relapse
Leukaemia	CVST, PRES, focal crbral arteriopathy of childhood	CVST? anticoagulate acutely and in relapse
Hypoglycaemia (Fig 18.2 d)	Hypoglycaemia (Fig 18.2 d)	Glucose
Epilepsy	Subtle seizures, EEG may show, e.g. Rolandic spikes	Consider anticonvulsants
Hypertensive encephalopathy	Hypertensive encephalopathy	Slow reduction blood pressure
Migraine e.g. hemiplegic	Family history, headache, EEG shows unilateral slowing	May respond to calcium-channel blockers, phenytoin, or acetazolamide
Metabolic conditions		
Ornithine transcarbamylase ↑NH_3 deficiency	Unilateral cerebral oedema (Fig 18.2 f)	Lower ammonia, appropriate diet
Mitochondrial (MELAS?)	MRI: parieto-occipital lesions not typical of AIS (Fig 18.2e); high lactate	Consider arginine

Table 18.1 (continued) Aetiology, differential diagnosis, investigation, and management in the child with suspected stroke

Aetiology	Features	Treatments
Moyamoya	Preceding transient ischaemic attacks in some cases, may be a family history or clues to an underlying diagnosis	Revascularization
Lacunar stroke with normal vascular imaging	Exclude PFO using transoesophageal or bubble ECHO or TCD	Long-term aspirin; consider closure of PFO after randomized controlled trials have evaluated

AIS, arterial ischaemic stroke; AVM, arteriovenous malformation; CT, computed tomography; CTV, computed tomographic venography; DWI, diffusion-weighted imaging; ECHO, echocardiography; EEG, electroencephalography; MRI, magnetic resonance imaging; MRV, magnetic resonance venography; PFO, persistent foramen ovale; PRES, posterior reversible encephalopathy syndrome; TCD, transcranial Doppler ultrasonography; CSVT, cerebral sinovenous thrombosis.

Pathology and causation

Perinatal AIS

Risk factors for neonatal stroke include maternal status (primiparity, history of infertility) and the following disorders: preeclampsia; alloimmune and autoimmune disorders; exposure to infection (e.g. prolonged rupture of membranes, chorioamnionitis); monochorionic diamniotic twinning; in utero drug exposure (e.g. cocaine); placental disorders (e.g. thrombosis, abruption, or infection); fetal/neonatal disorders (e.g. congenital heart disease, infection, vasculopathy including maldevelopment such as arteriovenous malformations; trauma and catheterization); hypoxia-ischaemia; and dehydration. Placental embolism is likely to be the origin in many but is difficult to prove.

Most perinatal strokes occur in the territory of the middle cerebral artery. There is a left-sided predominance of lesions, which may be related to the haemodynamics of a patent ductus arteriosus, or easier transfer from the left common carotid. Infants born preterm tend to have multifocal lesions involving the cortical or lenticulostrate branches of the middle cerebral artery, but infants born at term tend to have occlusions of the main trunk of the middle cerebral artery.

AIS in infancy

Half the incident cases of stroke in infancy are seen in association in children who already have a diagnosis of a chronic disease, particularly congenital heart disease or SCD (Figure 18.1 f). Focal arteriopathy is a common pathology and trauma and infection are common triggers (Fullerton et al. 2015) (Figure 18.1 b, c). Evidence of recent infection with neurotropic viruses, including Herpes viruses such as *Varicella zoster* (chickenpox) (Elkind et al. 2016) (Figure 18.1 c) and Parvovirus B19 (Fullerton et al. 2017) may be found. Rare causes of arteritis, often inherited, e.g. *ACTA2* mutations (McCrea et al. 2019) and PHACES (posterior fossa abnormalities, haemangioma, arterial lesions, cardiac abnormalities, eye problems, sternal cleft) (Garzon et al. 2016), also contribute disproportionately in this age group. Traumatic dissection of the carotid or vertebral artery in the neck may occur after a young child falls with a pencil in the mouth (Figure 18.3) or in the context of vascular compression in non-accidental injury. A distinct clinicoradiological entity, termed mineralizing angiopathy with infantile basal ganglia stroke after minor trauma (Figure 18.1 e), is characterized by acute hemiparesis and hemidystonia in previously typically developing infants aged 6 to 24 months following a minor fall. CT shows bilateral mineralization of lenticulostriate arteries (Lingappa et al. 2014). Good neurodevelopmental outcomes have been reported, apart from those with stroke recurrence precipitated by minor head trauma

CVST

CVST in childhood is a rare but underrecognized disorder which causes obstruction of venous outflow leading to venous infarcts (Figure 18.1 g) with seizures and hemiparesis, intracranial haemorrhages (Figure 18.1 h) and increased ICP with VIth nerve palsies and eventually coma (see Chapter 17). CVST-related primary subarachnoid and subdural haemorrhage can occur. In neonates and in case of deep venous thrombosis there is also an association with intraventricular haemorrhage. Without treatment, thrombus extension with increased symptoms is common with neurological sequelae apparent in up to 40% of survivors and mortality approaching 10% (Dlamini et al. 2010). However, recurrence of CVST is less common than AIS in children (Kenet et al. 2007). CT and/or MRI including CT venography (CTV) or MR venography (MRV) and sequences detecting blood (SWI or T2*-weighted imaging) are mandatory for the diagnosis. Cerebral vein thrombosis may lead to central venous hypertension that may provoke multifocal infarcts and haemorrhages.

Stroke in neonates and infants with congenital heart disease

In congenital heart disease, neuroimaging may show focal infarcts preoperatively (40% in transposition of the great arteries). This may be due to prior atrial septostomy, hypotension at presentation, or perinatal events. Postoperatively, infarcts and haemorrhages are seen in 15% of cases. These arise from microemboli as bypass clamps or device closures are released. Extracorporeal membrane oxygenation and anticoagulation may predispose to haemorrhage. Low-flow cardiac conditions, for example a hypoplastic left heart, predispose to thrombus and embolic stroke and require anticoagulation and/or antiplatelet treatment. Paradoxical emboli with right-to-left shunting from the right side of the circulation in children may be seen with cyanotic heart disease.

Arterial stroke in neonates and infants with SCD

Symptomatic arterial stroke occurs under the age of 1 year in SCD, but this is rare, at least in part because of the protective effect of high haemoglobin F levels until the end of this period. However, silent cerebral infarction and vasculopathy have been well documented on MRI/magnetic resonance angiography (MRA) in this age group and are associated with delayed cognitive development as well as future stroke (Cancio et al. 2015). Transcranial Doppler screening is not usually recommended under the age of 2 years, in part because the normal range has not been established. Stroke and cerebral abscess may occasionally be embolic in relation to a patent foramen ovale in this age group (Figure 18.1 f). CVST and PRES (Figure 17.4 c2,3; Figure 18.2 a) may occur.

Aneurysm is very rare in this age group, but HS may occur after rapid transfusion or with the use of steroids. In children with SCD and acute neurological deficits, including transient ischemic attack, the American Society for Hematology Guideline Panel recommends blood transfusion within hours of presentation (DeBaun et al. 2020). When exchange transfusion is not available within 2 hours and haemoglobin is ≤8.5g/dL, simple transfusion should be commenced *slowly* to increase the haemoglobin to *no more than* 10.0g/dl. Hydroxyurea, which increases haemoglobin F, has been recommended in the USA from the age of 9 months and may reduce the prevalence of neurological complications (Nottage et al. 2016).

Investigations

See also Table 18.1.

Cranial ultrasound can be used in case of open fontanelle and is a sensitive method of detecting haemorrhage and periventricular strokes, but cortical ischaemic strokes seen on MRI are missed on ultrasound. *Computed tomography* (CT) does not show parenchymal infarction reliably within 24 hours of an ischaemic stroke, but may be required urgently to exclude haemorrhage (Figure 18.1 a). CT is sensitive for the calcification associated with mineralizing angiopathy (Figure 18.1 e) and occasionally other vascular abnormalities may be revealed, e.g. vein of Galen malformation or Sturge-Weber syndrome. CT may show venous sinus thrombosis (Figure 18.1 g and h), particularly post-contrast or with CT-venography (CTV). CTV and CT-arteriography may be the appropriate modality for making the diagnosis quickly in an affected child, although the radiation dose is relatively high. Ischaemic infarction may not be obvious within the first 24 hours on CT (Figure 18.1 b). *Magnetic resonance imaging* (MRI) is more sensitive and the method of choice in infants (Figure 18.1 c) to find other abnormalities, for example collaterals associated with moyamoya disease (Figure 18.1 d).

MRI using diffusion-weighted imaging (DWI) as well as T2-weighted sequences to demonstrate acute ischemic injury and MRA to identify some amount of arterial obstruction are mandatory to diagnose the stroke and exclude mimics (Figure 18.2). Increased DWI signal in ischemic brain tissue may observed within a few minutes after arterial occlusion. MRI with gradient echocardiogram or susceptibility-weighted imaging will exclude haemorrhage, and may reveal venous sinus thrombosis, and may be useful for documenting vascular abnormalities in more detail. In addition, MRV, extra- and intracranial arteriography (MRA) and sequences for fat-saturated T1-weighted MRI of the neck will usually either diagnose or exclude vascular disease. If there is no obvious arterial disorder involving the intracranial vessels on MR arteriography, venous sinus thrombosis should be investigated either with CTV or MRV and dissection in the neck vessels should be excluded using Doppler sonography, or if necessary conventional arteriography.

MRI is also the modality of choice for diagnosing conditions mimicking stroke, including PRES (Figure 17.4 c2,3; Figure 18.2a) and hemiplegic migraine (Figure 18.2 b) (DeLaroche et al. 2018).

Electroencephalography can be useful in demonstrating that focal signs are epileptic, e.g. benign Rolandic epilepsy with centrotemporal spikes, or migrainous (typically hemispheric slowing) in origin.

Echocardiography, ideally with bubble contrast during a Valsalva manoeuvre, to detect a significant right to left shunt at atrial or pulmonary level, should be undertaken in all children with stroke, whether or not they have another underlying condition such as sickle cell disease (Dowling et al. 2017). It is, however, rare for a previously undiagnosed cardiac lesion to be revealed and poor ventricular function is at least as common as patent foramen ovale on echocardiography. Bubble-contrast transcranial Doppler ultrasonography may also detect minor degrees of shunting. However, the need to close any patent foramen ovale found is currently very controversial.

Laboratory investigation of red-blood-cell indices is important, (ferritin levels or, if necessary, more detailed iron studies) since a substantial proportion of young children with cerebrovascular disease (particularly venous sinus thrombosis) have iron deficiency (Figure 18.1 g). It is more difficult to justify extensive prothrombotic screening, as any association with stroke in neonates and infants is controversial (Curtis et al. 2017). In addition, although prothrombotic disorders may be associated with the risk of recurrence (deVeber et al. 2019), this risk is very low in neonatal and presumed perinatal stroke, while there is no evidence base for treatment as randomized trials of secondary prevention have not yet been conducted. However, if there is a family history of a specific prothrombotic disorder (e.g. antithrombin deficiency), this should be excluded in the child.

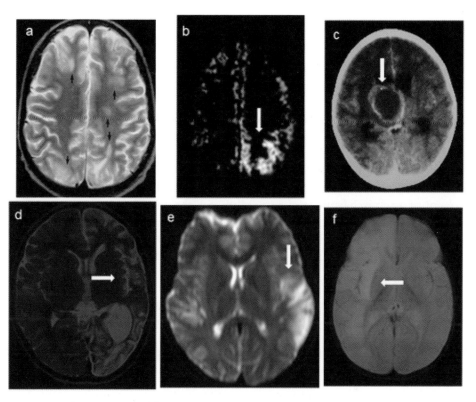

Figure 18.2 Stroke mimics. (a) MRI showing posterior reversible encephalopathy syndrome in a child with sickle cell anaemia and nephrotic syndrome who had acute visual loss and seizures; (b) diffusion-weighted MRI showing parieto-occipital abnormality in a patient with hemiplegic migraine and unilateral slowing on EEG; (c) cerebral abscess in a toddler with sickle cell anaemia and acute seizures; (d) hemispheric damage in a child with type 1 diabetes who had an acute hypoglycaemic episode; (e) abnormality in a nonvascular distribution in a child with mitochondrial encephalopathy and stroke-like episodes (MELAS); (f) unilateral oedema in a child with ornithine transcarbamylase deficiency.

Acute management (see Resources)

Appropriate management involves general supportive care or symptomatic measures, such as correction of dehydration and hypovolemia, which may reduce the risk of recurrence and improve outcome. If there is any reduction in level of consciousness the child requires emergency transfer to a centre in which emergency intervention can be undertaken. Imaging such as CT can be performed while transportation is organized but neuroimaging should not delay transfer. It is very important that principles of good emergency management of an affected child are followed, with attention to management of the airway, circulation, and any seizures.

Although there are resources, evidence-based guidelines for care that exist for adults do not exist for children presenting with AIS. When presenting early after a stroke, adult patients have several hyperacute interventional options available that have been studied for efficacy of thrombolysis and restoration of brain perfusion with intravenous administration of tissue plasminogen activator (tPA) and endovascular thrombectomy. However, children under 18 years have generally been excluded from hyperacute stroke interventional studies. The international multicentre study enrolling children ages 2 to 17 years with clinically and radiographically confirmed AIS within 3 hours of symptom onset to assess dose-determination, safety, and efficacy of IV tPA failed to recruit but the available observational evidence suggests that the risk of haemorrhage is low (Amlie-Lefond et al. 2020). As there are no randomized controlled trials of emergency management of acute ischaemic stroke in childhood, thrombolysis is not recommended for children under the age of 2 years. However, despite the absence of age-appropriate safety data or dosing guidelines, children who present with an acute stroke are sometimes treated with hyperacute therapy outside of the recommended guidelines for use of tPA.

Mechanical embolectomy in children with AIS or basilar thrombosis is described in small case series.

For HS secondary to structural abnormalities of the arteries, a decision may be made by the appropriate multidisciplinary team that vascular neurosurgery, such as clipping of an aneurysm, or stereotactic radiotherapy to obliterate an arteriovenous malformation, is the best management strategy.

Anticoagulation in neonates and infants with CSVT should be considered, as adult randomized controlled trials showed benefit in terms of mortality and morbidity, the risk of haemorrhage is low and observational data suggest that it is life-saving.

For acute AIS in infants, in view of the data from adults and the very low risk of complication (haemorrhage or Reye syndrome), most paediatricians give aspirin at a dose of 5mg/kg per day in the acute situation, while some anticoagulate with heparin and then with warfarin (see Resources). Very occasionally, children with a high risk of recurrent stroke may be suitable for interventional neuroradiological procedures, such as coils or stents, but in many settings, access to these skills will not be available.

Surgical decompression (Figure 18.3) may be life-saving if the patient is deeply unconscious.

Prevention of recurrence (see Resources)

The recurrence rate is high in referral centres and is more common in children with arteriopathies, isolated antithrombin deficiency, elevated lipoprotein, or more than

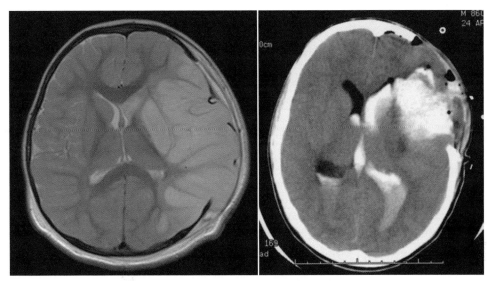

Figure 18.3 Surgical decompression in (left) ischaemic stroke secondary to carotid occlusion in a toddler who fell with a pencil in his mouth and (right) haemorrhagic stroke in a young child with sickle cell disease who was transfused rapidly after a fall in haemoglobin in the context of acute chest syndrome

one prothrombotic risk factor (deVeber et al. 2019). However, population-based studies suggest a lower risk, while screening for risk factors is expensive (Mallick et al. 2016). It is important to exclude or treat iron deficiency and to ensure all children have a healthy diet full of fruit and vegetables, a reduced fat intake, and plenty of exercise. Aspirin should continue at 5mg/kg or a reduced dose of 1 to 3mg/kg per day for at least 2 years, with expert advice before discontinuing. Recent cohort studies suggest that aspirin prophylaxis may have been associated with a reduction in the risk of recurrence, at least for cryptogenic anterior stroke and focal cerebral arteriopathy, but there have been no randomized controlled trials.

In venous sinus thrombosis in neonates and infants, anticoagulation is usually continued for 3 to 6 months and then discontinued, except in high-risk situations such as recurrence of nephrotic syndrome or exacerbation of inflammatory bowel disease, or inherited thrombophilia such as antithrombin deficiency, Prothrombin 20210, or Factor V Leiden.

Outcome

Mortality

Mortality for acute AIS is low: 1.5% for neonates and 3.1% for children, according to an International Paediatric Stroke Study (Beslow et al. 2018). Mortality is higher in those with both posterior and anterior infarction, as well as those with congenital heart disease. However, at least a third are haemorrhagic and case fatality for intracerebral haemorrhages can reach 46% (Laugesaar et al. 2010).

Over 50% of survivors of stroke have persistent neurological, cognitive, or psychiatric deficits and epilepsy is common, particularly after neonatal and presumed perinatal stroke (Laugesaar et al. 2010; Laugesaar et al. 2018; Kolk et al. 2011; Billinghurst et al. 2017; Lõo et al. 2018).

Rehabilitation

Some children make a very rapid recovery from stroke while others have considerable residual disability. Early rehabilitation by a skilled team (e.g. physiotherapist, occupational therapist, speech therapist, and psychotherapist) can make a big difference to the long-term outcome. Children may need an educational statement or be referred for special education when they start school, and they and their families need considerable support.

REFERENCES

Amlie-Lefond C, Shaw DWW, Cooper A, et al. (2020) Risk of Intracranial Hemorrhage Following Intravenous tPA (Tissue-Type Plasminogen Activator) for Acute Stroke Is Low in Children. *Stroke* 51:542–548.

Armstrong-Wells J, Johnston SC, Wu YW, et al. (2009) Prevalence and predictors of perinatal hemorrhagic stroke: results from the Kaiser pediatric stroke study. *Pediatrics* 123: 823–828.

Beslow LA, Dowling MM, Hassanein SMA, et al. (2018) Mortality after arterial ischemic stroke. *Pediatrics* 141: e20174146.

Billinghurst LL, Beslow LA, Abend NS, et al. (2017) Incidence and predictors of epilepsy after pediatric arterial ischemic stroke. *Neurology* 14; 88: 630–637.

Cancio MI, Helton KJ, Schreiber JE, Smeltzer MP, Kang G, Wang WC (2015) Silent cerebral infarcts in very young children with sickle cell anaemia are associated with a higher risk of stroke. *Br J Haematol* 171: 120–129.

Curtis C, Mineyko A, Massicotte P, et al. (2017) Thrombophilia risk is not increased in children after perinatal stroke. *Blood* 129: 2793–2800.

DeBaun M, Jordan LC, King AA, et al. (2020) American Society of Hematology 2020 guidelines for sickle cell disease: prevention, diagnosis, and treatment of cerebrovascular disease in children and adults. *Blood Adv* 4: 1554–1588.

DeLaroche AM, Sivaswamy L, Farooqi A, Kannikeswaran N (2018) Pediatric stroke and its mimics: limitations of a pediatric stroke clinical pathway. *Pediatr Neurol* 80: 35–41.

deVeber G, Andrew M, Adams C, et al. (2001) Cerebral sinovenous thrombosis in children. *N Engl J Med* 345:417–423.

deVeber GA, Kirton A, Booth FA, et al. (2017) Epidemiology and Outcomes of Arterial Ischemic Stroke in Children: The Canadian Pediatric Ischemic Stroke Registry. *Pediatr Neurol* 69:58–70.

deVeber G, Kirkham F, Shannon K, et al. (2019) Recurrent stroke: the role of thrombophilia in a large international pediatric stroke population. *Haematologica* 104: 1676—1683.

Dlamini N, Billinghurst L, Kirkham FJ (2010) Cerebral venous sinus (sinovenous) thrombosis in children. *Neurosurg Clin N Am* 21: 511—527.

Dowling MM, Quinn CT, Ramaciotti C, et al. (2017) Increased prevalence of potential right-to-left shunting in children with sickle cell anaemia and stroke. *Br J Haematol* 176:300—308.

Elkind MS, Hills NK, Glaser CA, et al. (2016) Herpesvirus Infections and Childhood Arterial Ischemic Stroke: Results of the VIPS Study. *Circulation* 33: 732—41.

Fullerton HJ, Hills NK, Elkind MS, et al. (2015) VIPS Investigators. Infection, vaccination, and childhood arterial ischemic stroke: Results of the VIPS study. *Neurology* 85: 1459—1466.

Fullerton HJ, Luna JM, Wintermark M, et al. (2017) Parvovirus B19 infection in children with arterial ischemic stroke. *Stroke* 48: 2875—2877.

Garzon MC, Epstein LG, Heyer GL, et al. (2016) PHACE Syndrome: consensus-derived diagnosis and care recommendations. *J Pediatr* 178: 24—33.e2.

Kenet G, Kirkham F, Niederstadt T et al. (2007) Risk factors for recurrent venous thromboembolism in the European collaborative paediatric database on cerebral venous thrombosis: a multicentre cohort study. *Lancet Neurol* 6:595-603.

Kirkham FJ, Zafeiriou D, Howe D, et al. (2018) Fetal stroke and cerebrovascular disease: Advances in understanding from lenticulostriate and venous imaging, alloimmune thrombocytopaenia and monochorionic twins. *Eur J Paediatr Neurol* 22: 989—1005.

Kirton A, deVeber G, Pontigon AM, et al. (2008) Presumed perinatal ischemic stroke: Vascular classification predicts outcomes. *Ann Neurol.* 63: 436—43.

Kirton A, Shroff M, Pontigon AM, deVeber G (2010) Risk factors and presentations of periventricular venous infarction vs arterial presumed perinatal ischemic stroke. *Arch Neurol* 67: 842—848.

Kolk A, Ennok M, Laugesaar R, et al. (2011) Long-term cognitive outcomes after pediatric stroke. *Pediatr Neurol* 44: 101—109.

Laugesaar R, Kolk A, Uustalu U, et al. (2010) Epidemiology of childhood stroke in Estonia. *Pediatr Neurol* 42: 93—100.

Laugesaar R, Vaher U, Lõo S, et al. (2018) Epilepsy after perinatal stroke with different vascular subtypes. *Epilepsia Open* 3: 193—202.

Lee J, Croen LA, Backstrand KH, et al. (2005) Maternal and infant characteristics associated with perinatal arterial stroke in the infant. *JAMA* 293: 723—729.

Lingappa L, Varma RD, Siddaiahgari S, Konanki R (2014) Mineralizing angiopathy with infantile basal ganglia stroke after minor trauma. *Dev Med Child Neurol* 56: 78—84.

Lõo S, Ilves P, Männamaa M, et al. (2018) Long-term neurodevelopmental outcome after perinatal arterial ischemic stroke and periventricular venous infarction. *Eur J Paediatr Neurol* 22: 1006—1015.

McCrea N, Fullerton HJ, Ganesan V (2019) Genetic and environmental associations with pediatric cerebral arteriopathy. *Stroke* 50: 257—265.

Mallick AA, Ganesan V, Kirkham FJ, et al. (2014) Childhood arterial ischaemic stroke incidence, presenting features, and risk factors: a prospective population-based study. *Lancet Neurol* 13:35—43.

Mallick AA, Ganesan V, Kirkham FJ, et al. (2016) Outcome and recurrence 1 year after pediatric arterial ischemic stroke in a population-based cohort. *Ann Neurol* 79: 784–793.

Nottage KA, Ware RE, Aygun B, et al. (2016) Hydroxycarbamide treatment and brain MRI/MRA findings in children with sickle cell anaemia. *Br J Haematol* 175: 331–338.

Resources

DeBaun M, Jordan LC, King AA, et al. (2020) American Society of Hematology 2020 guidelines for sickle cell disease: prevention, diagnosis, and treatment of cerebrovascular disease in children and adults. *Blood Adv* 4: 1554–1588.

Ferriero DM, Fullerton HJ, Bernard TJ, et al. (2019) Management of Stroke in Neonates and Children: A Scientific Statement From the American Heart Association/American Stroke Association. *Stroke* 50: e51–e96.

Golomb MR, MacGregor DL, Domi T, et al. (2001) Presumed pre- or perinatal arterial ischemic stroke: risk factors and outcomes. *Ann Neurol* 50: 163–168.

Ganesan V, Kirkham FJ. Stroke and cerebrovascular disease in childhood. ICNA series of monographs in Child Neurology, MacKeith Press, 2011.

Monagle P, Chan AKC, Goldenberg NA, et al. (2012) Antithrombotic therapy in neonates and children: antithrombotic therapy and prevention of thrombosis, 9th ed: American College of Chest Physicians Evidence-Based Clinical Practice Guidelines. *Chest* 141 (Suppl. 2): e737S–e801S.

RCPCH. Stroke in childhood — clinical guideline for diagnosis, management and rehabilitation. Available at https://www.rcpch.ac.uk/resources/stroke-childhood-clinical-guideline-diagnosis-management-rehabilitation

Acute neurological illness with fever: meningitis, encephalitis, and infective space-occupying lesions

Rachel Kneen and Charles Newton

Key messages

- Central nervous system (CNS) infections are neurological emergencies. The outcome is improved by early recognition and appropriate management.
- Clinical features are useful but cannot be used to predict the risk of CNS infections. Therefore appropriate investigations are needed, especially a lumbar puncture (LP) if no contraindications exist.
- The findings of cerebrospinal fluid (CSF) analysis are very useful for children with suspected CNS infections. All children should have an LP unless an established contraindication exists (Box 19.1).
- CSF analysis in both meningitis and encephalitis usually shows a pleocytosis; but it can be normal, especially if the LP was done early in the illness (Table 19.1).
- An LP postponed because of previous contraindications still adds important diagnostic information.

- In encephalitis, brain imaging findings are useful, but computed tomography (CT) can be normal, especially in the early stages of the illness. Magnetic resonance imaging is more sensitive but may not be available in many settings.
- The list of pathogens causing CNS infections is extensive, but careful history taking and examination can help establish the correct diagnosis.
- The causes of CNS infections vary geographically. Local knowledge is important to understand the individual risks of particular pathogens.
- An immunocompromised child with a CNS infection may have a subtle presentation. Clinical suspicion needs to be high in these patients. Different pathogenic organisms also need to be considered.

Common errors

- Failing to investigate a child with a prolonged 'postictal phase' after an assumed febrile seizure (see Chapter 20).
- Diagnosing febrile seizures in epilepsy (e.g. Dravet syndrome; see Chapter 20).
- Failing to properly investigate a child with symptoms suggestive of a CNS infection (in particular, not doing an LP when no contraindications exist).
- Failing to appreciate that a child may have a CNS infection for other reasons including: discounting the parents' history that their child is excessively irritable, a bit confused or subdued, has a change in personality, or is 'not quite right'. It is usually a mistake to ignore parents' opinions.
- Relying on cranial imaging (especially CT) to rule out raised intracranial pressure: CT may be normal in a child with an impending brain herniation syndrome. Clinical skills must be used to look for and to identify brain herniation syndromes.
- Overtreating children with aciclovir for herpes simplex virus (HSV) encephalitis when they have a pre-existing neurological disorder (especially those with epilepsy and/or cerebral palsy) plus a nonspecific viral infection; observe and investigate rather than immediately starting aciclovir.
- Overtreating children with aciclovir for HSV encephalitis when there is another definite cause for their encephalopathy, such as a head injury or drug overdose.
- Discounting a possible infective space-occupying lesion because there is no fever or history of fever: symptoms and signs can be subtle.

When to worry

Acute problems

- Infants are at risk of an acute deterioration for many reasons (see section

> on acute bacterial meningitis); they must be carefully monitored to identify and manage complications.
> - Intensive care has complications: infants with CNS infections can develop venous thrombosis with or without pulmonary embolism, aspiration pneumonia, feeding difficulties, nutritional deficiencies, ventilator- and possible tracheostomy-dependence, critical illness neuropathy, or myopathy.
>
> Chronic problems in the recovery phase due to brain injury include:
>
> - Ongoing seizures (epilepsy).
> - Chronic raised intracranial pressure (often with a ventriculoperitoneal shunt).
> - Movement disorders, including dystonia and spasticity, new physical disabilities, communication and swallowing difficulties needing therapists and orthotists.
> - Nutritional needs and feeding difficulties (nasogastric tube-feeding or percutaneous endoscopic gastrostomy feeding may be needed).
> - New learning difficulties and behavioural problems.

INTRODUCTION TO NEUROLOGICAL INFECTIOUS DISEASES

The topic of neurological infections in infants is important because, unlike many other neurological disorders, specific and potentially life-saving treatments can be given. There are several ways of thinking about this group of disorders, but perhaps the most useful is to classify them into presenting clinical syndromes, then to consider specific causative organisms or other pathologies. Some organisms can cause more than one neurological syndrome. The key neurological syndromes that will be discussed here include meningitis, encephalitis, and space-occupying lesions (SOLs; abscesses). There can be considerable overlap between the presentations of these syndromes. Febrile seizures are covered in Chapter 20 and congenital brain infections in Chapter 22.

DEFINITIONS

Meningitis is defined as inflammation of the brain meninges, characterized clinically by inflammatory cells in the cerebrospinal fluid (CSF). Typically, the infant is febrile and fully conscious with signs of meningeal irritation, but he/she may be encephalopathic in severe cases (see section on clinical features below). In this situation, the term meningoencephalitis is used.

Encephalitis is the inflammation of the brain parenchyma. This is strictly a pathological diagnosis, but unless a brain biopsy or postmortem is carried out, surrogate markers, such as CSF pleocytosis seen during microscopy or abnormal findings on brain magnetic resonance imaging (MRI), are used. Typically, the infant is febrile and encephalopathic with an altered level of consciousness or a behavioural change. The infant may also have signs of meningeal irritation (see section on clinical features) and have focal neurological symptoms or signs.

Infective SOLs include brain abscesses and extra-axial collections of pus. Lesions may be single or multiple depending on the cause. Typically, the infant is febrile and will have focal neurological symptoms or signs, but not in all cases (see below). There may be underlying medical problems which provide the source of infection for the SOL; e.g., congenital cardiac abnormalities, ear/nose/throat infection, septicaemia (particularly if there are any catheters, or intravenous or arterial lines present).

Children who are immunocompromised may present with milder or atypical symptoms and signs for any of these infective neurological syndromes. These infants may not even be febrile. A careful history should be taken to establish whether an infant could be immunocompromised, particularly if their illness is unexplained. This includes asking the mother about risk factors for human immunodeficiency virus (HIV).

ACUTE BACTERIAL MENINGITIS

Incidence and aetiology

The incidence of meningitis during infancy, particularly during the neonatal period, is higher than during any other period of the lifespan. The causative organisms are dependent upon age. During the neonatal period, Group B *Streptococcus*, *Escherichia coli*, and *Listeria monocytogenes*, but also other organisms, particularly gram-negative organisms such as *Citrobacter* species, can cause devastating meningitis, often complicated by the formation of abscesses. Although the organisms that most commonly cause acute bacterial meningitis (ABM) in older infants can cause ABM in neonates, these organisms are relatively rare. In infants aged 1 to 3 months the above organisms become less common, and by the age of 4 months *Streptococcus pnemoniae*, *Haemophilus influenzae*, and *Neisseria meningitidis* are the predominant organisms.

Clinical features

Classic symptoms include a triad of a short history of fever, headache, and neck stiffness. Caution is needed because a young infant may have a low or unstable body temperature; also, an infant cannot localize pain so is likely to be irritable in place of complaining of a headache. There may be associated photophobia, but this cannot usually be detected in an infant.

Signs

- Petechial or purpuric rash in cases caused by meningococcus.

- Bulging anterior fontanelle.

- Meningism (i.e. neck stiffness Brudzinski and Kernig signs) may be absent in the first year of life or no more than a subtle reluctance to flex neck.

- Altered level of consciousness in severe cases.

- Seizures (focal or generalized) in 30%.

- Focal neurological signs: cranial nerves 15%, other 10%.

- Septicaemic shock, multiorgan involvement, deranged clotting, especially meningococcal infection.

Infants, especially those who are immunocompromised, may not display typical features. A high index of suspicion is needed and a lumbar puncture (LP) should be undertaken unless there is a specific contraindication (see Box 19.1). Infants with tuberculous (TB) meningitis may have a more chronic presentation. They may also present with signs of hydrocephalus or raised intracranial pressure (see section on TB meningitis).

Differential diagnosis

Other infections: viral (aseptic) meningitis (see below). Beware of diagnosing viral meningitis in a child who has received antibiotics which may lower CSF white cell count in ABM; other bacterial meningitis including listeria, cryptococcal, or TB (see below); other infections including Lyme disease (borelliosis), fungal meningitis, brucellosis, rickettsial infections, and parasitic infections.

Non-infectious disorders: some drugs, such as trimethoprim-sulfamethoxazole, ampicillin, intravenous immunoglobulin, nonsteroidal anti-inflammatory drugs; autoimmune diseases, such as collagen vascular diseases or other autoimmune diseases (rare in infancy); Aicardi–Goutières syndrome (see also Chapter 17, and Table 23.1); malignant meningitis, i.e. meningitis due to a malignant neoplastic process.

Investigations

CSF examination by LP is essential, except in the presence of a specific contraindication (Box 19.1), when ABM is suspected. See Table 19.1 for the typical changes seen in the CSF in infants with various infective neurological disorders.

Box 19.1   Contraindications to lumbar puncture

☑ Glasgow Coma Scale score* <9 or deteriorating level of consciousness

☑ Signs of raised intracranial pressure, including:

  ☑ Dilated pupils or absent pupillary response to light

  ☑ Hypertension >95th centile for age or bradycardia <60/min

  ☑ Abnormal respiratory pattern

  ☑ Papilloedema

  ☑ Abnormal posturing, especially decerebrate or decorticate posturing[†]

  ☑ Absent oculocephalic (doll's eye) reflex

☑ Other focal neurological signs: hemi-/monoparesis, abnormal plantar responses, ocular palsies

☑ Glasgow Coma Scale score <13 and convulsive seizures that are recent (in preceding 30min) or prolonged (lasting >30min)

☑ Focal or tonic seizures (is it decerebrate or decorticate posturing, not a seizure?)

☑ Strong suspicion of meningococcal infection (typical purpuric rash in an ill child)

☑ State of shock

☑ Local superficial infection in lumbar region

☑ Disordered blood coagulation

See also www.nottingham.ac.uk/paediatric-guideline/Guideline%20algorithm.pdf(see Resources list).

*See Table 17.1.
[†]See Figure 19.1.

Cranial imaging is often normal in a child with suspected meningitis. Clinical features, rather than imaging, must be used to determine whether it is safe to do an LP. Computed tomography (CT) is only needed if there are clinical contraindications to an LP (see Box 19.1) and waiting for CT to inform decisions can cause unnecessary delays in investigation and treatment. .

Request a CT or brain MRI if the child is encephalopathic or has focal neurological symptoms or signs. This is necessary to make an alternative diagnosis (e.g. an infective SOL, arterial ischaemic stroke, or encephalitis) and is abnormal in approximately 30% of cases; give contrast if possible. In meningitis, the meninges usually enhance, and infective SOL will usually also enhance. However, radiologists are often reluctant to give gadolinium to infants. Imaging may also be useful in the management of a child with definite meningitis if they become encephalopathic or deteriorate in other ways, or if a complication of the infection is suspected at a later stage of management.

Table 19.1 Typical cerebrospinal fluid (CSF) findings in central nervous system infections

	Viral meningo-encephalitis	ABM	TB meningitis	Fungal	Normal
Opening pressure	Normal—high	High	High	High—very high	Age <1 year, <5cm
Colour	Clear	Cloudy	Cloudy/yellow	Clear/cloudy	Clear
Cells/mm^3	Normal—high 0—1000	High—very high 1000—50 000	Mild elevation 25—500	Normal—high 0—1000	<5
Differential	Lymphocytes	Neutrophils	Lymphocytes	Lymphocytes	Lymphocytes
CSF/plasma glucose ratio	Normal	Low	Low—very low (e.g. <0.3)	Normal—low	66%*
Protein (g/L)	Normal—high 0.5—1	High >1	High High—very high 1.0—5.0	Normal—high 0.5—5.0	<0.5

Normal values: a bloody tap will falsely elevate the CSF white cell count, and protein. To correct for a bloody tap, a very approximate estimation can be derived by subtracting one white cell for every 700 red blood cells/mm^3 in the CSF, and 0.1g/dL of protein for every 1000 red blood cells.

*Although a normal CSF glucose ratio is quoted as 66%, only values <50% are likely to be significant.

Some important exceptions

- In viral CNS infections, an early lumbar puncture may give predominantly neutrophils, or there may be no cells in early or late lumbar punctures. In patients with acute bacterial meningitis (ABM) that have been partially pretreated with antibiotics (or patients <1 year old) the CSF cell count may not be very high and may be mostly lymphocytes.

- TB meningitis may have predominant CSF polymorphs early in the infection.

- *Listeria monocytogenes* can give a similar CSF picture to TB meningitis, but the history is shorter.

- CSF findings in bacterial abscesses range from near normal to purulent, depending on location of the abscess, and whether there is associated meningitis or rupture.

- A cryptococcal antigen test (CRAG) and Indian ink stain should be performed on the CSF of all patients in whom cryptococcus is possible

Investigation on CSF obtained at LP

- Measure opening pressure using a manometer or an intravenous 'giving set' (narrow-gauge, flexible plastic tubing) and a tape measure to measure the vertical height above the LP needle to which the column of CSF in the tube rises.

- Send CSF for microscopy, culture and sensitivities, glucose (with paired plasma sample), protein, and lactate.

- Rapid antigen testing may be possible for several bacteria (*S. pneumoniae, N. meningitidis, H. influenzae*).

- Polymerase chain reaction (PCR) may be possible for several bacteria (*S. pneumoniae, N. meningitidis, H. influenzae*).

- Save (freeze) a sample in case further investigations are needed.

- Send CSF for PCR for enterovirus, adenovirus, and HSV if viral meningitis is suspected.

- Consider sending CSF for PCR for viruses shown in the section on viral encephalitis (VE) as well (see below) if the child is encephalopathic.

- Send for Ziehl–Neelsen staining and TB culture (see below) if TB meningitis is suspected. Ideally, a 2 to 5ml sample is needed to improve yield.

Blood investigations

- Full blood count and differential white cell count (may show low or high white cell count, left shift, atypical white cells, low or high platelets).

- Blood culture.

- C-reactive protein, renal and liver function studies.

- Rapid bacterial antigen testing (*S. pneumoniae, N. meningitidis, H. influenzae*).

- Clotting/coagulation studies if the child appears ill or has a petechial rash.

- Chest X-ray or imaging of the sinuses may be helpful, depending on clinical features.

- Freeze serum for specific antibody tests. A convalescent sample will also be needed 3 weeks after the onset of the illness. A decision about which organisms to test for can be made at a later date.

Treatment

Meningitis during infancy, particularly during the neonatal period, should be treated aggressively. In particular, it is good practice to start appropriate antibacterial and antiviral therapy when there is a reasonable suspicion of meningitis and before the results of bacterial culture or PCR testing are known. Provided that cultures are obtained prior to starting treatment, it is also good practice to stop antibacterial and antiviral therapy when the results are available and show no evidence of infection. Since it is difficult to distinguish between viral meningoencephalitis and bacterial meningitis in neonates, give both antibacterial and antiviral (e.g. aciclovir) treatment. Antibacterial treatment needs to cover a wide range of organisms including the gram-positive and gram-negative organisms; consider the possibility of antibiotic resistance using all available local information.

Recommended antimicrobial regimens include ampicillin and an aminoglycoside such as gentamicin. However, resistance of *Escherichia coli* to ampicillin has been reported. Cefotaxime is often added, although resistance to this antibiotic has also been reported.

Antimicrobial treatment for confirmed infection should last for 14 to 21 days in neonatal meningitis and the antimicrobials may need to be adjusted in the light of culture and sensitivity results. Repeating the LP 24 to 72 hours after onset of treatment may help with management. There is little evidence that corticosteroids improve the outcome in neonatal meningitis.

Supportive care is important for

- maintaining blood pressure to ensure adequate cerebral perfusion,

- careful fluid management,

- correction of electrolyte disorders,

- respiratory support, that may be needed, and

- management of seizures with phenobarbital, benzodiazepines, or phenytoin, although it can be difficult to ensure appropriate levels.

Complications

Acute: raised intracranial hypertension and progression to a brainstem herniation syndrome (see Figure 19.1), effusions and empyema, acute symptomatic seizures, cerebritis, abscess formation, hydrocephalus, electrolyte disturbances (particularly a low sodium or a metabolic acidosis), venous sinus thrombosis leading to cerebral infarction.

Chronic: intellectual disability or learning difficulties, behavioural problems, hemiplegia, spastic quadriplegia, dystonia, spasticity, hearing or visual loss, epilepsy. Seizures may be focal or multifocal and may be refractory to medical treatment (see Chapters 16 and 20). Always test hearing early in the recovery phase since early detection increases options for treatment.

CHRONIC BACTERIAL MENINGITIS

Chronic bacterial meningitis is uncommon during the neonatal period, although fungal infections are associated with neonates requiring intensive care.

TB meningitis occurs in infancy, either as a separate clinical syndrome or as part of miliary TB. Most infants present with fever, vomiting, cough, and impaired consciousness. Seizures are common. A bulging fontanelle is noticeable in younger infants; paresis or opisthotonus may occur and should lead to consideration of TB. TB and fungal infections can be transmitted during pregnancy, although congenital meningitis is uncommon. Diagnosis is often based upon a high index of suspicion, history of contacts, positive tuberculin test, and evidence of TB in other organs, particularly in the lungs.

Laboratory investigations

- Hyponatraemia is common.

- CSF pleocytosis, usually <1000 cells/mm^3, mostly lymphocytes (Table 19.1).

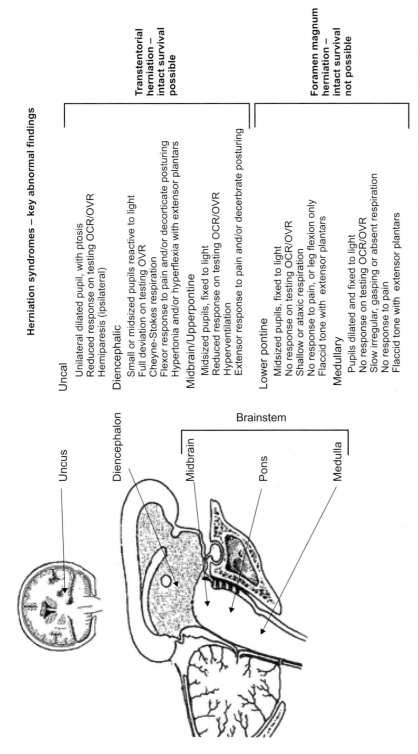

Herniation syndromes – key abnormal findings

Uncal
Unilateral dilated pupil, with ptosis
Reduced response on testing OCR/OVR
Hemiparesis (ipsilateral)

Diencephalic
Small or midsized pupils reactive to light
Full deviation on testing OVR
Cheyne-Stokes respiration
Flexor response to pain and/or decorticate posturing
Hypertonia and/or hyperflexia with extensor plantars

Midbrain/Upperpontine
Midsized pupils, fixed to light
Reduced response on testing OCR/OVR
Hyperventilation
Extensor response to pain and/or decerebrate posturing

Lower pontine
Midsized pupils, fixed to light
No response on testing OCR/OVR
Shallow or ataxic respiration
No response to pain, or leg flexion only
Flaccid tone with extensor plantars

Medullary
Pupils dilated and fixed to light
No response on testing OCR/OVR
Slow irregular, gasping or absent respiration
No response to pain
Flaccid tone with extensor plantars

Transtentorial herniation – intact survival possible

Foramen magnum herniation – intact survival not possible

Uncus

Diencephalon

Brainstem
Midbrain
Pons
Medulla

Figure 19.1 Mid-sagittal section of brain showing anatomy and key abnormal findings of midline herniation syndromes, and (above) coronal section showing herniation of the uncus of the temporal lobe. This compresses the third nerve (to cause a palsy of CNIII), and the contralateral cerebral peduncle (to cause an ipsilateral hemiparesis). OCR, oculocephalic (doll's eye) reflex; OVR, oculovestibular (caloric) reflex.

- Increased CSF protein.

- Decreased CSF glucose.

- Acid-fast bacilli are often not seen and culture is often not positive.

- PCR can be helpful in reliable laboratories.

- CT or MRI and cranial ultrasound commonly show hydrocephalus and, less often, basal enhancement and/or infarction of the basal ganglia.

Treatment

Isoniazid, rifampicin, streptomycin, and pyrazamide should be started with dexamethasone since the latter reduces neurological sequelae. The streptomycin, pyrazinamide, and dexamethasone are given for 2 months, and the isoniazid and rifampicin for 18 months.

Ventriculoperitoneal shunting is often required for hydrocephalus.

Outcome

Mortality is high and neurological sequelae are common.

FUNGAL MENINGITIS

Fungal meningitis, particularly cryptococcal meningitis, commonly occurs in immunocompromised hosts and may be the first sign of an acquired immune deficiency syndrome (AIDS)-defining illness. It is seen in immunocompromised infants. The other fungi that commonly cause meningitis are *Candida albicans* and *Coccidioides immitis*. It is reported in immune-competent infants as well.

The presentation may be more insidious than TB, presenting with respiratory distress, not tolerating feeds, and/or abdominal distension in low-birthweight infants. Fundoscopic examination may reveal disseminated Candida. CNS signs may occur, but the meningitis is often detected during a screen for sepsis. The organisms may be seen with fungal stains of the CSF, but the organism is usually isolated from other parts of the body, and meningitis is suspected from the pleocytosis.

Treatment

Candida: amphotericin B in combination with flucytosine.

Cryptococcus: amphotericin B and flucytosine for 6 to 10 weeks in HIV-negative patients. For HIV-positive patients, amphotericin B and flucytosine for 2 weeks and then fluconazole for 10 weeks.

Outcome

The mortality rate is very high and sequelae are common in those that survive.

VIRAL (ASEPTIC) MENINGITIS

Incidence and aetiology

The epidemiology depends on geography, climate, and vaccination coverage. Epidemics can occur and new viruses can emerge. Viral meningitis is common, but children are not usually 'toxic' nor do they have multiorgan failure or clotting derangements. Mild elevation of the liver enzymes or pancreatic enzymes can occur with some viruses.

A specific diagnosis is often not found, but the yield can be increased by sending stool/rectal swabs and throat swabs for culture in a viral culture medium (see below).

The most common agents are

- *Enteroviruses*: (85%) including echovirus, coxsackie, and poliovirus. All may cause diffuse rashes with or without more of the following specific features:

  o Echovirus: conjunctivitis, myositis.

  o Coxsackie: hand, foot and mouth disease, myocarditis, pericarditis, pleurisy.

  o Poliovirus (very rare if vaccination coverage is good): isolated meningitis or meningitis before onset of typical paralytic disease.

  o Parechovirus: similar features to enterovirus but usually neonates or young infants CSF may be acellular.

- *Mumps*: parotitis, pancreatitis (with elevated amylase and lipase), hearing loss.

- *Herpes viruses*:

  o Herpes simplex virus (HSV) type 1: usually no cold sores or skin lesions found. Usually a primary infection. For details about congenital herpes infections, see Box 20.1

  o Varicella zoster virus (VZV): may have typical chicken pox rash with fluid-filled blisters.

  o Epstein—Barr virus (EBV): pharyngitis, lymphadenopathy, splenomegaly, atypical peripheral lymphoctyes, may have abnormal liver-function tests (uncommon in infancy).

  o Cytomegalovirus (CMV): may have abnormal liver-function tests and retinitis (uncommon unless immunocompromised).

- Human herpes viruses (HHV) 6 and 7: roseola infantum ('slapped-cheek' rash), febrile seizures.

- *Measles*: typical confluent rash, lymphadenopathy, conjunctivitis, pneumonitis (rare if vaccination coverage is good).

- *Adenovirus*: conjunctivitis, respiratory infection, or gastroenteritis.

- *Lymphocytic choriomeningitis virus*: subacute illness with orchitis, myocarditis, parotitis, alopecia. Requires contact with rodents.

- *Arboviruses* (requires an infected mosquito or tick bite): not found in Northern Europe, consider if patient has travelled to South or Southeast Asia (Japanese encephalitis, dengue), all other continents (West Nile, Zika virus).

Clinical features

See section above on ABM. Altered level of consciousness is very uncommon.

Investigations

If viral meningitis is suspected, an LP is essential. A contraindication is very unlikely to exist (Box 19.1). See Table 19.1 for the typical changes seen in the CSF in viral meningitis.

CSF analysis: see section on ABM. Similar CSF tests are needed in an infant with suspected viral meningitis.

Other investigations: see section on ABM. Similar investigations are needed in an infant with suspected viral meningitis. It is very unlikely that an infant will need cranial imaging. It is also useful to send a throat swab and a rectal swab or a stool sample for *viral* isolation (note: viral culture medium needed). A serum sample should be saved to compare with a convalescent sample taken 3 weeks after the onset of the illness.

Differential diagnosis: see section on ABM.

Treatment: for uncomplicated viral meningitis, no specific treatment is needed. Full recovery usually occurs within 2 weeks, although some patients may have post-viral fatigue syndrome (rare in infancy). HSV meningitis is accompanied by encephalitis and specific treatment is required (see next section). Always test hearing after recovery.

ENCEPHALITIS

Encephalitis in infancy is uncommon but the incidence in infants is higher than in older children. Encephalitis can broadly be divided into infectious and immune mediated causes. Even if appropriate investigations are undertaken, a definite diagnosis is only found in approximately 50% of cases. The most common causes of sporadic VE in infants are HSV type 1, enterovirus, and VZV. In some parts of the world, arboviruses or rabies virus are more common. The epidemiology depends on the geography, climate, and vaccination coverage. Epidemics can occur and new viruses can emerge.

It is very important to identify and treat an infant with VE due to HSV type 1 as the outcome is better if the child is treated early in the illness. The differential diagnosis of encephalitis is quite wide (see below).

Most common causes of VE in infancy

The list is very similar to that given for viral meningitis above. Other specific details are given below.

Herpes viruses

HSV type 1 is the most common sporadic cause of VE in the western setting. In an infant this is usually a primary infection, but despite this, the presence of the typical herpes blistering rash, cold sores, or gingivostomatitis is unusual. Seizures and focal neurological signs are common. Presentation may be with a subtle, behavioural presentation and low-grade fever in older children and the immunocompromised.

HSV in neonates. The fetus is usually infected during delivery. Rarely, there is postnatal infection from close contacts (usually HSV type 1). Some 50% to 75% of cases are type 2 and the remainder type 1. Asymptomatic infection is common in the mother, but unusual in the infant. Infants born preterm are more frequently affected. Fetal scalp electrodes are a risk factor. Damage is caused by inflammation and lysis of cells. Many features are similar to other congenital infections, including what is known as TORCH (toxoplasmosis, other [infections], rubella, CMV, and HSV). Severe cases have multiorgan involvement with a predilection for the reticuloendothelial system (anaemia, jaundice, haemorrhages). Specific features include vesicular mucocutaneous lesions (often over the site of viral entry), conjunctivitis, and keratitis. If infection is localized to the CNS (without visceral involvement), symptom onset is later (second or third week of life). CNS abnormalities include meningoencephalitis and/or multifocal, severe and diffuse, seizures/coma, and a bulging fontanelle (see also Table 19.1).

VZV

VZV can have many neurological manifestations including postinfectious cerebellitis (common, but not in the first year of life), meningitis, an acute encephalitis (rare), and reactivation syndromes including large- and small-vessel vasculitis (see below) or neuropathies causing brainstem encephalitis including Ramsay—Hunt syndrome (facial palsy, hearing impairment/vertigo, and rash affecting ear canal and palate) or involvement of other cranial nerves including ophthalmic shingles. Those with VE caused by VZV may have a concomitant VZV rash or this may appear later. The virus lies dormant in ganglia along the entire neuroaxis. Reactivation can lead to an encephalitis. In the immunocompetent host this causes a large-vessel vasculitis leading to a stroke syndrome (see Chapter 18). This is common in infants and can occur up to several months after the primary infection. An immunocompromised host is more likely to get a small-vessel vasculitis leading to a progressive encephalitis. VZV is also associated with acute disseminated encephalomyelitis (ADEM), but this is very uncommon in the first year of life.

HHV 6 and 7

HHV 6 and 7 encephalitis mainly affects young children (<2 years old) during a primary infection. It usually causes a milder VE with febrile seizures and the typical roseola/ 'slapped-cheek' rash seen with HHV 6. Both viruses can be reactivated in the immuno-compromised.

Arboviruses

These are the most common cause of VE worldwide and are also 'emerging' diseases in previously unaffected geographical areas, but the identity of the specific virus depends on geography and the presence of the specific transmitting vector. Seizures are common.

Some specific virus types cause a movement disorder with Parkinsonian-like features and a flaccid paralysis 'polio-like illness' with anterior horn cell involvement. The arbovirus most likely to affect the Commonwealth of Independent States in Central and Eastern Europe and Central Asia is the tickborne encephalitis *flavivirus*. This virus is unlikely to affect infants because of lack of exposure, but in older children and adults a flaccid paralysis affecting the upper limbs and neck is seen. The clinical signs are similar to motor neuron disease. Some patients are also reported to have developed repeated and regular myoclonic seizures affecting the limbs. Patients from South or Southeast Asia may have *dengue encephalitis*. Most patients also have the typical vascular abnormalities seen in dengue haemorrhagic fever.

Enteroviruses

Enteroviruses commonly affect neonates and infants. Brainstem features are common. Epidemics with *enterovirus 71* strain are reported in the Asian Pacific region. These children may also have myocarditis. The D68 strain can cause outbreaks of CNS infection and acute flaccid myelitis: the outcome for paralysis is poor.

Measles virus

Causes four neurological syndromes: acute illness with the infection (the EEG is abnormal in a high proportion of 'uncomplicated' measles); acute ADEM-like illness within weeks of infection; a subacute progressive encephalitis affecting the immunocompromised around 6 months after primary infection; and subacute sclerosing pan encephalitis (SSPE), which presents years later (i.e. outside infancy) and is even rarer if immunization rates are high.

Influenza types A and B (including H1N1 'swine flu' strain)

Different neurological presentations are described, from mild encephalopathy with seizures to more severely affected cases with ADEM, malignant brain oedema syndrome, and acute necrotizing encephalopathy (ANE) (see Chapter 17). These are rare in infants.

Rotavirus

Infants with rotavirus gastroenteritis can present with clusters of seizures and this may not be associated with fever. Some cases reported with positive PCR for rotavirus ribonucleic acid (RNA) in CSF and there may be a CSF pleocytosis (usually <100 cells/ml). The outcome is good.

Non-viral causes of encephalitis

The neurological syndrome of encephalitis (as described in the definitions section above) can also be caused by acute and chronic bacterial infections such as *S. pneumoniae* and *Mycobacterium tuberculosis* but also by immune-mediated mechanisms.

Clinical features

Classically, there is a short history of fever, irritability, lethargy, encephalopathy, and sometimes seizures. Focal neurological signs are often identified. Multiorgan failure or clotting abnormalities are uncommon but mild elevation of the liver enzymes or pancreatic enzymes can occur with some viruses. A specific diagnosis is often not found, but as with the investigation of children with viral meningitis, the yield can be increased by sending stool, rectal, or throat swabs for culture (see above).

There may also be a subtler presentation with behavioural change, excessive sleepiness, or lethargy for a few days. Eventually the child may have a seizure, but the early symptoms may be dismissed by healthcare professionals. This is particularly the case for VE caused by HSV type 1; therefore, VE should be considered in an infant with this presentation, particularly if the infant could be immunocompromised.

Differential diagnosis

The differential diagnosis of VE includes the same disorders shown in the section on ABM above, but other disorders to consider include:

- metabolic encephalopathy: particularly mitochondrial disorders, fatty acid oxidation defects, and urea-cycle defects (see Chapters 15, 16, and 29). Also, acquired metabolic disorders of blood biochemistry (e.g. high or low sodium, low calcium, low blood glucose);

- trauma (especially inflicted traumatic brain injury; see Chapter 17);

- spontaneous brain haemorrhage (more common in neonates than older infants) or acute arterial stroke (see Chapter 18);

- exacerbation of seizures in a child with established epilepsy or non-convulsive status epilepticus (often occurs with nonspecific viral infections). Or febrile infection-related epilepsy syndrome (FIRES), a devastating non-encephalitic epileptic encephalopathy (very rare in infancy);

- endocrine disorders: consider a new presentation of diabetes mellitus (rare in infants);

- toxins: accidental ingestion or poisoning; and

- CNS vasculitis: very rare indeed in infancy. Vasculitis may be associated with systemic connective tissue disorders, such as systemic lupus erythematosus or primary CNS vasculitis.

Investigations

Many of the investigations needed for VE are the same as for ABM or viral meningitis (see sections on ABM and viral meningitis above). LP is mandatory and is still useful after treatment is started as CSF HSV PCR can still be positive up to 10 days after treatment with aciclovir. Failure to get CSF analysis may result in unnecessary prolonged treatment with aciclovir.

For HSV type 2 in a neonate, examination of vesicular fluid/skin scrapings is useful; histology: multinucleated giant cells or intranuclear inclusions seen, or electron microscopy: viral particles identified.

Viral isolation from throat, stool, urine, and CSF (viral culture media swabs needed). Serology is less useful as the IgM response may be delayed.

CSF findings are similar to those of viral meningitis, although the protein count may be up to 6g/L (see Table 19.1). It may be normal if an LP is performed in the first 48 hours of the illness. Repeat LP if VE is still strongly suspected and the first CSF analysis is normal.

PCR for viral DNA/RNA is possible for many viral infections (seek local advice for which are offered) but may be negative if the LP is undertaken less than 2 days or more than 10 days after the onset of the illness. Send CSF for PCR for HSV 1 and 2 and VZV initially, as VE caused by these viruses responds to treatment with aciclovir. Store CSF for further tests if these are negative. Viral isolation is sometimes possible.

Measurement of IgM response to specific viruses in the CSF is also possible and may confirm the diagnosis, even if viral PCR is negative. Discuss with a clinical virologist, if possible.

Brain imaging

CT is usually the first-line investigation, but CT can be normal in up to 30% of cases, especially in the early stages of the illness. Abnormal areas will show as hypodensities with or without patchy haemorrhage. MRI is the investigation of choice as the sensitivity is good and diffusion-weighted images are particularly helpful for identifying early changes.

- HSV type 1: most commonly gives an abnormal signal (often with haemorrhage) in the temporal lobes, insular cortex, frontal lobes, and thalami. Meningeal enhancement is also often present. Midline shift may be present if significant cerebral oedema is apparent. However, appearances may be atypical, especially in infants and children.

- HSV type 2: CT and ultrasound may identify multifocal parenchymal abnormalities.

- VZV: may have multiple abnormal areas of signal in the grey and white matter representing vasculitis and infarction. These may be in an arterial distribution in a case associated with viral reactivation.

- Enteroviruses: may have an abnormal signal isolated to the brainstem, dentate nucleus of the cerebellum, or thalami.

- Arboviruses: may have an abnormal signal in the basal ganglia and thalami.

- Rotavirus: usually normal.

- Influenza A and B: depends on the clinical syndrome associated with the virus; may be normal or have focal changes but is more likely to have changes consistent with ADEM or ANE.

Electroencephalography shows diffuse slowing of the background in all cases. Epileptiform focal abnormalities may also be seen and periodic lateralizing epileptiform discharges (PLEDs) may be present later in the illness in HSV type 1 encephalitis (Figure 19.2). PLEDs are not specific and may occur in SOL or other focal brain abnormalities.

Brain biopsy has become unnecessary for this diagnosis since the advent of PCR for viral DNA/RNA. However, it might need to be considered if the findings could change clinical management, for example if considering microabscesses from an embolic source, TB or a parasitic or fungal infection, vasculitis, or distinction between an infective SOL or a malignant process (see section below on SOL).

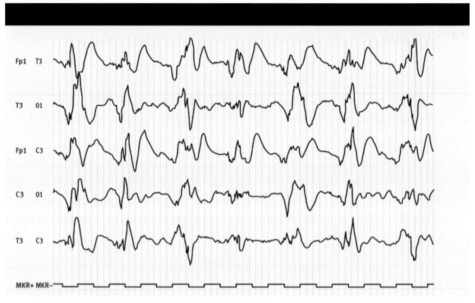

Figure 19.2 Electroencephalography showing left-sided periodic discharges every 2 seconds in herpes simplex virus type 1 encephalitis. (Reprinted from Kneen and Solomon, 2008 with permission from Elsevier.)

Treatment

Proven HSV 1 and 2: intravenous aciclovir for 21 days. Monitor renal function. If relapse occurs, re-treat and consider prophylaxis with valaciclovir or oral aciclovir for 90 days (although there is no published randomized controlled trial to support this).

Use of steroids in VE is controversial. Some anecdotal evidence of improvement in outcome is reported. Consider using a 3- to 5-day pulse of methylprednisolone or dexamethasone in severe cases with raised intracranial pressure. Consider surgical decompression in cases where raised intracranial pressure is refractory to medical treatment. There are no other specific antiviral treatments currently used for VE.

Prognosis

Prognosis depends on the cause and the severity of the clinical illness at presentation. In VE caused by HSV type 1, the prognosis depends upon the time interval before treatment was started, with mortality reduced by 40% in HSV type 1 if aciclovir is given promptly. Neurorehabilitation is often needed in a multidisciplinary setting. Patients who have had VE caused by HSV type 1 often experience severe memory problems. In neonates with HSV type 2, the mortality is highest (30–60%) for those with disseminated infection and is lower (15%) in those with isolated CNS disease. There are high levels of sequelae in survivors of both groups.

ADEM

All forms of immune-mediated parainfectious CNS disorders are very rare in the first year of life.

ADEM (see Chapter 17) occurs in the first year of life very rarely. Its diagnosis relies on brain imaging with MRI being the most sensitive imaging modality (see Chapter 8) but it may not be available in all settings.

AUTOIMMUNE ENCEPHALITIS

Autoimmune encephalitis (AE), also known as immune-mediated encephalitis, is an increasingly recognized aetiology of acute neurological and/or psychiatric disorders in adults and children.

Epidemiology

Its *prevalence* has been reported to be similar to that of infective encephalitides of all types (11.6/100 000) or the subgroup of viral infective encephalitides (8.3/100 000). The *incidence* rates of AE and infectious encephalitis were 0.8/100 000 and 1.0/100 000 person-years respectively (Dubey et al. 2018). Its clinical manifestations are broad and include seizures, movement disorders, behaviour and mood changes, psychosis, catatonia, memory/cognitive impairment, autonomic dysfunction, and altered level of consciousness.

Diagnosis

Stingl, Cardinale, and Van Mater, 2018 propose that a diagnosis of possible AE may be considered when patients present with

- An acute or subacute (<3 months) history of working memory deficits, altered mental state, or psychiatric symptoms.

- At least one of the following additional abnormalities:

    o   New-onset focal neurological signs.

    o   Seizures.

    o   White blood cell count >5 cells/ml in CSF.

    o   MRI abnormalities suggestive of encephalitis.

- Other causes have been excluded.

AE is associated with an increasing number of autoantibodies including voltage-gated potassium channel complex (anti-LGI1 and Caspr2), N-methyl-D-aspartate receptor (see Figure 17.4 b1 for an illustrative MRI), glutamate decarboxylase, AMPA receptors, and GABA; however, many cases are seronegative. Oligoclonal bands are sometimes detectable in paired serum and CSF. The presence of paraneoplastic antibodies is very rare in children and infants and AE is very rare in the first year of life.

Treatment

The general framework for treatment may be divided into first-line, second-line, and maintenance therapy. Patients treated early for AE have a better response to treatment than those treated late. If there is a strong clinical suspicion of the diagnosis, treatment may need to be started before the results of antibody testing is known and is, in any case, warranted in some antibody-negative cases. First-line therapy is steroids (methyl-prednisolone 30mg/kg [max dose 1gm] daily × 3–5 days). In severe and intractable cases, intravenous immunoglobulin (IVIG, 2gm/kg over 2 days) or plasma exchange (which should not be undertaken <3 days after IVIG) may be helpful as additional first-line treatments (Stingl, Cardinale, and Van Mater, 2018).

If patients respond promptly to these therapies, all of which have a rapid onset of action and relatively low associated risk, the use of prolonged 'maintenance' immunosuppression, or second-line agents, may not be necessary. However, if patients are not showing improvement or are deteriorating, escalation to second-line therapy is warranted. The timing of such escalation is not established, but for patients requiring inpatient care, it may be undertaken if the child is not improving within 10 to 14 days of initiating first-line therapy. This scenario is very rare in infants. Second-line therapies include rituximab and cyclophosphamide, mycophenolate, mofatil or azathioprine which are considered higher risk medications given their longer duration of action and greater immunosuppressive effects (Stingl, Cardinale, and Van Mater, 2018).

Supportive treatment

Patients may need treatment for agitation: as required or regular benzodiazepines can be helpful (e.g. lorazepam). Antiepileptic drugs may be needed (e.g. levetiracetam).

Antipsychotic medication should be avoided in patients with catatonia as malignant hyperpyrexia can emerge. Some patients may need intensive care support during the acute stage to manage agitation or severe movement disorders. Neurorehabilitation may be needed if recovery is protracted.

MALARIA

Malaria is caused by the infection of Plasmodium species, of which only two *Plasmodium falciparum* and *Plasmodium vivax* are associated with neurological manifestations. *P. falciparum* is the most common parasitic infection of the CNS, with children living in sub-Saharan Africa accounting for 75% of the infections. *P. vivax* is more commonly seen in Asia, Oceania, and, to a lesser extent, South America. Both infections are increasingly seen in infants who travel to malaria endemic areas.

Malaria should be suspected in any infant who has visited or even transiently landed at an airport in a malarious area within the last 3 months and develops CNS symptoms such as irritability, seizures, and changes in mental status. Vomiting and to a lesser extent diarrhoea are common. Fever is usually present, although its absence does not exclude the diagnosis. Falciparum malaria is more severe than vivax malaria. Both present with seizures, but coma (cerebral malaria) is a feature of falciparum malaria.

Neurological complications of falciparum malaria

The main manifestations neurological manifestations are seizures, prostration, agitation, impaired consciousness, including deep coma (cerebral malaria). These complications are often associated with metabolic acidosis, severe anaemia, renal failure, and pulmonary oedema, which may make the prognosis worse. Seizures are common and many occur when the child is apyrexial. They are often complex in that many are repetitive (more than one during the acute illness), focal, or prolonged. Prostration is common (i.e. the infant is unable to sit unsupported) and is often associated with metabolic dysfunction.

Malaria with impaired consciousness is the most severe neurological manifestation but is difficult to diagnose in infancy since the World Health Organization (WHO) has adopted strict criteria which include: (1) a patient is unable to localize a painful stimulus (such as pressure on the sternum) at least 1 hour after the last seizure; (2) asexual parasites are present in the peripheral blood; and (3) other causes of encephalopathy (e.g. meningitis, encephalitis, or hypoglycemia) are excluded (WHO, 2014). Any infant with *P. falciparum* infection and disturbed consciousness should be treated for cerebral malaria. Features of malaria retinopathy (retinal hemorrhages, retinal whitening, colour changes in the vessels, and, less frequently, papilloedema) increases the sensitivity of the diagnosis in the malaria endemic area. Meningism may be present, such that cerebral malaria cannot be differentiated clinically from bacterial meningitis.

A history of seizures is common and often precipitate the lapse into coma. Raised intracranial pressure is common and manifests with bulging fontanelle, brainstem signs, sluggish and dilated pupils, and/or decerebrate posturing. The liver and spleen are often enlarged. Spontaneous bleeding from the gastrointestinal tract occurs in nonimmune individuals.

Laboratory investigations

Rapid diagnostic tests such as the immunochromatographic test for *P. falciparum* histidine-rich protein 2 and lactate dehydrogenase have become widespread and are the investigation of choice. The asexual parasites can be detected on thick or thin blood films, stained with Giemsa or Field stains, but this requires more expertise. The lack of a detectable parasitaemia does not exclude the diagnosis of cerebral malaria, since the parasites may be sequestered within the deep vascular beds, or chemoprophylaxis may have suppressed the parasitaemia. Thus, blood smears need to be examined every 6 hours for 48 hours to exclude this infection.

Hypoglycaemia and a lactic acidosis are common and if severe, associated with a poor prognosis. Hyponatraemia is usually caused by salt depletion, but some cases may be caused by inappropriate antidiuretic hormone secretion. Hypoxaemia is associated with pulmonary oedema. Renal impairment is common and may progress to renal failure. Anaemia is usually present, caused by haemolysis (raised unconjugated bilirubinaemia, low haptoglobin concentration). Thrombocytopaenia is common but rarely severe enough to cause bleeding. Fibrin degradation products are raised, but laboratory features of frank disseminated intravascular coagulation are uncommon.

The CSF is usually acellular and if a pleocytosis is found other diagnoses such as encephalitis should be considered, although cerebral malaria cannot be excluded. CSF lactate concentrations are raised, but total protein and glucose concentrations are usually normal. Blood cultures may detect bacteraemia particularly caused by gram-negative organisms. Urinary tract infections occur.

Management

Antimalarial therapy

Antimalarial therapy is the only treatment that improves outcome. Parasites resistant to antimalarial drugs require complicated treatment and the recommendation is that a combination of antimalarials with different actions should be used. For severe malaria, parental artemesinin compounds are the recommended first-line drugs (Table 19.2), since they are more parasiticidal and have less side effects than the cinchinoid alkaloids (quinine and quinidine).

Table 19.2 Drug treatments for malaria

Drug	Route	Loading dose	Maintenance dose
Artesunate	IV/IM	2.4mg/kg	1.2mg/kg after 24h, then 1.2mg/kg/day for 7 days
Artemether	IM	3.2mg/kg	1.6 mg/kg/day for a minimum of 5 days
Quinidine gluconate	IV	15mg base/kg (24mg/kg salt) in normal saline over 4h or 6.25mg base/kg (10mg salt/kg) over 2h	75mg base/kg (12mg salt/kg) infused over 4h, every 8–12h with ECG monitoring then 0.0125mg base/kg/min (0.02mg salt/kg/min) as a continuous infusion for 24h
Quinine dihydrochloride	IV	20mg salt/kg over 2–4h	10mg salt/kg every 8–12h, until able to take orally
Quinine dihydrochloride	IM	20mg salt/kg (dilute IV formulation to 60mg/ml) given in 2 injection sites (anterior thigh)	10mg salt/kg every 8–12h until able to take orally

IV, intravenous; IM, intramuscular; ECG, electrocardiogram.

Artesunate is the favoured drug, since it can be administered intravenously or intramuscularly and is associated with less neurotoxicity in animal models, and has reduced mortality in adults with severe malaria (WHO, 2014).

Other antimalarial drugs

Other antimalarial drugs should be combined with the parenteral antimalarials to prevent the emergence of resistant parasites, usually given during the recovery phase.

Atovaquone-proguanil (Malarone) and Mefloquine can be used.

Supportive treatment

Children with impaired consciousness should be admitted to an intensive care unit, since they require close monitoring (WHO, 2014). Most children die within 24 hours, before the antimalarials have had time to work. Blood glucose and fluid balance should be measured every 6 hours, parasitaemia and haematocrit every 12 hours. Electrolytes, tests of renal function, albumin, calcium, phosphate, and blood gases should be performed at least daily during the acute stages.

Fluid balance is critical in severe malaria, as many children are hypovolaemic, but over-aggressive fluid therapy can precipitate pulmonary oedema and aggravate intracranial hypertension. Renal function needs to be carefully monitored because acute renal failure is a common cause of death in nonimmune patients. Patients with pulmonary oedema or adult respiratory distress syndrome require supplemental oxygen and positive pressure ventilation, with positive end expiratory pressure to maintain adequate oxygenation, and diuretics or hemofiltration to correct the fluid overload.

Blood transfusions should be considered when the haematocrit falls toward 20%, or the child has evidence of cardiovascular compromise. The role of exchange transfusions in the management of cerebral malaria is controversial, but most authorities recommend exchange transfusion in patients who have a parasitaemia in excess of 10% or who are deteriorating in spite of conventional treatment (WHO, 2014). Vitamin K and cryoprecipitate should be administered if a patient has a bleeding diathesis. Seizures must be treated promptly with a benzodiazepine drug, and a prophylactic anticonvulsant, such as phenytoin or phenobarbital, should be used if they recur. Neuroimaging should be done to exclude brain swelling before an LP is performed. If brain swelling is detected, intracranial pressure monitoring should be considered. Steroids appear to be deleterious, increasing the incidence of bleeding without any beneficial effect on outcome.

Secondary bacterial infections should always be suspected. Blood, urine, and CSF should be sent for culture and repeated examinations of the chest should be performed since aspiration or hypostatic pneumonia is common. Broad-spectrum antimicrobial treatment should be started as soon as a complicating infection is suspected.

Outcome

The mortality of cerebral malaria in nonimmune individuals ranges from 15% to 26%, with patients usually dying within the first 4 days of the illness, often from renal failure or pulmonary oedema. African children have a similar mortality rate but most die within 48 hours of admission, often with brainstem signs suggestive of transtentorial herniation.

Neurological sequelae occur in about 5% of nonimmune individuals with cerebral malaria and include cranial nerve lesions, extrapyramidal tremor, polyneuropathy, epilepsy, or psychiatric manifestations. In African children, sequelae are more common and more severe. Neurological deficits occur in 11%, with hemiparesis, quadriparesis, ataxia, and cortical blindness the most common sequelae. Up to 24% of African children have impaired cognitive function, particularly in memory, executive functions, and language, following cerebral malaria and complex seizures (Kihara, Carte, and Newton, 2006). Epilepsy occurs in about 10% of children 2 to 4 years after the admission with cerebral malaria (Christensen and Eslick, 2015). This figure is likely to be greater with longer follow-up.

INFECTIVE SOLS

Brain abscesses or extra-axial collections can be caused by bacteria, fungi, or parasites with the most common causal organisms in infancy being staphylocci (*Staphyloccus aureus* and other staphylococcal species), *Streptococcus* (aerobic and anaerobic), and *H. influenzae*. Anaerobic organisms such as bacteroides, *Streptococcus milleri*, and *Fusobacterium species* are also commonly found. CNS TB should be considered. Fungi (*Aspergillus species*) and parasites have also been reported. Approximately 40% of abscesses will contain mixed flora.

They may be caused by haematogenous or local spread and be single or multiple. Localization is related to an underlying predisposing factor, with those spreading in the blood found in a distribution that reflects the cerebral blood supply, usually the middle cerebral artery. There may also be a haematogenous venous spread from the sinuses to the frontal lobes. There may be direct invasion from infections of the sinuses or middle ear and these infections tend to cause abscesses in the temporal lobes or cerebellum.

Risk factors

- Infancy: infective SOLs are more common in infants than older children.

- Congenital heart disease.

- Sinus or ear infections.

- Poor dental hygiene (very rare in infancy).

- Immunosuppression.

- Presence of a ventriculoperitoneal shunt.

- Skull fracture.

- Dermal sinuses or other channel to the CNS from head, neck, or back.

- Complication of bacterial meningitis.

- Following aspiration of a foreign body (very rare in infancy).

Clinical features

Irritability and fever are typical with a focal neurological deficit that depends on location of lesion(s). In infancy, the fontanelle can bulge and the head circumference can increase rapidly. There may be irritability or lethargy or a reduced level of consciousness, but children can appear surprisingly well and present with progressive macrocephaly. Raised intracranial pressure and brain herniation syndromes can develop.

Acute neurological decompensation and signs of meningitis may supervene if the abscess ruptures into the ventricular system.

Laboratory investigations

- There may be nonspecific haematological markers of infection with elevated peripheral white cell count, erythrocyte sedimentation rate, and C-reactive protein.

- Blood cultures are rarely positive.

- A cardiac assessment including an echocardiogram should be undertaken.

- CSF examination (LP) is contraindicated due to the risk of brain herniation syndromes.

- Drainage of a suspected abscess may be required for SOL over 2cm in diameter. Needle biopsy sampling of SOL under 2cm may also be helpful to confirm the diagnosis of infection, obtain sensitivities to antibiotics, and exclude other diagnoses. This clearly requires access to appropriate neurosurgical expertise and equipment, preferably including stereotactic guidance equipment.

Cranial imaging

Cranial ultrasound may be useful in a neonate. CT is useful and will detect most SOLs, but lesions in the posterior fossa or temporal lobe may be missed. Contrast should be given as extra-axial collections can be missed on an unenhanced CT scan and ring enhancement of lesions is characteristic. MRI is the modality of choice, with and without contrast if possible. Diffusion-weighted MRI and magnetic resonance spectroscopy can also be helpful in differentiating a single parenchymal lesion from a tumour.

Differential diagnosis

- Brain tumour.

- Intraparenchymal haemorrhage.

- Lymphoma or an isolated single demyelinating lesion are included in the differential diagnosis but are very unlikely to occur in infancy.

Treatment

Small lesions (<2cm in diameter) or those in whom the causative organism has been identified may be amenable to medical treatment with antimicrobials. Surgical drainage followed by prompt initiation of empirical broad-spectrum empirical antimicrobial therapy is often needed (usually for 6 weeks, but longer in the immunocompromised). Surgical specimens should be sent for histology and for microbiology investigations.

Typical first-choice antibiotics would include a third-generation cephalosporin and metronidazole, but advice should be sought from the infectious diseases team. If an associated foreign body, such as a central line or ventriculoperitoneal shunt, is found, it should be removed.

Outcome

Depends on the severity and location of parenchymal damage. Neurorehabilitation is often necessary (see above) as 40% of children have neurological sequelae and 25% have epilepsy.

ACKNOWLEDGEMENT

We are grateful to the authors of Chapter 17, Tiina Talvik, Fenella Kirkham, Tuuli Metsvaht, and Inga Talvik, for drafting the section of this chapter on autoimmune encephalitis and its treatment.

REFERENCES

Christensen SS, Eslick G (2015) Cerebral malaria as a risk factor for the development of epilepsy and other long-term neurological conditions: a meta-analysis. *Trans R Soc Trop Med Hyg* 109: 233–238.

Dubey D, Pittock SJ, Kelly CR, et al. (2018) Autoimmune encephalitis epidemiology and a comparison to infectious encephalitis. *Ann Neurol* 83: 166–177.

Kihara M, Carte JA, Newton CRC (2006) The effect of Plasmodium falciparum on cognition: A systematic review. *Trop Med Int Health* 11: 386–397.

Stingl C, Cardinale K, Van Mater H (2018) An update on the treatment of pediatric autoimmune encephalitis. *Curr Treat Options in Rheum* 4: 14–28.

WHO (2014) Severe Malaria. *Trop Med Int Health* 19 (Suppl. 1): 7–131.

Resources

Barbagallo M, Vitaliti G, Pavone P, Romano C, Lubrano R, Falsaperla R (2017) Pediatric autoimmune encephalitis. *J Pediatr Neurosci* 12: 130–134.

Dale R, Gorman MP, Lim M (2017) Autoimmune encephalitis in children: clinical phenomenology, therapeutics and emerging challenges. *Curr Opin Neurol* 30: 334–344.

Kim KS (2010) Acute bacterial meningitis in infants and children. *Lancet Infect Dis* 10: 32–42.

Kneen R, Michael BD, Menson E, et al. (2012) Management of suspected viral encephalitis in children. Association of British Neurologists and British Paediatric Allergy, Immunology and Infection Group National Guidelines. *J Infect* 64: 449–77.

Kneen R, Solomon T (2008) Management and outcome of viral encephalitis in children. *J Paediatr Child Health* 18: 7-16.

Paediatric Accident and Emergency Research Group. Management of the child with a decreased conscious level. An evidence-based guideline. Available at https://www.nottingham.ac.uk/paediatric-guideline/Guideline%20algorithm.pdf

Sheehan JP, Jane JA, Ray DK, Goodkin HP (2008) Brain abscess in children. *Neurosurg Focus* 24: E6.

Visintin C, Mugglestone MA, Fields EJ, et al. (2010) Management of bacterial meningitis and meningococcal septicaemia in children and young people: summary of NICE guidance. *BMJ* 340: c3209 (https://www.nice.org.uk/guidance/%20CG102/Guidance/pdf/English).

CHAPTER 20

Postneonatal epileptic seizures

Hans Hartmann and J Helen Cross

Key messages

- Differentiate epileptic seizures from nonepileptic paroxysmal events. Home videos demonstrating an event can be extremely helpful.
- Manage infants with simple febrile seizures expectantly.
- Treat an infant with status epilepticus vigorously.
- Recognize possible underlying structural causes, infectious, genetic, or metabolic disorders in infants presenting with epileptic seizures.

Common errors

- Diagnosing epilepsy in an infant with nonepileptic paroxysmal events.
- Treating infants with sodium-channel disorders with the wrong anti-seizure drugs.

When to worry

- When seizures occur in clusters or the infant goes into status epilepticus.
- When there are persistent focal signs.
- When the infant does not adequately regain consciousness following a seizure.
- When the infant shows developmental plateau or regression.

DEFINITIONS

The following definitions and classifications have been developed and approved by task forces of the International League Against Epilepsy (ILAE). They are operational definitions, specifically worded to optimize patient management.

Epileptic seizures are transient and fully reversible events involving a disturbance of neurological function. Epileptic seizures are caused by abnormal, excessive activity of a, more or less, extensive population of cerebral neurons (Fisher et al. 2005). They need to be differentiated from nonepileptic seizures, considered in Chapter 21. Although most information will be derived from a description of events, this differentiation can be supported by electroencephalography (EEG) demonstrating (or not) epileptic discharges, i.e. temporary paroxysmal changes in EEG activity. Most epileptic seizures are brief, lasting only seconds to a few minutes. Following a seizure, the infant may be drowsy and, in case of a focal motor seizure, transiently show a hemiparesis (Todd paresis).

Status epilepticus (SE) refers to abnormally prolonged seizures. It is a condition that can have long-term consequences, including neuronal death, neuronal injury, and alteration of neuronal networks, depending on the type and duration of seizures (Trinka et al. 2015).

Epilepsies are diseases of the brain defined by any of the following conditions: (1) at least two unprovoked (or reflex) seizures occurring >24 hours apart; (2) one unprovoked (or reflex) seizure and a probability of further seizures similar to the general recurrence risk (at least 60%) after two unprovoked seizures, occurring over the next 10 years; (3) diagnosis of an epilepsy syndrome (Fisher et al. 2017).

Epilepsy syndromes are clinical entities that can reliably be identified by a cluster of electroclinical characteristics: seizure type(s), age at onset, family history of epilepsy, and EEG features (Berg et al. 2010).

Epileptic encephalopathy refers to a condition where 'the epileptic activity itself contributes to severe cognitive and behavioural impairment above and beyond that expected from the underlying pathology and that these can worsen over time' (Berg et al. 2010). If in an infant with epilepsy, it can be assumed that the developmental consequences arise directly from the effect of the underlying cause, e.g. a genetic variant, in addition to the effect of the frequent epileptic activity on development, this disorder may be labelled developmental and epileptic encephalopathy (Scheffer et al. 2017).

EPILEPTIC SEIZURES

Seizure classification

Epileptic seizures can be classified as generalized onset or focal onset, depending on the manifestations at seizure onset. Figure 20.1 summarizes the 2017 classification of seizures by the ILAE (Fisher et al. 2017).

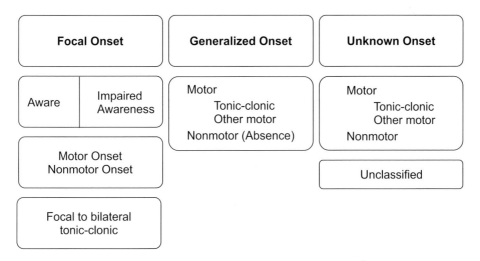

Figure 20.1 International League Against Epilepsy classification of seizure types. (Basic version, adapted from Fisher et al. 2017 with permission from the International League Against Epilepsy.)

Generalized onset epileptic seizures are conceptualized as originating at some point within, and rapidly engaging, bilaterally distributed networks. Such bilateral networks can include cortical and subcortical structures, but do not necessarily include the entire cortex (Berg et al. 2010).

Focal onset epileptic seizures are conceptualized as originating within networks limited to one hemisphere. They may be discretely localized or more widely distributed. Focal seizures may originate in subcortical structures. Descriptors for focal seizures include the following:

- without impairment of awareness;

- with impairment of awareness (traditional terminology: complex partial seizures);

- motor or non-motor symptoms;

- evolving to a bilateral, convulsive seizure involving tonic—clonic or tonic and clonic components (traditional terminology: secondarily generalized seizures).

Some phenomena that can typically be observed during seizures, according to the ILAE glossary of descriptive terminology for seizure semiology, are shown in Table 20.1. An online diagnostic manual containing extensive teaching material including videos of different seizure types can be accessed via the ILAE website (https://www.ilae.org/education/diagnostic-manual).

Table 20.1 Phenomena that may typically be observed during seizures

Term	Description
Absence, typical	Sudden onset, interruption of ongoing activities, a blank stare, possibly a brief upward deviation of the eyes
Absence, atypical	An absence seizure with changes in tone that are more pronounced than in typical absence or the onset and/or cessation is not abrupt
Atonic	Sudden loss or diminution of muscle tone without apparent preceding myoclonus or tonic event
Automatism	A coordinated motor activity usually occurring when cognition is impaired. This often resembles a voluntary movement
Autonomic seizure	Distinct alteration involving cardiovascular, pupillary, gastrointestinal, sudomotor, vasomotor, and thermoregulatory functions
Aura	Subjective ictal phenomenon
Awareness	Knowledge of self or environment
Clonic	Jerking, either symmetric or asymmetric, i.e. regularly repetitive and involves the same muscle groups
Dystonic	Sustained contractions of both agonist and antagonist muscles producing athetoid or twisting movements which may produce abnormal postures
Epileptic spasms	Sudden flexion, extension, or mixed flexion-extension of predominantly proximal and truncal muscles that is usually more sustained than a myoclonic movement but not as sustained as a tonic seizure. Epileptic spasms frequently occur in clusters. Infantile spasms are the best known form, but spasms can occur at all ages
Fencer's posture seizure	Focal motor seizure type with extension of one arm and flexion at the contralateral elbow and wrist

Table 20.1 (continued)   Phenomena that may typically be observed during seizures

Term	Description
Figure-of-4 seizure	Upper limbs with extension of the arm (usually contralateral to the epileptogenic zone) with elbow flexion of the other arm, forming a figure-of-4
Behavioural arrest	Pause of activities, freezing, immobilization
Myoclonic	Sudden, brief (<100ms) involuntary single or multiple contraction(s) of muscles(s) or muscle groups. Myoclonus is less regularly repetitive and less sustained than is clonus
Myoclonic—atonic	A generalized seizure type with a myoclonic jerk leading to an atonic motor component (previously called myoclonic—astatic)
Myoclonic tonic—clonic	One or a few jerks of limbs bilaterally, followed by a tonic—clonic seizure. The initial jerks can be considered to be either a brief period of clonus or myoclonus (common in juvenile myoclonic epilepsy)
Sensory seizure	Perceptual experience not caused by appropriate stimuli in the external world
Versive	Sustained, forced conjugate ocular, cephalic, and/or truncal rotation or lateral deviation from the midline

(Adapted from Fisher et al. 2017 with permission from the International League Against Epilepsy)

CLINICAL APPROACH TO AN INFANT PRESENTING WITH A FIRST SEIZURE

Questions to be asked

Was the seizure epileptic or does the infant have a nonepileptic paroxysmal disorder (see Chapter 21)?

Was the seizure possibly provoked by an acute illness, such as a febrile illness or infection?

Is there evidence for an underlying chronic illness?

Is the child in a stable condition following the seizure?

Examinations always indicated following a first nonfebrile seizure

- Blood pressure.

- Finger-prick blood test to exclude hypoglycemia if the child is drowsy after the seizure.

- Electrocardiogram.

Examinations that may be indicated following a first nonfebrile seizure

To exclude central nervous system (CNS) infection, perform lumbar puncture, including cerebrospinal fluid (CSF) cell count and differential cell count, glucose (paired with serum glucose preferably from sample taken immediately before lumbar puncture), lactate, protein. Herpes simplex virus polymerase chain reaction should always be undertaken in infants with focal seizures because of the importance of early treatment with aciclovir. Further studies regarding other neurotropic viruses may be indicated. Bacterial culture should be performed whenever meningitis is suspected. To exclude electrolyte disturbance, measure plasma concentrations of sodium, calcium, and magnesium and if abnormal, assess the likely cause in the context of the wider electrolyte and clinical picture.

Imaging studies

Such studies are usually *not* indicated following a first seizure if the child subsequently is well unless there is evidence of trauma or hemorrhaging, or the child had a first nonfebrile seizure with focal signs.

EEG

EEG is usually indicated following a first nonfebrile seizure in infancy, whereas EEG is usually *not* indicated following a first simple febrile seizure (see Figure 20.2 and Figure 20.3).

FEBRILE SEIZURES

Febrile seizures are age-related events affecting approximately 3% of children between the ages of 6 months and 5 years. It is important to characterize a febrile seizure as either simple or complex because complex febrile seizures are associated with a less good prognosis.

Criteria for simple febrile seizures include the following:

- generalized tonic–clonic seizure,

- duration of less than 15 minutes,

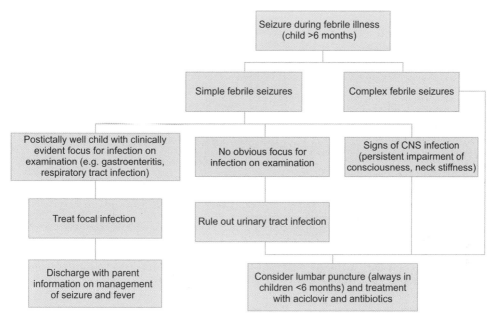

Figure 20.2 Management of a child following a first seizure during a febrile illness. CNS, central nervous system.

- no recurrence within the next 24 hours,

- no focal features during or after seizures (approximately 30% of febrile seizures are focal).

Criteria for complex febrile seizures include the following:

- prolonged seizures lasting 15 minutes or more,

- repetitive febrile seizures in clusters (two or more within 24h),

- seizures with focal features at onset or after the event.

Most febrile seizures are brief, lasting 3 to 6 minutes. However, in 8% they are longer than 15 minutes and become febrile status epilepticus (SE). Children with febrile SE show an increased risk for developing epilepsy. Recurrences of simple febrile seizures occur in 30% to 50% of cases. They are more common in those with a first-degree relative who has had febrile seizures and in those experiencing a first febrile seizure under 1 year of age. The overall risk for epilepsy developing after a febrile seizure is 3%. While it is only 1% to 2% in infants who experience a simple febrile seizure, it increases to 15% in children having complex febrile seizures, according to how many and which risk factors they carry.

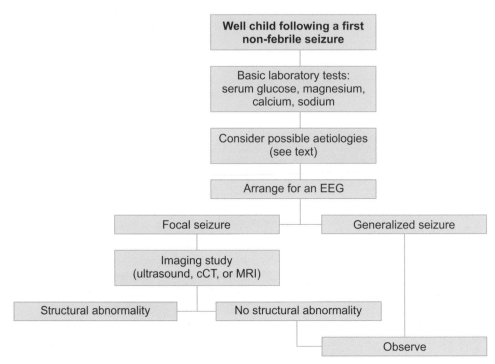

Figure 20.3   Management of a child following a first nonfebrile seizure. EEG, electroencephalography; cCT, cranial computed tomography; MRI, magnetic resonance imaging.

The intellectual and behavioral outcome following febrile seizures is good. The subsequent psychomotor development of children who were typically developing before the onset of febrile seizures is normal and children perform as well as other children at school.

Acute management of an infant with a febrile seizure

Long-lasting febrile seizures (>10min) are a medical emergency. If a febrile seizure has lasted longer than 5 minutes, emergency services should be called and pharmacological treatment should be given in the form of either rectal diazepam (5mg for children <12kg, 10mg for children ≥12kg), buccal midazolam (2.5mg at age 6–12 months or 5mg at 1–5 years), or nasal midazolam (0.3mg per kg up to a maximum of 10mg), depending on availability and national guidelines. If in the hospital, intravenous benzodiazepines should be used as first-line treatment. Additionally, antipyretics should be given.

Prevention and management of recurrence of febrile seizures

Antipyretic therapy in infants with a history of febrile seizures does not reduce the recurrence risk. Therefore, antipyretic therapy should be used, as in children without history of febrile seizures, to comfort the child and help avoid dehydration. Continuous prophylactic treatment with anti-seizure medication is not recommended for children with febrile seizures. In case of a further febrile seizure, parents should be advised to:

- place the infant on their side or stomach,

- give emergency medication (see above) if the febrile seizure has not ceased within 5 minutes, and call for professional medical assistance if this does not stop the seizure or the child does not fully regain consciousness.

Other situation-related seizures

Seizures may also occur in relation to CNS system metabolic disorders, trauma, and infections (see Chapters 15, 17, and 19). In most of these situations the infant will usually show signs of an underlying acute illness before the seizure, suffer serial seizures, or not recover completely following the seizure.

Neurocysticercosis is a common cause of focal seizures in some regions e.g. 17% of children presenting with focal seizures in Western Nepal (Rao et al. 2017). This is a treatable cause of epilepsy and, although rare in infancy, needs to be considered in the context of the local disease prevalence when an infant presents with a first afebrile seizure. There may be associated signs of raised intracranial pressure. CT and MRI reveal single, or occasionally multiple, cystic lesions and serology confirms the diagnosis. Cysticidal drugs (e.g. abendazole) are the mainstay of treatment.

STATUS EPILEPTICUS

Whereas traditionally a seizure going on for more than 30 minutes or a series of seizures without complete recovery of consciousness in between was defined as SE, this has now been replaced by an operational definition, the purpose of which is to help improve treatment efficacy (Trinka et al. 2015). According to the new definition, SE is a condition resulting either from the failure of the mechanisms responsible for seizure termination or from the initiation of mechanisms which lead to abnormally prolonged seizures (defined by their continuation beyond time point t1). It is a condition that can have long-term consequences (if continuing beyond time point t2), including neuronal death, neuronal injury, and alteration of neuronal networks, depending on the type and duration of seizures. Treatment should be initiated at t1, and aim to terminate SE before t2, in order to avoid possible long-term consequences. Nevertheless, CSE requires a vigorous diagnostic work-up and pharmacological treatment. Therefore, in CSE, t1 has been defined as 5 minutes, and t2 as 30 minutes (Trinka et al. 2015).

Since any seizure type can progress to SE, a wide range of clinical symptoms can be observed. Clinically it is important to distinguish 'convulsive', (i.e. tonic–clonic, tonic or clonic SE [CSE]), from non-convulsive SE (NCSE). CSE is a life-threatening emergency. In population-based studies, the incidence of CSE has been calculated as 14.5 in 100 000 per year. Outcome, including mortality, further episodes of CSE, development of epilepsy, and neurodevelopment, strongly depends on the aetiology. It is reassuring that in a population-based study all deaths occurring in SE could be attributed to severe underlying diseases such as meningitis and neurodegenerative disorders (Chin et al. 2008). Nevertheless, CSE requires a vigorous diagnostic work-up and pharmacological treatment.

CSE can occur in the context of a febrile illness or without fever. In febrile CSE, it is important to exclude CNS infection before CSE can be attributed to a prolonged febrile seizure. Differential diagnosis of afebrile CSE includes

- acute electrolyte imbalance, including hypoglycaemia, hypocalcaemia, and hypo-magnesaemia,

- acute head injury,

- intracranial haemorrhage,

- stroke,

- drug overdose,

- intoxication,

- hypoxia,

- infections, including neurocysticercosis or congenital infections,

- seizures secondary to preexisting neurological abnormality, including CNS malformation, previous brain injury, and cerebral palsy,

- metabolic diseases, or

- epilepsy-related.

Diagnostic investigations in an infant with new-onset CSE should always include serum electrolytes, blood sugar, EEG, imaging (CT or MRI), a lumbar puncture, if there are signs of infection, and urine toxicology, if there is a possibility of intoxication. In an infant with previously known epilepsy, investigations should include blood concentrations of anti-seizure drugs and electrolytes and an EEG. Additionally, the possibility of an acute infectious disorder causing CSE independently of the previously known epilepsy needs to be considered.

Various treatment protocols have been suggested for prolonged seizures and CSE, including in the World Health Organization's downloadable 2016 Paediatric Emergency, Triage, Assessment and Treatment guideline (WHO, 2016). A treatment algorithm is given in Figure 20.4. Generally, benzodiazepines are used as first-line drugs. In the pre-hospital setting, either rectal diazepam or buccal / nasal midazolam is used. In hospital, treatment should be continued via intravenous access and as initial treatment, a second dose of benzodiazepines is suggested. Lorazepam has been shown to be more effective in terminating the seizure than other benzodiazepines. Most treatment protocols suggest observation periods of 10 minutes between medications. A maximum of two doses of benzodiazepines should be given prior to the next stage. Second-line medications then include phenobarbital, phenytoin, and sodium valproate. Levetiracetam 40mg/kg given IV was recently reported to be at least as effective as phenytoin in this context (Lyttle et al. 2019).

In children with a history suggestive of Dravet syndrome, phenytoin should be avoided, because its action on sodium channels can result in a worsening of the epileptic condition, although some children prior to the diagnosis may have been seen to respond appropriately. Caution should also be exercised with sodium valproate if a metabolic disorder is suspected. If the second-line medication is not successful, the infant needs to be transferred to an intensive care unit and further management may include thiopental or continuous midazolam infusion.

NCSE is characterized by a cognitive or behavioral change (ranging from mild confusion to coma) coupled with evidence of seizure activity on EEG that has changed from baseline. It can be either generalized (i.e. absence SE), or focal. It is extremely uncommon in the first year of life but may occur in the context of genetic or structural epilepsies, underlying metabolic encephalopathies, or acute symptomatic seizures following trauma or hypoxic-ischemic encephalopathy. Cerebral function monitoring may be helpful to diagnose NCSE and treatment should focus on possible treatment of any underlying disorder in addition to anti-seizure drugs. Definitions of t1 and t2 with regard to treatment remain less clear than with CSE, whether successful treatment of NCSE will result in improved developmental outcome is unclear.

EPILEPSIES WITH ONSET IN THE FIRST YEAR OF LIFE

The incidence of epilepsy is age-specific, being highest in young children and elderly people. During the first year of life, the incidence is around 82.1 per 100 000 children (Eltze et al. 2013). Epilepsy syndromes are also age-specific. The seizure type and epilepsy may be more dependent on the child's age than on the underlying pathology. In an infant with recurrent unprovoked seizures, an attempt should be made to classify the epilepsy, according to the 2017 ILAE classification, considering the type of seizures, underlying aetiology, and associated comorbidities (Scheffer et al. 2017). Diagnosis of

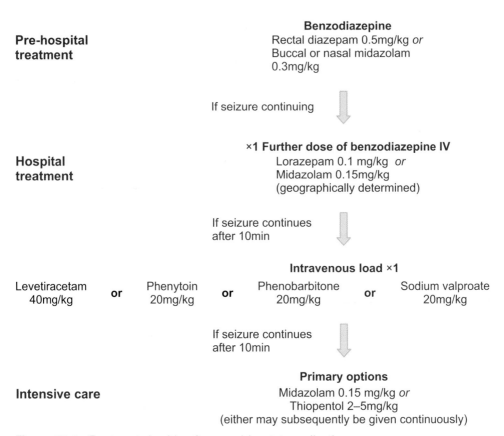

Pre-hospital treatment

Benzodiazepine
Rectal diazepam 0.5mg/kg *or*
Buccal or nasal midazolam
0.3mg/kg

If seizure continuing

Hospital treatment

×1 Further dose of benzodiazepine IV
Lorazepam 0.1 mg/kg *or*
Midazolam 0.15mg/kg
(geographically determined)

If seizure continues after 10min

Intravenous load ×1

Levetiracetam 40mg/kg **or** Phenytoin 20mg/kg **or** Phenobarbitone 20mg/kg **or** Sodium valproate 20mg/kg

If seizure continues after 10min

Intensive care

Primary options
Midazolam 0.15 mg/kg *or*
Thiopentol 2–5mg/kg
(either may subsequently be given continuously)

Figure 20.4   Treatment algorithm for convulsive status epilepticus

an underlying aetiology may influence treatment, and exact classification of an epilepsy may help the early recognition of comorbidities.

Aetiology

Causes of epilepsy recognized by the 2017 ILAE classification include:

- *Structural:* these include acquired disorders such as stroke, trauma, and infection. They may also be of genetic origin (e.g. tuberous sclerosis, many malformations of cortical development). As we currently understand it, here there is a separate disorder interposed between the genetic defect and the epilepsy.

- *Genetic:* the epilepsy is the direct result of a genetic variant(s) in which seizures are the core symptom of the disorder. A genetic cause may be known, as in some channelopathies, or presumed, as in the majority of patients with idiopathic generalized epilepsies. 'Genetic' is not synonymous with 'inherited', for example in 50% of patients with an autosomal-dominant disorder, the pathogenic variant is due to a de novo variant.

- *Infectious:* these include, among others, neurocysticercosis, tuberculosis, human immunodeficiency virus (HIV), cerebral malaria, subacute sclerosing panencephalitis, cerebral toxoplasmosis, and congenital infections such as Zika virus and cytomegalovirus. Whereas signs of infection may be obvious in some, epilepsy may be the only presenting sign, especially in neurocysticercosis. Infectious causes may be amendable to specific treatments and therefore are important to recognize.

- *Metabolic:* many inborn errors of metabolism affecting the CNS present with acute symptomatic seizures, and some with epilepsy.

- *Immune:* epilepsies may be caused by autoantibodies targeting neuronal antigens, such as the *N*-methyl D-aspartate receptor, and present with epilepsy.

- *Unknown cause:* the nature of the underlying cause is, as yet, unknown. It may have a fundamental genetic defect at its core as yet undetermined or it may be the consequence of a separate as yet unrecognized disorder (Scheffer et al. 2017).

In infants, structural, genetic, and metabolic causes are frequent, and may influence treatment. Genetic causes, in particular, are now frequently identified. This has added to our understanding of epilepsy in infants and the concept of developmental and epileptic encephalopathies. Very often, an unfavorable development of an infant with epilepsy is not entirely attributable to the epileptic activity or prolonged seizures but also to the effect of the underlying disorder itself. For example, development in patients with Dravet syndrome, due to pathogenic *SCN1A* variants, may be hindered by inadequate treatment; but even if an infant is diagnosed early and only has a moderate epileptic burden, development will not always be favourable.

If a specific clinical syndrome is frequently associated with a pathogenic variant of a single gene, this is sometimes used as a descriptor (e.g. *CDKL5* encephalopathy). However, the same clinical picture may also be caused by another genetic defect, and a single gene may be associated with different clinical phenotypes (e.g. *SCN1A*). Therefore, currently both electroclinical and causative descriptors are used in parallel.

Most causes of neonatal seizures can also cause epilepsy in infancy and therefore causes of neonatal seizures must continue to be considered in infants older than 28 days. Late presentations of pyridoxine-dependent epilepsy, pyridoxal phosphate-dependent epilepsy, or other inborn errors of metabolism (see Chapter 15) do occur.

Clinical approach to an infant with epilepsy

Questions to be asked

Can the seizure type be clearly described?

At what age did seizures start?

Is there a family history of epilepsy?

Was there anything remarkable during pregnancy, birth, or the immediate postnatal period?

Was the infant's development typical until the manifestation of the epilepsy?

Have the seizures affected the infant's development?

Physical examination should especially include

- Measurement and determination of centiles for body length, weight, and head circumference.

- Cutaneous abnormalities, especially hypo- or hyperpigmented areas; check for areas of hypopigmentation using Wood's light (ultraviolet light wavelength c. 365nm), also check for nevus flammeus affecting face or scalp.

- External abnormalities, including external genitalia.

- Hepato- or splenomegaly or other features of a storage disorder.

- Possible dysmorphism.

- Neurological examination and developmental assessment.

- Eye-movement disorder.

Diagnostic procedures must include

- EEG, preferably also sleep EEG.

- Ophthalmological examination of the retina (fundus).

- MRI, unless the underlying pathology is known.

Metabolic investigations may, in selected cases, include

- Blood gas analysis.

- Serum glucose and lactate.

- Plasma amino acids, plasma homocysteine.

- Acyl carnitine profile.

- Plasma very-long-chain fatty acids.

- Urinary organic acids, mucopolysaccharides, and oligosaccharides.

- CSF protein, glucose (paired with serum glucose from a sample taken immediately prior to lumbar puncture) and lactate, amino acids, neurotransmitters, folates, pterins.

- Plasma pipecolic acid and urinary alpha-amino-adipic semialdehyde (if late-onset vitamin B6-dependent epilepsy is considered).

Genetic investigations may, in selected cases, include

- Karyotyping.

- Microarray.

- Epilepsy panels.

- Whole exome sequencing.

EPILEPSIES WITH ONSET DURING THE NEONATAL PERIOD OR EARLY INFANCY

The 2010 ILAE report (Berg et al. 2010) differentiates syndromes by age at onset. Electroclinical syndromes with onset during the neonatal period include benign familial neonatal seizures (BFNS), early myoclonic encephalopathy (EME), and early infantile epileptic encephalopathy (EIEE; Ohtahara syndrome). Seizures in BFNS are limited to the neonatal period and this is discussed in Chapter 16. EME and EIEE are further discussed here as the impact of the seizures in these conditions is protracted throughout infancy.

EIEE (Ohtahara syndrome)

Children typically present during the first weeks of life with tonic epileptic spasms and other seizures including partial and myoclonic seizures. EEG shows a suppression-burst pattern during wakefulness and sleep. Infants usually become inactive and floppy, and they do not show developmental progress. During the course of the disease, infants usually show severe neurological abnormalities such as a cerebral palsy. EIEE is often associated with cortical malformation or structural brain injury. Rarely, underlying metabolic aetiologies may be identified. More recently, genetic causes have been described. The epilepsy usually does not respond to antiepileptic treatment and in about 75% of cases it evolves into West syndrome at 2 to 6 months of age.

EME

As with EIEE, EME seizures may start during the first weeks of life. However, the predominant seizure type is erratic myoclonia, which may be both epileptic and nonepileptic. The EEG also shows a suppression-burst pattern. In contrast to EIEE, underlying metabolic disorders are often identified, especially nonketotic hyperglycinaemia and other amino acid disorders. The clinical course of the disorder is severe, with infants developing neurological abnormalities and developmental arrest. Antiepileptic treatment is usually not effective.

EPILEPSIES WITH ONSET IN INFANCY

The following epileptic syndromes typically start during infancy.

West syndrome

West syndrome is an age-related epileptic encephalopathy affecting children between the ages of 3 months and 24 months, characterized by a specific seizure type referred to as epileptic spasms. Children usually present with the abrupt onset of head and arm jerks, both flexor and extensor, lasting 0.2 to 2 seconds. Occurrence of spasms is usually associated with or preceded by development arrest or regression and most infants subsequently show developmental impairments. A clustering of spasms is often seen and may especially occur after sleep/wake transition. The infant may become upset and cry during the events which appear to impair consciousness only briefly. Most infants subsequently show developmental impairments. The diagnosis of West syndrome is confirmed by EEG showing hypsarrhythmia (high-voltage, chaotic, and asynchronous pattern with multifocal epileptiform discharges) but this may be present only in an EEG recording made when the child is asleep. West syndrome is seen with many underlying aetiologies and associated conditions, including those listed in Box 20.1.

Investigations need to be directed to exclude any specifically treatable disorder as soon as possible. These include especially some metabolic diseases or intoxications. The prognosis of West syndrome depends mainly on the aetiology but there is also evidence that rapid recognition and control of seizures will improve outcome (O'Callaghan et al. 2018).

If no specifically treatable disorder can be identified, then treatment of West syndrome can be attempted with hormonal therapy (adrenocorticotropic hormone or oral prednisolone), with or without vigabatrin. Compared with that seen following hormonal therapy alone, the rate of early cessation of seizures has been lower following vigabatrin treatment and higher following hormonal therapy plus vigabatrin in randomized controlled trials. Longer-term epilepsy outcomes or developmental outcomes appear to be similar after any of these three treatments options, even in those with no identifiable aetiology whose outcomes might most readily be improved by rapid control of

---

Box 20.1 Underlying aetiologies and associated conditions seen in West syndrome

☑ Genetic
  - ○ Chromosomal abnormalities (trisomy 21)
  - ○ X-linked disorders (e.g. ARX, CDKL5)
  - ○ Other autosomal dominant and recessive disorders

☑ Structural
  - ○ Neurocutaneous disorders, especially TSC
  - ○ Hypoxic-ischaemic encephalopathy
  - ○ Congenital infections
  - ○ Trauma
  - ○ Disturbed brain development with malformations related to
      - abnormal proliferation of neurons of glia
      - abnormal neuronal migration
      - abnormal cortical organization
  - ○ Intracranial haemorrhage
  - ○ Infection

☑ Metabolic
  - ○ Pyridoxine dependency
  - ○ Nonketotic hyperglycinaemia
  - ○ Peroxisomal disorders
  - ○ Amino acid disorders, especially untreated phenylketonuria
  - ○ Organic acid disorders, especially glutaric acidaemia type 1
  - ○ Biotinidase deficiency
  - ○ Mitochondrial disorders

ARX, aristaless-related homeobox; CDKL5, cyclin-dependent kinase-like 5; TSC, tuberous sclerosis complex.

---

seizures (O'Callaghan et al. 2018). This failure to demonstrate longer-term benefits of rapid seizure control may possibly be due to early switching of infants in whom cessation of seizures was not achieved early to other drug treatments. Vigabatrin is the drug of choice in tuberous sclerosis where it seems to be especially effective.

Self-limiting infantile familial and nonfamilial seizures

Self-limiting familial infantile seizures are characterized by clusters of seizures with an age at onset of 3 to 20 months (peak 5–6 months). Seizures are usually brief and predominantly focal with motor arrest, impairment of consciousness, staring, and automatisms. Between the seizures the infants behave typically. The EEG will show abnormalities only during a seizure; the interictal EEG is normal. Patients respond extremely well to low dosages of carbamazepine, valproate, or phenobarbitone, which can be withdrawn after 1 year.

Dravet syndrome (severe myoclonic epilepsy in infancy)

This is an epilepsy syndrome of lifelong duration with onset in early infancy. Clinically it is characterized by three stages:

1. Infants develop typically until early-onset febrile seizures occur mostly between 3 months and 12 months, often febrile SE. Fever after vaccinations may trigger seizures but this does not alter the natural history of the condition (McIntosh et al. 2010).

2. Subsequently, with a peak age at onset of 12 months, they develop febrile and nonfebrile clonic seizures, myoclonic seizures, atypical absences with some impairment of consciousness, often accompanied by myoclonic jerks and head drops, and complex focal seizures. SE is common. Children show impairment of cognitive function and ataxia.

3. Later, children show intellectual disability, and tonic–clonic seizures often persist.

In about 80% of infants with Dravet syndrome, variants of a gene encoding a sodium-channel protein (*SCN1A*) can be found. This is very important because many anti-seizure drugs act by inhibiting the function of sodium channels. These drugs (phenytoin, carbamazepine, oxcarbazepine, and lamotrigine) should be avoided for seizures suggestive of Dravet syndrome because they may aggravate seizures, promote SE, and worsen developmental outcome.

Myoclonic epilepsy in infancy

This is an age-specific epilepsy presenting in infancy. It is characterized by brief myoclonic jerks affecting head, eyeballs, upper extremities, and the diaphragm. Jerks can be single or clustered and may be elicited by tactile or acoustic stimuli.

Consciousness is usually not disturbed. The interictal EEG is usually normal, and the ictal EEG may show generalized spikes or polyspikes. Whereas the myoclonic seizures usually remit during early childhood, 10% to 20% of children may show generalized tonic–clonic seizures later. Antiepileptic treatment with valproate or levetiracetam is usually effective.

Epilepsy in infancy with migrating focal seizures (EIMFS)

This is a rare disorder usually starting within the first months of life. Children present with unprovoked seizures showing both motor and autonomic symptoms occurring in clusters. Seizures are characterized by 'migration' of the focality +/- of the EEG during the seizure. Evolution to bilateral convulsive seizures is common. It is important to recognize this disorder because of the extremely poor prognosis. Regardless of treatment, most children go on to show a wide spectrum of seizure types and developmental regression. In some patients, genetic variations have been found in epilepsy genes such as KCNT1 or SCN8A.

TREATMENT OPTIONS FOR EPILEPSY IN THE FIRST YEAR OF LIFE

Medical treatment

Infants with epilepsy will usually require medical treatment. Treatment with anti-seizure drugs should be considered after a second epileptic seizure. If a structural (e.g. brain tumour) or metabolic (e.g. phenylketonuria) cause for the epilepsy can be identified, this needs to be treated appropriately. If the cause for epilepsy is genetic or unknown, or if causative treatment of a structural or metabolic epilepsy is not possible or unlikely to be successful, antiepileptic treatment should be initiated. Valproate should be avoided when an underlying metabolic cause remains likely. Therapeutic principles are summarized in Table 20.2.

Surgical treatment

Surgery is an option for infants who have epilepsy as the result of a unilateral structural abnormality. All infants with a unilateral structural abnormality should be referred for surgical assessment where available, regardless of response to treatment in view of the high risk of relapse and consequence of seizures on neurodevelopmental progress. However, at the very least, it should be considered when two drugs have been tried without achieving seizure freedom, especially if there is evidence of West syndrome or another epileptic encephalopathy.

Alternative therapies

Ketogenic diet therapies (KDT) may be an option for infants who do not respond to first- or second-line medical treatment and in whom surgical treatment is not an option. KDT have consistently been described as beneficial in, among other disorders,

Table 20.2 Therapeutic principles of the treatment of epilepsy

Epilepsy or epileptic syndrome	First-line treatment	Second-line treatment	Comments
Structural	CBZ, OXC	LTG, VPA, corticosteroids	
Metabolic			Treatment generally according to the underlying cause
West syndrome	Prednisolone +/-VGB (but VGB first choice in patients with tuberous sclerosis)	VGB, KDT	
Self limiting infantile familial and non-familial seizures	CBZ, OXC	PB	Treatment may be stopped at age 1 year
Dravet syndrome	VPA	Clobazam, stiripentol	Avoid CBZ, OXC, LTG, PHT
Myoclonic epilepsy in infancy	VPA, levetiracetam		Treatment may be stopped after 1 year
Malignant migrating seizures in infancy	Bromide, KDT		Consider quinidine if *KCNT1* gene variant

CBZ, carbamazepine; LTG, lamotrigine; OXC, oxcarbazepine; PB, phenobarbitone; PHT, phenytoin; VGB, vigabatrin; KDT, ketogenic diet therapies; VPA, valproate; KCNT1, potassium sodium-activated channel subfamily T member 1.

glucose transporter 1 deficiency syndrome (GLUT1D), pyruvate dehydrogenase deficiency (PDHD), West syndrome, Ohtahara syndrome, and tuberous sclerosis complex. Because of possible unwanted effects and risks, especially in infants, its use should be restricted to specialized units.

REFERENCES

Berg AT, Coryell J, Saneto RP, et al. (2010) Revised terminology and concepts for organization of seizures and epilepsies: report of the ILAE Commission on Classification and Terminology, 2005–2009. *Epilepsia* 51: 676–685.

Chin RF, Neville BG, Peckham C, Wade A, Bedford H, Scott RC. (2008) Treatment of community-onset, childhood convulsive status epilepticus: a prospective, population-based study. *Lancet Neurol* 7: 696–703.

Eltze CM, Chong WK, Cox T, et al. (2013) A population-based study of newly diagnosed epilepsy in infants. *Epilepsia* 54: 437–445.

Fisher RS, van Emde Boas W, Blume W, et al. (2005) Epileptic seizures and epilepsy: definitions proposed by the International League. Against Epilepsy (ILAE) and the International Bureau for Epilepsy (IBE). *Epilepsia* 46: 470—472.

Fisher RS, Cross JH, D'Souza C, et al. (2017) Instruction manual for the ILAE 2017 operational classification of seizure types. *Epilepsia* 58: 531—542.

Lyttle MD, Rainford NEA, Gamble C et al. (2019) Levetiracetam versus phenytoin for second-line treatment of paediatric convulsive status epilepticus (EcLiPSE): a multicentre, open-label, randomised trial. *Lancet* 393: 2125-2134. https://doi.org/10.1016/S0140-6736(19)30724-X

McIntosh AM, McMahon J, Dibbens LM, et al. (2010) Effects of vaccination on onset and outcome of Dravet syndrome: retrospective study. *Lancet Neurol* 9: 592—598.

O'Callaghan FJK, Edwards SW, Alber FD, et al. (2018) Vigabatrin with hormonal treatment versus hormonal treatment alone (ICISS) for infantile spasms: 18-month outcomes of an open-label, randomised controlled trial. *Lancet Child Adolesc Health* 2: 715—725.

Rao KS, Adhikari S, Gauchan E, et al. (2017) Time trend of neurocysticercosis in children with seizures in a tertiary hospital of western Nepal. *PLoS Negl Trop Dis* 11: e0005605.

Scheffer IE, Berkovic S, Capovilla G, et al. (2017) ILAE classification of the epilepsies: Position paper of the ILAE Commission for Classification and Terminology. *Epilepsia* 58: 512—521.

Trinka E, Cock H, Hesdorffer D, et al. (2015) A definition and classification of status epilepticus — Report of the ILAE Task Force on Classification of Status Epilepticus. *Epilepsia* 56: 1515—1523.

WHO (2016) Updated guideline: Paediatric emergency triage, assessment and treatment: care of critically-ill children. Geneva: WHO. Available at http://www.who.int/maternal_child_adolescent/documents/paediatric-emergency-triage-update/en/

Resources

Fisher RS, Cross JH, French JA, et al. (2017) Operational classification of seizure types by the International League Against Epilepsy: Position Paper of the ILAE Commission for Classification and Terminology. *Epilepsia* 58: 522—530.

International League Against Epilepsy. Diagnostic manual. https://www.ilae.org/education/diagnostic-manual

Kossoff EH, Zupec-Kania BA, Auvin S, et al. (2018) Optimal clinical management of children receiving dietary therapies for epilepsy: Updated recommendations of the International Ketogenic Diet Study Group. *Epilepsia Open* 3: 175—192.

Novotny EJ Jr, Koh S (2017) Early-life epilepsies and the emerging role of genetic testing. *JAMA Pediatr* 171: 863—871.

van der Louw E, van den Hurk D, Neal E, et al. (2016) Ketogenic diet guidelines for infants with refractory epilepsy. *Eur J Paediatr Neurol* 20: 798—809.

Wilmshurst JM, Gaillard WD, Vinayan KP, et al. (2015) Summary of recommendations for the management of infantile seizures: Task Force Report for the ILAE Commission of Pediatrics. *Epilepsia* 56: 1185—1197.

Yoong M, Chin RFM, Scott RC (2009) Management of convulsive status epilepticus in children. *Arch Dis Child Educ Pract Ed* 94: 1—9.

CHAPTER 21

Nonepileptic paroxysmal disorders in infancy

John BP Stephenson and Alla Nechay

Key messages

- Most paroxysmal events are nonepileptic.
- Most — but not all — are benign.
- Precise description and a video of events are of most value for diagnosis.
- Most do not require medications of any kind.
- Psychological support and reassurance of the family is the main treatment.

Common errors

- To use electroencephalography between episodes to decide whether it is epilepsy.
- To give antiepileptic medications ('anticonvulsants') without being certain that the infant has epilepsy.
- To give other 'brain medicines' of no proven value.

When to worry

- Suspicion that the intracranial pressure might be high.
- Episodes of stiffness with startle (hyperekplexia).
- All episodes occur when only the mother is present.
- *Note*: all these are rare.

BREATH-HOLDING SPELLS (PROLONGED EXPIRATORY APNOEA)

Definition

An episode in response to pain or annoyance that begins with grunting expiration followed rapidly by deep cyanosis with loss of consciousness and rigid extension. After an inspiratory groan, the infant or toddler is briefly dazed and usually cries on regaining consciousness. In English this is usually called a cyanotic breath-holding spell (CBHS).

Clinical approach

If there are jerks or nonepileptic spasms they are irregular. The diagnosis is made from the clinical history. It may be difficult to distinguish this type of reflex syncope from reflex anoxic seizures/reflex asystolic syncope, but this distinction is not important.

What is important is *not to make the diagnosis of epilepsy for this condition*: epileptic seizures are never directly provoked by discomfort or frustration.

Note: when we talk about anoxic seizures, we mean events that look like epileptic seizures but are due to lack of oxygen or oxygenated blood going to the brain. By contrast, epileptic seizures occur when there is sudden, excessive hypersynchronous neuronal activity. For this reason, cerebral activity is markedly reduced in an anoxic seizure due to syncope, whereas cerebral activity is markedly increased in an epileptic seizure.

Management

Reassurance that episodes will terminate spontaneously is most important. Parents are often very frightened by what they see and need support. No medication or other treatment is of any value. Remission usually occurs before school age. In cases of iron deficiency anaemia and high-frequency CBHS, iron therapy may result in reduction in the frequency of episodes.

REFLEX ANOXIC SEIZURES (OR REFLEX ASYSTOLIC SYNCOPE)

Definition

An episode of stiffening and loss of consciousness in response to pain or surprise, especially an unexpected bump on the head, assumed to be due to reflex arrest of cardiac action, i.e. reflex asystole.

Clinical approach

Episodes of reflex anoxic seizure resemble episodes of cyanotic breath-holding, except that there is no more than mild cyanosis, and the latency between the stimulus (pain or surprise) is shorter, maybe only 10 seconds. The children are often described as going grey or looking as if they had died.

Management

If there is any concern that there might be a long QT syndrome it is wise to obtain a 12-lead electrocardiogram to confirm that the QT interval corrected for heart rate (QTc) is normal. Reassurance about the excellent prognosis is the key to management.

ANOXIC-EPILEPTIC SEIZURES WITHOUT EPILEPSY

Definition

Anoxic-epileptic seizures (AES) are a rare sequence of two paroxysmal events when a true epileptic seizure follows a triggering nonepileptic syncope. In most cases the trigger for the true epileptic seizures is a neurally mediated syncope with either reflex asystole (reflex anoxic seizures) or prolonged expiratory apnoea (CBHS).

Clinical approach

The duration of the triggering syncope (the anoxic seizure) is usually less than 30 seconds. The resultant epileptic seizure usually lasts more than 2 minutes (sometimes up to 40min). In most cases the triggered epileptic seizures are reported as clonic. Sometimes the epileptic component resembles a myoclonic absence. Syncope-triggered epileptic seizures are easily distinguished from the much more common anoxic seizures in that

- AES are long, many minutes rather than less than 1 minute in duration, and

- the jerks in AES are rhythmic rather than irregular.

The syncopes and epileptic component typically remit in preschool years and are not usually associated with learning disability. Most children with AES do not have epilepsy, that is, their epileptic seizures are only provoked by syncopes. Any individual with AES usually has simple syncopes leading only to anoxic seizures and only a minority of syncopes trigger epileptic seizures (Horrocks et al. 2005). Videos of AES are available at www.jle.com/medline.md?issn=1294-9361&vol=6&iss=1&page=15.

Management

Because AES are uncommon in most affected children, rescue medication, such as a benzodiazepine, is commonly sufficient to abort the epileptic component. If anti-epileptic drugs (AED) are prescribed for children with frequent AES, they may abolish the epileptic component of AES, however, the syncopes will not change.

TONIC ATTACKS WITH ACUTELY RAISED INTRACRANIAL PRESSURE

Synonyms include extensor posturing (e.g. in meningitis, encephalitis, hydrocephalus).

Definition

Although clonic epileptic seizures (with rhythmic jerking) may occur in infections of the central nervous system or acute hydrocephalus, it is important to recognize tonic attacks in which there is stiffening in extension because these usually indicate dangerously high intracranial pressure.

Clinical approach

It can be argued that lumbar puncture is contraindicated in this situation but that is debatable. The important point in management of this situation is not to give AED, in particular, not to give rectal or intravenous diazepam.

Management

It is wise to treat the infection; consider mannitol and perhaps other ways of safely lowering intracranial pressure and avoid AED such as diazepam.

IMPOSED UPPER AIRWAYS OBSTRUCTION

Definition

Episodes are covertly induced by the mother by occluding the infant's airway (synonym: smothering). Only rarely is the father the perpetrator.

Clinical approach

The mother presents as a very caring, competent, concerned parent. Episodes always begin in her presence and the onset is never observed by others, but the mother shows the limp pale cyanosed infant to neighbours or friends or nurses or doctors. She often becomes skilled at cardiopulmonary resuscitation. The diagnosis depends on an absolutely precise history. This may be very difficult to obtain as no one else sees the suffocation by hand, pillow, cling-film, or by pressing the infant's face against the mother's bosom. If the infant is in hospital and nurses are charting episodes it is essential to determine whether what is written on the 'seizure chart' is a direct observation of the nurse or a transcription of what the mother has told the nurse. This disorder may be regarded as a dangerous form of fabricated or induced illness by carers.

Management

If the mother is separated from the infant or *constantly* observed, the episodes will cease. Multidisciplinary assessment may well recommend involvement of psychiatry, social services and specialist police services (see Chapter 17 on inflicted traumatic brain injury).

ALTERNATING HEMIPLEGIA OF CHILDHOOD

Definition

Alternating hemiplegia of childhood (AHC) is a disease of early childhood, typically presenting with attacks of hemiplegia of one or another side or bilaterally symmetrical. Hemiplegias usually start at 6 to 18 months of age, typically accompanied by autonomic phenomena, but stiffening (tonic episodes) and bouts of nystagmus (which may be unilateral) commonly begin in the neonatal period or soon after.

Clinical approach

Paroxysms of hemiplegia and/or tetraplegia happen once or twice per week and may be accompanied by tonic or dystonic episodes, disorders of eye movements (episodic strabismus, monocular nystagmus), choreoathetosis, crying and autonomic presentations. Episodes always disappear with sleep and are absent after awaking. nonepileptic symptoms in children with AHC include developmental impairment, muscular hypotonia, choreoathetosis, and ataxia. Hot and warm baths, strong emotions, and physical fatigue may provoke attacks of AHC. Usually the disease progresses, at least during initial period.

Epilepsy is also present in about half of children with AHC. Seizures are completely different from the episodes of weakness but may happen at the same time. AHC is primarily caused by mutations in the *ATP1A3* gene; very rarely, a mutation in the *ATP1A2* gene is involved in the condition. Special investigations are not informative, but taking into account that moyamoya disease is thought to be a possible cause of this condition, brain magnetic resonance imaging (with or without magnetic resonance angiography) will be necessary.

Differential diagnosis

- Partial epilepsy with Todd paresis,

- Hemiplegic migraine,

- Paroxysmal dyskinesia,

- Mitochondrial encephalomyopathy, lactic acidosis, and stroke-like episodes (MELAS),

- Vascular abnormalities (including moyamoya disease).

Management

Blockers of calcium channels (flunarizine or, when flunarizine is not available, cinnarizine) may be effective in prophylaxis of episodes of AHC. Benzodiazepines may be effective in aborting episodes of AHC and reduce the frequency of events. Limitation of provoking factors is recommended.

HYPEREKPLEXIA

Definition

Hyperekplexia (or stiff baby syndrome, or startle disease) is a rare genetic disorder in which there is excessive startle. In the neonatal period the infant is both stiff and easily startled, with excessive brainstem reflexes, including a positive nose-tapping test.

Clinical approach

Hyperekplexia is easy to overdiagnose as all infants may show startle. If there is a positive family history of dominantly inherited startle with sudden falls then the diagnosis is not too difficult. With no family history one must be very careful and precise. Affected neonates not only startle excessively to sounds but have prominent head-retraction reflex on tapping the tip of the nose, immediately followed by a flexor spasm. This response to a nose tap does not habituate, so that repeated nose taps elicit repeated head retraction and flexor spasms. A dangerous complication is severe apnoeic syncope (accompanied by severe quivering stiffness) that may be fatal if untreated.

Management

If possible, DNA should be obtained for analysis of the hyperekplexia genes. Medical staff, nurses, and parents should be taught the Vigevano manoeuvre: if the infant becomes stiff and apnoeic, he/she is flexed by bringing the head towards the feet. Oral clonazepam is usually helpful, but the condition often spontaneously improves in the first year.

BENIGN NEONATAL SLEEP MYOCLONUS

Definition

Flurries of myoclonia that only occur during sleep with onset in the neonatal period, usually between day 1 and day 16.

Clinical approach

Benign neonatal sleep myoclonus (BNSM) is a common condition occurring in perhaps 2% of the general population and in nearly 70% of infants of opioid-dependent mothers. The only harm that may come to the infant is if a diagnosis of epilepsy is wrongly made: if AED are given, the myoclonus worsens and intensive care may be needed. It is, thus, most important that all doctors who deal with neonates are very familiar with BNSM, and preferably have seen videos of the condition.

The myoclonus appears as flurries of myoclonia affecting the limbs (though rarely the face). The flurries last no more than 0.5 seconds and to the casual observer look like a single jerk. Bouts of jerking may continue for up to 30 minutes or more but cease if the infant wakes up or is made to wake up. They may be triggered by rocking the infant.

Management

No investigations are required. In particular, an electroencephalogram (EEG) is not indicated nor any type of brain scan or blood test. No AED ('anticonvulsants') must ever be given. The parents should be reassured that the jerkings are harmless and will probably cease by age 3 months (rarely up to 10 months or so).

FEJERMAN SYNDROME: SHUDDERING, BENIGN NONEPILEPTIC INFANTILE SPASMS, BENIGN MYOCLONUS OF EARLY INFANCY

Definition

Isolated or repeated movements involving the upper limbs that may be shudders, spasms, or jerks or even loss of tone, of a nonepileptic nature.

Clinical approach

The history will be of a typically developing infant having sudden movements of the upper limbs and upper body that may occur singly or occur in clusters. These movements may be shudders (resembling a shiver) or spasms (resembling epileptic infantile spasms) or jerks (that look like myoclonus). Sometimes there is loss of tone (as in negative myoclonus or an astatic epileptic seizure). The infant is not disturbed by these events (which only occur in the awake state) and if there is a series or cluster, the cluster terminates if the infant is distracted. No developmental regression occurs and after a while – perhaps some months – episodes cease.

Management

No investigations are usually required, but a home video – for instance using a mobile phone – may be very helpful in clarifying the diagnosis. A further advantage of a home video is that it may be shown to a more experienced paediatric neurologist to confirm your impression.

INFANTILE MASTURBATION/GRATIFICATION

Definition

Rhythmic repetitive lower limb movements, in particular, thigh adduction, accompanied by a 'distant' or absorbed facial appearance.

Clinical approach

Infantile masturbation is highlighted because it has been often mistaken for epilepsy due to its usual presentation with paroxysmal movements of a recurrent character. Infantile masturbation can also mimic other conditions such as abdominal pain, paroxysmal dystonia, and dyskinesia. Masturbatory activity in infants and young children is difficult to recognize because it has a spectrum of different behaviour patterns, which often do not involve manual stimulation of the genitalia. Resulting misdiagnosis may then lead to unnecessary investigations and treatment. The condition is more often seen in females than in males. Usually it starts at under 1 year of age. Episodes are often observed when the child is sitting in a car seat, when he/she is bored or tired, and in relation to sleeping.

During episodes of masturbation, children exhibit different types of behaviour: dystonia-like posturing of different parts of the body, grunting, flushing, and sweating; rocking may also be observed in these children. Episodes may last from several seconds up to several hours, sometimes many times per day. Children never lose consciousness during the events and can be distracted from the activity by parents, although sometimes unwillingly. Careful history-taking is an important key to the diagnosis.

Management

Home-video recording is of most help in understanding the nature of the episodes and extremely important for the prevention of unnecessary investigations and treatment of these children. Parents prefer the term 'gratification' (or even benign idiopathic infantile dyskinesia) to infantile masturbation as there is less social stigma attached to these terms. It is debatable whether these episodes, which involve predominantly the lower limbs rather than the upper limbs, are different in nature from Fejerman syndrome.

PAROXYSMAL TORTICOLLIS

Definition

Paroxysmal torticollis of infancy is a benign disorder characterized by recurrent and transient episodes of cervical dystonia of unknown aetiology.

Clinical approach

Episodes of head tilt to one or other side are often accompanied by vomiting, pallor, ataxia, and irritability, settling spontaneously within hours or days. The disorder, which disappears within the first few years of life, is often misinterpreted and the child undergoes numerous pointless tests.

Management

Investigations are usually not informative, although, rarely, *CACNA1A* mutations have been detected. Usually head tilt becomes less prominent after infancy, being replaced by vertigo and eventually by migraine headaches.

SUMMARY AND CONCLUSIONS

In this chapter we have given brief descriptions of most of the common nonepileptic conditions that may occur in infants. We have concentrated on conditions (not necessarily disorders) that may be confused with epilepsy. Most are seen in otherwise typically developing infants, although some, if not all, may be seen in those with slow development or with development that is outside the range of typical development from normal variation.

The important point that we emphasize is that such nonepileptic conditions should not be misdiagnosed as epilepsy (the definition of which includes the presence of recurrent unprovoked epileptic seizures). In particular, it is essential not to prescribe antiepileptic medications (i.e. 'anticonvulsants') nor sedatives, nor other brain-altering drugs. Exceptions to this rule are the rare disorders AHC in which flunarizine (or, when flunarizine is not available, cinnarizine) may help, and hyperekplexia, in which clonazepam is the treatment of choice.

It should be borne in mind that in almost all the conditions we describe in this chapter, the only harm that may come to the infant comes from the doctor — paediatric neurologist or otherwise — who does not recognize the nonepileptic nature of the events and prescribes medications that may impair the infant's brain function. This chapter aims to prevent such unfortunate iatrogenic consequences.

Home video, nowadays often taken on a mobile phone, greatly assists in the diagnosis of many of these conditions. Once an event has been captured on video, this may also be viewed by other paediatric neurologists with more experience. Other investigations such as EEG and brain imaging should be used with great care and caution, as false positives are frequent. Diagnosis should be *clinically* based on your skills as a doctor.

REFERENCES

Horrocks IA, Nechay A, Stephenson JBP, Zuberi SM (2005) Anoxic-epileptic seizures: observational study of epileptic seizures induced by syncopes. *Arch Dis Child* 90: 1283—1287.

Resources

Mineyko A, Whiting S, Graham GE (2011) Hyperekplexia: treatment of a severe phenotype and review of the literature. *Can J Neuro Sci* 38: 411—416.

Stephenson JBP (1990) *Fits and Faints*. London: Mac Keith Press.

Stephenson J, Breningstall G, Steer C, et al. (2004) Anoxic-epileptic seizures: home video recordings of epileptic seizures induced by syncopes. *Epileptic Disord* 6: 15—19. http://www.jle.com/medline.md?issn=1294-9361&vol=6&iss=1&page=15

Uldall P, Alving J, Hansen LK, Kibaek M, Buchholt J (2006) The misdiagnosis of epilepsy in children admitted to a tertiary epilepsy centre with paroxysmal events. *Arch Dis Child* 91: 219—221.

CHAPTER 22

Microcephaly, including congenital infections

Alasdair PJ Parker, Vlatka Mejaški-Bošnjak, and Richard FM Chin

Key messages

- Identify and classify a small head.
- Investigate microcephaly in a logical and efficient manner.
- Manage children with microcephaly with multidisciplinary support.

Common errors

- Inaccurate assessment of head circumference.
- Failing to measure head circumference in parents/siblings.
- Intervening in a typically developing infant with a smaller head circumference.

When to worry

- Seizures in association with microcephaly.
- Other focal neurological or systemic signs.
- Loss of developmental milestones.
- Successive plots of occipitofrontal head circumference cross the centiles downwards.
- Dysmorphic features.

DEFINITION

Microcephaly is defined as an occipitofrontal circumference (OFC) that is significantly less than that of typically developing children of the same sex, age, and ethnicity. It is a clinical sign — an estimate of brain size — and not a diagnosis. There are many possible aetiologies, among which are genetic, neurometabolic disorders, and brain injury. It can be categorized by aetiology, in relation to growth parameters (proportionate or disproportionate), or by time of onset (Woods and Parker, 2013). Here we use the last of these classifications.

According to this classification, microcephaly can be primary, i.e. when brain growth is reduced during pregnancy, or secondary/acquired, i.e. when head circumference is within standardized limits at birth, but then fails to grow as expected (Ashwal et al. 2009; Woods and Parker, 2013). Studies suggest that primary microcephaly is a result of decreased neurogenesis, while acquired microcephaly results from a decrease in dendritic complexity and impaired myelination.

In about 41% of cases, the aetiology of microcephaly remains unknown and although many of these 'unknown' cases are thought to be genetic, the exact genetic variant may not be found.

MEASUREMENT

Head circumference should be measured with a non-stretchable tape across the occiput and the supraorbital ridges, above the ears, midway between the eyebrows and the hairline. Take the measurement three times or until you get a consistent value (Harris, 2015).

Microcephaly can be defined as either 2 or 3SD below the mean, or below the 0.4th centile, i.e. 2.67SD below the mean (Woods and Parker, 2013).

Different OFC charts are available, but it is important to use the same chart for the same child over time. Ethnicity-based head circumference charts are not widely available.

We recommend investigating microcephaly when the head circumference is less than the 0.4th centile or whenever a child with a head circumference below the 2nd centile (−2SD) has significant risk factors from history or examination to suggest an underlying disease process that needs further clarification. This approach will increase investigation yield and the likelihood of diagnosing the pathology (Woods and Parker, 2013).

Serial measurements over time are more informative than single ('spot') measurements because they provide a time trend. For example, a decelerating rate of growth of OFC is typical of some metabolic disorders.

It is also important to record the parental head circumferences, which can prompt the clinician to think of benign familial microcephaly. If no head circumference at birth is available, serial OFC measurements can provide a clue. Consecutive OFC measurements that create a curve parallel to a centile suggest primary microcephaly, whereas those that show a drop or a plateau are more typical of secondary microcephaly.

CONSULTATION

Families will often be unaware of the microcephaly and/or the implications, so it is important to build a rapport with them. The consultation should be structured around the child, ideally both parents should be present. You may consider having a nurse or other members of the multidisciplinary team present who may be involved in the care of the child later on (Seregni and Parker, 2018).

A comprehensive history should include the following points:

- *Antenatal history:* suspected or proven maternal infections during pregnancy, e.g. TORCH (toxoplasma, other, rubella, cytomegalovirus, herpes), Zika, other rashes, or pyrexia of unknown source; fetal exposure to alcohol, medications (e.g. maternal antiepileptic medications) or other drugs (e.g. heroin or cocaine); maternal medical problems (e.g. human immunodeficiency virus [HIV], phenylketonuria, autoimmune conditions, thyroid disease, malnourishment); placental insufficiency; antenatal scan abnormalities and in utero growth abnormalities (disproportionate fetal growth, intrauterine growth restriction [IUGR]); travel history during pregnancy (e.g. Zika areas); and maternal abdominal injury (Tables 22.1 and 22.2).

- *Birth history:* need for resuscitation, hints towards perinatal asphyxia or stroke (e.g. seizures).

- *Medical history:* including seizures, hypoglycaemia, and relevant systems review.

- *Concerns around hearing and vision.*

- *Development milestones:* in gross/fine motor, social, and language domains; school attendance, academic progress, and social communication.

- *Family history:* including history of neurological or metabolic conditions and premature deaths.

- *Parental consanguinity.*

Anthropometric measurements of height/length, weight, and nutritional status are essential parts of the assessment, because microcephaly can be isolated or associated with growth failure or short stature in syndromes such as Seckel and Rubinstein-Taybi syndromes. Similarly, chromosomal breakage disorders, such as Bloom syndrome or Fanconi anaemia, present with growth restriction unresponsive to nutritional supplementation.

In particular, it is important to inspect:

- *Facial features:* ears (e.g. low-set), characteristic nose shape (e.g. upturned nose and flat nasal bridge in fetal alcohol disorders), philtrum, chin, hypo- or hypertelorism (e.g. Wolf-Hirschhorn syndrome), eyebrows (e.g. arched eyebrows which meet in the middle suggest synophrys in Cornelia De Lange syndrome), teeth (e.g. a single maxillary incisor is associated with holoprosencephaly).

- *Head shape, sutures, and fontanelles:* the anterior fontanelle closes at between 10 months and 24 months of age. Premature closure is associated with craniosynostosis, late closure is associated with syndromes like Rubinstein-Taybi, or chromosomal abnormalities (e.g. trisomy 21 or cri du chat [5p deletion]).

- *Spine for scoliosis and limbs for dysplasia.*

- *Skin, nails, and hair* (e.g. hypertrichosis in Cornelia De Lange syndrome); chromosomal breakage disorders (e.g. severe photosensitivity in Cockayne syndrome).

- *General physical examination* should also include abdominal palpation (hepato/splenomegaly can be suggestive of metabolic disorders or congenital infection) and cardiovascular assessment.

- *Any stereotypic repetitive midline movements that could suggest Rett syndrome where there is postnatal slowing of head circumference.*

A full neurological examination is essential, as microcephaly can be associated with motor dysfunction. Tone, power, and reflexes should, therefore, be assessed and the examiner should be on the lookout for movement disorders such as dystonia or dyskinesia.

An ophthalmology assessment is crucial to identify clues, e.g. chorioretinitis (TORCH intrauterine infection) or cataract (metabolic disorder); similarly, *a hearing assessment* is essential (congenital infections).

Finally, *observe the parents/siblings*, their facial features, and their head circumferences (Seregni and Parker, 2018).

PRIMARY MICROCEPHALY

Primary microcephaly is present before 36 weeks gestational age, if this was not recorded then birth values are used (Ashwal et al. 2009). The earlier in pregnancy that microcephaly is identifiable, the worse the expected outcome.

The damaging effect of different viruses on brain growth, particularly when acquired by the mother in the latter part of the first trimester, is well known (Ledger, 2008). The TORCH infections continue to cause concern, but some are becoming less prevalent thanks to public health interventions such as vaccination (e.g. rubella). Although TORCH analysis may be the only virological investigation, many other infections can cause microcephaly (the 'O' in TORCH); e.g. HIV and more recently, Zika in the first trimester (Table 22.1) (Chantry, Byrd, and Englund, 2003; Merfeld et al. 2017; de Araújo et al. 2018).

Teratogens, such as alcohol, recreational drugs, and medications, may reduce head size, or it can be genetically driven (Table 22.2) (Keegan et al. 2010). Other causes of primary microcephaly include prenatal injury (e.g. strokes).

Table 22.1 Illustrative disorders in clinical practice

Type/ syndrome	Features	Comments
Primary with no other signs		
Benign familial	AD; small OFCs in family members with typical development, function typically, proportionately small body size, typical development; normal MRI	Review development at a later point
AR	Nonprogressive intellectual disability, normal neurological examination; slight reduction in white matter	Gene panel testing
With growth restriction		
Seckel	AR; IUGR, postnatal dwarfism, bird-like face	Genetics opinion
With other dysmorphic features — Mendelian inheritance disorders		
Cornelia de Lange	Long eyelashes, bushy eyebrows, and synophrys (joined eyebrows); short stature. Gastrointestinal and behaviour problems	Genetics opinion and targeted testing
With other dysmorphic features — copy number variants		
Trisomy 18 (Edwards)	Prominent occiput, talipes equinovarus, or rocker bottom feet, congenital heart disease	Microarray/CGH

Table 22.1 (continued)   Illustrative disorders in clinical practice

Type/ syndrome	Features	Comments
Secondary		
With dysmorphic features — Mendelian inheritance disorders		
Rubenstein–Taybi	AD; short stature, severe learning difficulties, broad first digits, malignancies	Dysmorphology database, clinical/molecular genetics
With dysmorphic features — with copy number variants		
Miller–Dieker	Lissencephaly and dysmorphism	Microdeletion on short arm of chromosome 17
Without dysmorphic features — with Mendelian inheritance disorders		
Rett	Female infant development and head size normal until 6–18 months, then regression, loss of purposeful hand movements, and decreased head growth; hand stereotypies and breathing irregularities	Deletion or CNV in *MECP2*
With inborn error of metabolism		
Smith–Lemli–Opitz	AR; syndactyly of the second and third toes, cleft palate, learning difficulties, behaviour problems	High 7 dehydrocholesterol levels
Phenylketon-uria	Progressive neurological/motor signs and learning disability	Raised phenylalanine
With neurological signs		
Aicardi–Goutières	AR; seizures, chilblains, intellectual disability; calcified basal ganglia	Abnormal interferon in plasma and CSF, molecular genetics
Cockayne	AR; deafness, photosensitivity, retinitis pigmentosa, facial change	DNA-repair defect studies and molecular genetics

AD, autosomal dominant; AR, autosomal recessive; CNV, copy number variant; CSF, cerebrospinal fluid; IUGR, intrauterine growth restriction; MRI, magnetic resonance imaging; OFC, occipitofrontal circumference.

Table 22.2 Acquired/environmental causes of microcephaly in infancy

Cause	Clinical or imaging features	Comment/management
Perinatal infections		
CMV	Common intrauterine infection affecting 1% of liveborn neonates by vertical mother—fetus transmission (most do NOT have brain injury). At birth: IUGR, sepsis-like syndrome, marked microcephaly, and chorioretinitis. Permanent sequelae in 40—58% of infants with symptomatic infection: SNHL (+ + +) intellectual disability, seizures, psychomotor delay, ASD neuroimaging. CT: periventricular calcification, MRI: alteration of white matter, cortical dysgenesis (polymicrogyria), cerebellar hypoplasia in early-onset infection, anterior temporal leukomalacia/cysts	Tests: positive IgM, IgG, and evidence of either PCR-CMV DNA of amniotic fluid or urine or serum or neonatal blood spot at birth. Therapy: antiviral drug: ganciclovir IV for 6 weeks might improve hearing outcomes Passive immunization of pregnant infected females Active immunization under investigation
HSV	Occurs in 1/3000 deliveries due to peripartum transmission, caused by HSV-2, but may not cause brain injury. Triad of cutaneous, neurological (microcephaly, spasticity, seizures), eye (chorioretinitis, microphthalmia) findings present at birth; brain CT/MRI reveal multiple areas of haemorrhagic necrosis	Tests: HSV DNA in CSF by PCR at birth. Therapy: aciclovir. Risk of transmission during third trimester can be reduced by Caesarean section delivery
Toxoplasmosis	Prevalence in neonates of 0.08%, often asymptomatic and may not cause brain injury. Severe neonatal disease: `sepsis-like syndrome', chorioretinitis. Long-term morbidity: severely impaired vision, spasticity, intellectual disability, microcephaly, hydrocephalus, seizures, SNHL. Neuroimaging reveals disseminated calcifications in caudate nuclei, choroid plexus, subependymal calcification (CT), MRI detects active inflammatory lesions	Tests: antenatal IgM, PCR on amniocentesis fluid at 16—18 weeks. Therapy: sulfadiazine, pyrimethamine therapy. Antepartum screening available; education programmes focus on handling raw meat with protective gloves, avoiding outdoor cats

Table 22.2 (continued)   Acquired/environmental causes of microcephaly in infancy

Cause	Clinical or imaging features	Comment/management
Rubella	Nowadays very uncommon in the Western world as result of vaccine-induced elimination of wild rubella viral transmission. Confirmed infection in first trimester of pregnancy results in damage of 50—90% of the fetuses: 'sepsis-like syndrome', meningoencephalitis. Permanent manifestation: intrauterine/postnatal IUGR, congenital heart disease, SNHL, visual impairment (cataracts, microphthalmia, retinopathy), microcephaly	Tests: positive IgM, IgG, and evidence of either PCR-viral DNA of amniotic fluid or urine or serum or neonatal blood spot at birth. Therapy: universal infant immunization with live attenuated MMR virus vaccine; targeted vaccination of adolescent females
HIV	Weight, length, OFC growth are all affected in HIV-infected children. (HIV 'wasting syndrome'). Decrements in OFC are early and sustained	Tests: HIV-screening should be used in high risk population of pregnant females (IV drug abusers); RNA-PCR
Zika	Zika virus (ZIKAV), an RNA flavivirus transmitted by Aedes mosquitoes, exhibiting tropism for neuronal progenitor cells (NPCs) inducing cell cycle arrest, apoptosis, and differentiation defects in the CNS was first reported in Brazil. Prenatal maternal ZIKAV infection causes congenital defects: ocular e.g. macular scarring and focal pigmentary retinal mottling, arthrogryposis, and especially microcephaly. Brain abnormalities include calcification, ventriculomegaly, malformation of cortical development (lissencephaly and polymicrogyria). The most severe cases of ZIKAV-associated microcephaly correlate with maternal infection during the first trimester	Tests: widespread brain calcification in the periventricular, parenchymal, thalamic basal ganglia areas, and evidence of cell migration abnormalities on prenatal fetal and neonatal cranial ultrasound, CT, or MRI scans. Confirmation: reverse transcription-PCR to identify ZIKAV RNA; capture-IgM ELISA in amniotic fluid, CSF, and serum for IgM antibodies. Prevention strategies: elimination of mosquito breeding areas; personal protective measures: preventing mosquito bites among pregnant females applying insect repellent, wearing long-sleeve shirts/trousers, and using mosquito nets

Table 22.2 (continued)   Acquired/environmental causes of microcephaly in infancy

Cause	Clinical or imaging features	Comment/management
Toxins		
Alcohol	Fetal alcohol spectrum disorders, teratogenic effect on developing fetus, in 1–3/1000 newborn infants; both moderate and high level of alcohol intake in early pregnancy result in altered fetal growth and morphogenesis. Characteristic facial phenotype, microcephaly, growth deficiency, delayed development, and intellectual disability (most common non-genetic cause of intellectual disability), ASD. Neuroimaging: overall reduction in brain volume and central nervous system disorganization, structural abnormalities of corpus callosum, caudate, hippocampus, brain malformation. MRI shows regional increases in cortical thickness, and disorganization of white matter	No specific therapy. Elimination of alcohol intake preconceptionally. See also Chapter 26
Heroin and methadone	The incidence of low birthweight among newborn infants of heroin-addicted females is approximately 50%, mostly due to IUGR. 40% are microcephalic. Unfavourable outcome is often related to associated factors: poor prenatal care, maternal undernutrition, intrauterine infections (HIV). 10–35% of children of methadone users are of low birthweight, of whom 40% are small for age. Low average mean developmental scores. Both heroin and methadone addiction sharply increase risk for SIDS and seizures, but seizures are more common in methadone exposure.	Tests: toxicology screen Characteristic withdrawal syndrome observed among about 60% of passively addicted newborn infants present within first 24h in 65%: coarse tremulousness (quite dramatic), irritability, hypertonus, excessive sucking, diarrhoea, sweating Treatment: supportive therapy, narcotic agent, phenobarbital

Table 22.2 (continued)   Acquired/environmental causes of microcephaly in infancy

Cause	Clinical or imaging features	Comment/management
Cocaine	A commonly misused drug. Pregnancy may be complicated by spontaneous abortion, preterm birth, placental abruption, fetal asphyxia, IUGR, stillbirth (increased catecholamines, vasoconstriction, derangements of homeostasis of neurotransmitters). Often polydrug use and biomedical risk factors (poor maternal nutrition, stress). Neonatal morbidity: tremulousness/lethargy, excessive startle responses, neonatal seizures. Microcephaly is the most common brain abnormality. Long-term morbidity: SIDS, epilepsy, CP, neurobehavioural deficits, developmental delay, learning difficulties, visual problems (optic nerve hypoplasia/atrophy coloboma). Neuroimaging: intracranial haemorrhage, hypoxic-ischaemic lesions, cerebral infarction, disturbance of midline prosencephalic development and neuronal migration	Screening: determination of cocaine metabolite in meconium/gastric aspirate/urine. No specific pharmacological intervention is warranted in neonatal period. Prevention of cocaine exposure in utero (socioeconomics and education)
Tobacco	Increased prevalence of smoking among youngest and oldest pregnant females particularly of lower educational achievement Higher rate of pregnancy complication: placental insufficiency, fetal growth restriction	Education of females of childbearing age remains the most important method of prevention

Table 22.2 (continued)   Acquired/environmental causes of microcephaly in infancy

Cause	Clinical or imaging features	Comment/management
Perinatal hypoxic-ischaemic/haemorrhagic brain injury		
HIE	1—2/1000 live births at term experience HIE and 0.3/1000 have significant neurological residua (CP, intellectual disability, epilepsy, sensory impairments, behavioural problems). Temporal characteristics, severity of hypoxia-ischaemia and gestation determine the type of resulting neuropathology: selective neuronal necrosis (cortical, basal ganglia/thalamus, brainstem), parasagittal cerebral, focal and multifocal cerebral injury. Neuroimaging: cranial ultrasound (basal ganglia, multifocal ischaemic injury) in neonatal age and early infancy. MRI is modality of choice (diffusion-weighted in first days) for assessment and follow-up of structural reorganization	Tests: CSF-/blood-/brain-specific isomer of creatine kinase, lactate acid, uric acid, magnesium, interleukin-6 EEG: voltage suppression/slowing, 'burst-suppression' Therapy: monitor glucose level, control of seizures, neuroprotection (see text)
PVL	PVL is the major form of brain injury and leading cause of chronic neurological disability in survivors of preterm birth. In 25% of survivors born preterm, major consequences are CP and visual impairments. By school age, 25—50% manifest a broad spectrum of cognitive and learning difficulties. Predilection for periventricular white matter (focal cystic necrotic lesions, diffuse disturbances of myelination). Predisposing factors include hypoxia, ischaemia, and maternal—fetal infection	Tests: cranial neonatal brain ultrasound/MRI. Therapy: supportive care, prevention of neonatal complications, treatment of infection. Neuroprotection (see text)

ASD, autism spectrum disorder; CMV, cytomegalovirus; CP, cerebral palsy; CT, computed tomography; EEG, electroencephalography; HIE, hypoxic-ischaemic encephalopathy; HIV, human immunodeficiency virus; HSV, herpes simplex virus; IUGR, intrauterine growth restriction; IV, intravenous; MMR, measles, mumps, rubella; MRI, magnetic resonance imaging; PCR, polymerase chain reaction; PVL, periventricular leukomalacia; SIDS, sudden infant death syndrome; SNHL, sensorineural hearing loss.

Primary microcephaly can be further classified according to the following associated clinical signs:

- Growth restriction (or dwarfism), either proportionate (e.g. Bloom syndrome) or disproportionate (e.g. Seckel syndrome).

- Dysmorphic features and/or congenital anomalies, including Mendelian disorders such as Cornelia De Lange syndrome or disorders with copy number variants such as Di George syndrome.

- Primary microcephaly as part of a wider disorder with additional clinical signs (e.g. metabolic disorders).

- Primary microcephaly with no other signs except early developmental impairment/intellectual disability; imaging reveals a brain which is reduced in size, with the cerebral cortex mostly affected. It is a diagnosis of exclusion, normally with an autosomal recessive cause (e.g. abnormal spindle-like microcephaly-associated protein [ASPM] genetic variations).

'BENIGN' FAMILIAL MICROCEPHALY

'Benign' familial microcephaly is a diagnosis of exclusion, occurring in a child with no abnormal features on history/examination. It is typically associated with a parent having normal learning ability, no neurological signs, and an OFC beneath the 2nd centile for adults. The value of this centile will vary between countries and ethnicities and has also been shown to vary with adult height. In the UK this centile creates an upper limit for microcephaly of approximately 52.6cm in adult females and 53.8cm in adult males (Cole, Freeman, and Preece, 1998). Some of these children may have mild intellectual disability or learning difficulties, which we discuss below, hence the label 'benign' should be used with caution.

SECONDARY MICROCEPHALY

Secondary microcephaly occurs when the OFC is normal at birth, but then fails to grow in proportion to the body (Ashwal et al. 2009; Woods and Parker, 2013). If current neurological development continues at the same rate as it has done in the past and there are dysmorphic features, then the most likely aetiology is genetic. In these cases, microcephaly can be caused by both Mendelian disorders with well-characterized dysmorphic features (e.g. Rubinstein-Taybi syndrome), or by less specific copy number variants that may be identified with microarray (e.g. Miller–Dieker syndrome with a microdeletion on the short arm of chromosome 17) (Rosman, Tarquinio, and Datseris, 2011).

Metabolic causes should be sought, particularly if there is progressive neurological deterioration, e.g. Smith–Lemli–Opitz syndrome – an inborn error of metabolism characterized by a defect of cholesterol synthesis. Usually, investigations are triggered by signs such as global developmental delay or refractory epilepsy, and microcephaly is a later finding; however, this group represents only 1% of the causes of microcephaly (von der Hagen et al. 2014; Seregni and Parker, 2018).

Several different genetic disorders can cause a similar phenotype to each other and present as secondary microcephaly, e.g. Aicardi–Goutières syndrome – an early-onset neurodegenerative 'interferonopathy' that mimics congenital infections.

Rett is a disorder characterized by developmental regression in childhood, slower head growth, and the loss of purposeful movements of the hands. It occurs almost exclusively in females – the inheritance is an X-linked dominant pattern with disease causing variants (mutations) in the *MECP2* gene.

Angelman syndrome may also account for postnatal head growth slowing, characteristic features, and neurological findings.

INVESTIGATIONS

Depending on the history, examination, and initial differential diagnosis, the clinician will decide to perform different investigations to guide towards a diagnosis. The algorithm in Figure 22.1 can provide some guidance on the process. In summary, when an environmental or perinatal disease process is suspected, or when there are neurological signs, magnetic resonance imaging (MRI) is recommended in the first instance. If, on the other hand, there is progressive neurological deterioration, biochemical investigations for metabolic conditions are recommended as the first step, with particular priority given to treatable disorders (e.g. phenylketonuria). Last, when dysmorphism suggests an underlying syndrome, genetic investigations should be prioritized. Very often, it will be hard to distinguish whether neurological, metabolic, or genetic factors underlie the disease process and more than one set of investigations will need to be carried out.

Congenital infections

Clinicians may have a low threshold for initiating TORCH testing, but in isolation this will not identify the cause, as the presence of an antibody can merely reflect the passive transfer of maternal immunoglobulins, or genuine infection that occurred only after the period when brain injury was likely to occur had passed (Mendelson et al. 2006). Viral testing should be targeted, and although likely to include TORCH, should also include consideration of rarer causes including HIV, Zika, and parvovirus B-19. Analysis of both antibody and viral levels can be challenging, and it is important to conclude that infection is the cause only if the clinical picture fits (e.g. typical pattern of intracranial calcification/white matter injury), with positive antibody testing and evidence that the infection was acquired at the correct period.

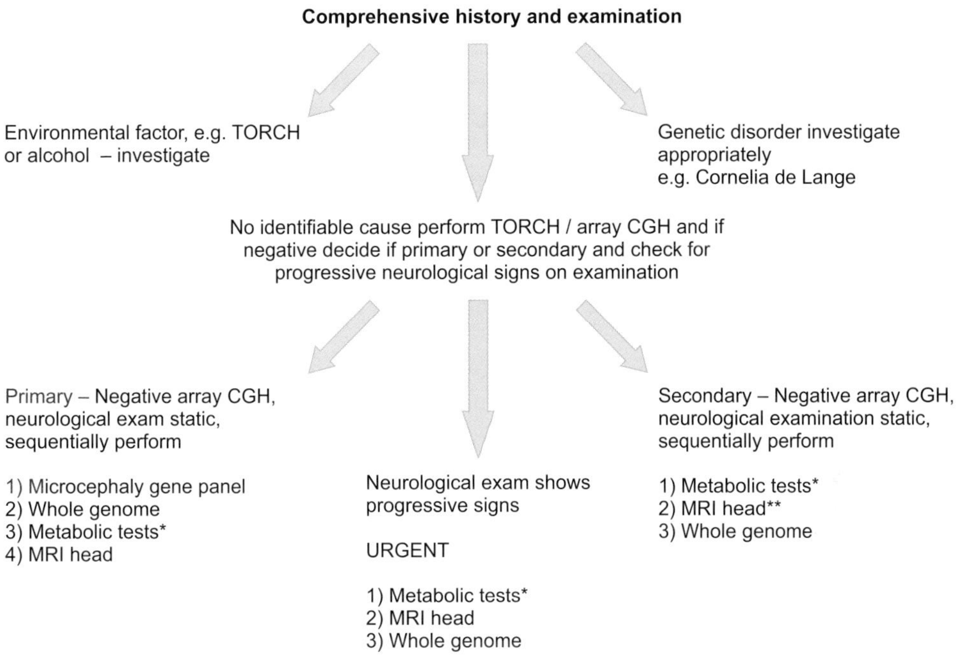

Comprehensive history and examination

Environmental factor, e.g. TORCH
or alcohol – investigate

Genetic disorder investigate
appropriately
e.g. Cornelia de Lange

No identifiable cause perform TORCH / array CGH and if
negative decide if primary or secondary and check for
progressive neurological signs on examination

Primary – Negative array CGH,
neurological exam static,
sequentially perform

1) Microcephaly gene panel
2) Whole genome
3) Metabolic tests*
4) MRI head

Neurological exam shows
progressive signs

URGENT

1) Metabolic tests*
2) MRI head
3) Whole genome

Secondary – Negative array CGH,
neurological examination static,
sequentially perform

1) Metabolic tests*
2) MRI head**
3) Whole genome

Figure 22.1   Practical algorithm of investigation
*See sections on secondary microcephaly/investigation discussing metabolic investigation.
**If craniosynostosis is being considered, computed topography may be more appropriate. CGH,
Comparative genomic hybridization; MRI, magnetic resonance imaging; TORCH, toxoplasma, other,
rubella, cytomegalovirus, herpes.

For example, a positive cytomegalovirus (CMV) antibody result on TORCH testing requires confirmation that the clinical picture is consistent with primary maternal CMV infection during the pregnancy, and preferably that there is evidence of actual virus present at birth by polymerase chain reaction (PCR) of the neonatal blood spot for fragments of CMV (or if the virus was cultured from urine obtained at birth). PCR for viruses including CMV is technically challenging, carrying a risk of false positive or false negative tests. Analysis of maternal serum at the beginning of pregnancy/after birth, if possible, can be very helpful in determining whether a PCR result is a true or false positive screen for CMV infection of the fetus. Finally, expert multidisciplinary discussion of all these factors is very helpful allowing a team decision as to whether congenital infection is the likely cause.

Genetic tests

Genetic tests are explained in Chapter 11. The physician should think very carefully before initiating any type of genetic testing, because of the following pitfalls:

- There is a significant chance that a true positive result will be distressing for family members and have direct implications for their own health (e.g. inherited contiguous gene deletions also involving oncogenic genes).

- An innocent variant may be mistakenly judged to be the cause of disease.

- Any cytogenetic or molecular genetic test can identify changes of uncertain significance, e.g. many smaller duplications in array results and many variants identified in whole genome sequencing (WGS). When the laboratory fails to identify a pathogenic variant, families often erroneously assume it is not a genetic disorder.

If the family understands the above issues and informed consent is obtained, then a clinician may request genetic investigations. If a clinician can suggest a phenotype-based genetic diagnosis, specific genetic tests for that condition can be performed. Comparative genomic hybridization (CGH)/microarrays, allowing detection of copy number variants of 50 000 to 500 000 bases and above (e.g. deletions or duplications) are an alternative. They are commonly used, but if they are not diagnostic, more detailed genetic investigations are needed. The next tier of investigation includes WGS, with either interrogation of a known panel of microcephaly genes only (or a linked panel such as metabolic) or the entire genome.

Close discussion with a clinical geneticist about the preferred genetic tests is highly recommended. All abnormal results should be assessed with a clinical geneticist to determine clinical significance before sharing with the patient and/or their family.

Imaging

Imaging is not mandatory in all children with microcephaly, especially if the OFC is between 3SD and 6SD below the mean, with no additional neurological features, or if a clear genetic diagnosis is identified.

If this is not the situation, MRI can be considered as it may identify structural abnormalities. MRI is recommended with an OFC >6SD below the mean for age or with neurological signs and symptoms such as hemiplegia or early-onset epilepsy.

In cases where a neurometabolic diagnosis, such as a mitochondrial disease, is suspected, magnetic resonance spectroscopy could be requested at the same time to look for a lactate peak.

Computed tomography is indicated when there is a clinical suspicion of bone structural abnormalities (such as craniosynostosis) or in congenital infections to look for micro-calcifications (Tarrant et al. 2009).

Biochemistry

Where the diagnosis is not elucidated by the above, plasma lactate, amino acids, ammonia, thyroid function, and urine organic acids should be assessed for inborn errors of metabolism. If there is high suspicion of a certain disorder, specific tests may be diagnostic (e.g. 7-dehydrochoelesterol for Smith–Lemli–Opitz syndrome). If the diagnosis is still unclear, in the absence of other signs, and after neurological/genetics opinions, then second line tests include: plasma/cerebrospinal fluid (CSF) glucose for GLUT1 deficiency, CSF lactate, creatine:guanadinoacetate profiles in urine or plasma for creatine disorders, and purine profile in urine for purine/pyrimidine disorders (Woods and Parker, 2013). If a diagnosis is still not reached, particularly in the presence of consanguinity, then the opinion of a specialist in metabolic disorders may help.

MANAGEMENT

The identification of microcephaly can be a challenging time for families. Particular concerns include the cosmetic appearance of a small skull, understanding that the head size reflects brain size, implications for learning/behaviour/social communication/seizures, recurrence risks, and testing pathway. The neurologist can reassure parents on most of these issues, many of which are pertinent to all children with intellectual disability.

The management will depend on aetiology. In the first instance, the clinician should focus on conditions where disease modification is available (e.g. phenylketonuria and some other inherited errors of metabolism). In most of the other cases, management will mainly be supportive and directed at treatment of the complications. In some cases, genetic counselling can be sought.

In the diagnosis and management of microcephaly, a multidisciplinary approach is crucial. Developmental paediatricians, ophthalmologists, audiologist, speech and language therapists, physio/occupational therapists, psychologists, as well as teachers and social workers should work closely in supporting children and their families. Referral by a coordinating paediatrician should be made to relevant team members, depending on the diagnostic questions (e.g. an audiology assessment is almost always needed) or therapeutic requirement (e.g. speech and language therapist) if there is delayed acquisition of language (Seregni and Parker, 2018).

Active management should focus on complications. Epilepsy is present in 40% of cases of microcephaly. Parents/carers should be educated on how to recognize seizures, even when epilepsy is not present at the point of diagnosis.

Ophthalmology as well as audiology assessments can help in both the identification of the underlying diagnosis (e.g. TORCH) and in the supportive care of the child; early identification of impairment allows early treatment.

Intellectual disability or learning difficulties are highly likely and individual developmental surveillance should be put in place for these children, with reassessment.

Whenever a syndrome is identified, the role of geneticists is important in providing prognostic likelihood of complications and counselling families around planning further pregnancies and risk of recurrence.

In families affected by 'benign' familial microcephaly, where comprehensive history and examination is otherwise unremarkable, we recommend that parents are counselled on how to arrange re-referral if any concerns arise regarding behaviour, learning, or seizures.

CONCLUSION

OFC measurement is an important part of the physical and neurological examination of children and should be regularly undertaken. A comprehensive history is essential, with a specific focus on pregnancy, perinatal, and family history. Classification into primary and secondary microcephaly may serve as a guide, although diagnosis can remain challenging and a multidisciplinary approach is recommended. If the aetiology is still unclear, first-line investigations include single gene testing if a single syndrome seems likely, otherwise: microarray, virology, MRI, and biochemistry. Modern genomic testing requires appropriate counselling for families, but is very useful. The management is usually supportive with a focus on rehabilitation strategies, with physio/occupational/speech/language therapists addressing comorbidities which may include epilepsy, and visual and hearing impairment. It is important to provide a supportive framework around the family, which may include developmental paediatricians, social workers, psychologists, and specialist nurses. Sometimes, a clear diagnosis for these children cannot be found despite prolonged investigations. In this case, it is important to offer reassurance and reassessment at a later point.

REFERENCES

Ashwal S, Michelson D, Plawner L, Dobyns WB (2009) Practice parameter: Evaluation of the child with microcephaly (an evidence-based review): report of the Quality Standards Subcommittee of the American Academy of Neurology and the Practice Committee of the Child Neurology Society. *Neurology* 73: 887–897.

Chantry CJ, Byrd RS, Englund JA (2003) Growth survival and viral load in symptomatic childhood human immunodeficiency virus. *Pediatr Infect Dis J* 22: 1038–1038.

Cole TJ, Freeman JV, Preece MA (1998). British 1990 growth reference centiles for weight, height, body mass index and head circumference fitted by maximum penalized likelihood. *Stat Med* 17: 407–29.

de Araújo TVB, Ximenes RAA, Miranda-Filho DB, et al. (2018) Association between micro-cephaly, Zika virus infection, and other risk factors in Brazil: final report of a case-control study. *Lancet Infect Dis* 18: 328—336.

Harris SR (2015) Measuring head circumference Update on infant microcephaly. *Can Fam Physician* 61: 680—684.

Keegan J, Parva M, Finnegan M, Gerson A, Belden M (2010) Addiction in pregnancy. *J Addict Dis* 29: 175—191.

Ledger WJ (2008) Perinatal infections and fetal/neonatal brain injury. *Curr Opin Obstet Gynecol* 20: 120—124.

Mendelson E, Aboudy Y, Smetana Z, Tepperberg M, Grossman Z (2006) Laboratory assessment and diagnosis of congenital viral infections: Rubella, cytomegalovirus (CMV), varicella-zoster virus (VZV), herpes simplex virus (HSV), parvovirus B19 and human immunodeficiency virus (HIV). *Reprod Toxicol* 21: 315—382.

Merfeld E, Ben-Avi L, Cerveny M, et al. (2017) Potential mechanisms of Zika-linked micro-cephaly. *Wiley Interdiscip Rev Dev Biol* 6: e273.

Rosman NP, Tarquinio DC, Datseris M, et al. (2011) Postnatal onset microcephaly: pathogenesis, patterns of growth, and prediction of outcome. *Pediatrics* 127: 665—671.

Seregni F, Parker APJ (2018) How to assess and support the child with microcephaly at secondary level. *Paediatr Child Health* 28: 468—473.

Tarrant A, Garel C, Germanaud D, et al. (2009) Microcephaly: A radiological review. *Pediatr Radiol* 39: 772—780.

von der Hagen M, Pivarcsi M, Liebe J, et al. (2014). Diagnostic approach to microcephaly in child-hood: a two-center study and review of the literature. *Dev Med Child Neurol* 56: 732—741.

Woods CG, Parker APJ (2013) Investigating microcephaly. *Arch Dis Child* 98: 707—713.

Resources

Baxter PS, Rigby AS, Rotsaert M, Wright I (2009) Acquired microcephaly: Causes, patterns, motor and IQ effects, and associated growth changes. *Pediatrics* 124: 590—595.

Boom JA (2017) Microcephaly in infants and children: etiology and evaluation. *UptoDate*. Available at https://www.uptodate.com/contents/microcephaly-in-infants-and-children-etiology-and-evaluation

Morris JK, Rankin J, Garne E, et al. (2016) Prevalence of microcephaly in Europe: population-based study. *BMJ* 354: i4721.

Raghuram K, Yang J, Church PT, et al. (2017) Head growth trajectory and neurodevelopmental outcomes in neonates born preterm. *Pediatrics* 140: e20170216.

Scott HJ, Kimberlin DW, Whitley RJ (2009) Antiviral therapy for herpes virus central nervous system infections: neonatal herpes simplex virus infection and congenital cytomegalovirus infection. *Antiviral Res* 83: 207—213.

Volpe JJ (2008) *Neurology of the Newborn*, 5th edn. Philadelphia: Elsevier.

CHAPTER 23

Macrocephaly, including hydrocephalus and brain tumours

Colin Kennedy

Key messages

- Distinguish a large head from an excessive rate of head growth.
- Manage typically developing infants with macrocephaly expectantly.

Common errors

- Diagnosing hydrocephalus without imaging.
- Diagnosing hydrocephalus without enlargement of lateral ventricles.
- Intervening in a typically developing infant with macrocephaly.
- Diagnosing craniosynostosis when the head shape is normal (unlikely).

When to worry

- Excessive rate of head growth.
- Marked separation of the cranial sutures.
- Lethargy, persistent unexplained vomiting, sunsetting.
- Focal neurological signs in association with macrocephaly.

DEFINITION

Macrocephaly (or macrocrania) can be defined as an occipitofrontal head circumference (OFC) more than three standard deviations above the mean level (i.e. >99.6th centile). Excessive rate of head growth (crossing centiles) is more likely to be associated with underlying pathology than a large head increasing in size appropriately (i.e. parallel to the centiles). Macrocephaly can be due to an increase in the volume of any cranial component.

CLINICAL APPROACH TO ASSESSMENT OF HEAD SIZE AND SHAPE

Head size

Measurement of OFC requires only a measuring tape, preferably a disposable paper tape, and a centile chart appropriate to the sex of the infant of head circumference against age. These are essential items for any neurologist and should both be carried by the examiner in all clinical settings. World Health Organization (WHO) centile charts for head circumference, height, and weight can be found in Appendix 1 at the end of the book.

Centile charts for head circumference do vary so that whichever growth standard is chosen, it is likely to lead to children being spuriously labelled as having abnormal head growth because the centiles in the reference population differ slightly from the centiles in the local population (Baxter, 2011; Wright et al. 2011). Providing that this caveat is remembered, the WHO 2007 head circumference growth standards (Appendix 1) are a suitable starting point.

As with length and weight, both measurements and centiles must be documented. Documentation in the medical records of OFC and centile, with date, forms part of the basic medical assessment of all infants, whether in the hospital or the community. This information can be very valuable, not only at the time but also later as evidence of the likely age at which abnormal growth first became evident. Measurement on more than one occasion enables determination of the growth rate. In both macro- and microcephaly (see Chapter 22), this often points the physician helpfully towards a diagnosis (e.g. birth asphyxia, congenital infection, hydrocephalus, brain tumour, possible inflicted injury, Rett, and other syndromes).

Head size is more closely related to parental head size than to the child's own weight or height. Genetic factors are the major determinant of head size in a well-nourished, typically developing infant. Parental head size and centiles give a clear indication of where the child's head size lies in relation to its genetic target. If only one parent is available to be measured, supply the family with a paper tape so they can inform the health team of a home measurement of the other parent.

Careful measurement of OFC avoids many unnecessary investigations in children with a familial tendency to small or large heads, including those with benign external hydrocephalus (see below). Rarely, a 'normal' head size may indicate excessive or insufficient head growth depending on the genetic target.

Signs that may be associated with macrocephaly or abnormal head shape

- Separation of the cranial sutures is a useful sign in obstructive hydrocephalus in young infants.

- Fullness and firmness of the anterior fontanelle can be useful additional signs, but are not quantifiable and occasionally misleading.

- A normally shaped head is unlikely to be seen in primary craniosynostosis.

- Ridging of the sutures (usually symmetrical either side of the ridge) is a sign of synostosis and must be distinguished from overlapping of the sutures, which can be a normal variant or seen after reduction of intracranial pressure or volume. In the latter case, the ridge has only one edge and relative movement between the bones can be felt by pressing on the lower of the bones that meet along the ridge. This is much easier to interpret than plain radiographs on which overlapping bones may cause a denser (i.e. higher attenuation) ridge compared with other parts of the skull, and thus mimic the appearance of ossification.

Investigation of macrocephaly

The first step is to consider whether, on the clinical assessment described above, there is

- no reason for concern,

- need for continued monitoring of head growth in the community, or

- need for special investigation.

Almost all intracranial causes can only be identified on cranial imaging. Ultrasound is good for defining the size of the cerebral ventricles but less good at describing the extracerebral and subdural spaces or abnormalities of the cerebral parenchyma.

Therefore, magnetic resonance imaging (MRI) or, if MRI cannot be accessed, computed tomography (CT), is needed to confirm ultrasound findings, except in cases of hydrocephalus, *where the cause is already known*, for example, intraventricular haemorrhage (IVH).

A list of causes of macrocephaly in infancy is given in Table 23.1. Head centile charts are shown in Appendix 1 at the end of this book.

Table 23.1 Causes of macrocephaly in infancy

Cause	Clinical or imaging feature	Possible other feature	Comment/ management
Cephalohaematoma	Boggy mass	May be calcified, not boggy, if chronic	NB: risk of infection if tapped
Extravasation of IV infusion into subcutaneous tissue	Recent scalp vein infusion	Pitting oedema	Stop infusion
Subdural haematoma	Consider inflicted injury	May be mimicked by traumatic CSF fistula	MRI, skeletal survey, eye exam if unexplained. Surgery only if very large or severe symptoms
Growing fracture	Cystic nontender mass, bony defect	Trauma with dural laceration	Surgical
Benign external hydrocephalus	Head size above mean at birth	Parental macrocephaly	See text. Outpatient observation; consider glutaric aciduria
Obstructive hydrocephalus	IVH	Infant born preterm; usually communicating	See text
	Aqueduct/fourth ventricle obstruction	Myelomeningocele, Dandy—Walker syndrome or other cerebral malformation, adducted thumbs	Surgical; consider genetics
	Infection; tumour; occasionally haemorrhage	Toxoplasma (perinatal); after bacterial meningitis	Also, chronic ventriculitis in infants born preterm
Megalencephaly	Parental macrocephaly	Developmentally typical	Syndromes (e.g. related to *PTEN* gene or *MCP4* or *PIK3CA* mutation) with dysmorphism and/or impairments

Table 23.1 (continued)   Causes of macrocephaly in infancy

Cause	Clinical or imaging feature	Possible other feature	Comment/ management
Rarer causes	Tumour mass effect	Vomiting, lethargy, or focal neurological signs	Often supratentorial
	Hydranencephaly		May appear surprisingly neurologically typical but not for long
	Walker—Warburg syndrome	Dysmorphic, eye and developmental impairments	ERG, molecular genetics
	Canavan disease	Irritability and white matter abnormality	Urine organic acids, see Chapter 29
	Alexander disease	Other neurodevelopmental or white matter abnormality	Molecular genetic testing for GFAP gene, see Chapter 29
	Neurocutaneous	Hypomelanosis of Ito*, NF1, MCAP	
	Vein of Galen malformation	Hydrocephalus, bruit	Interventional neuroradiology
	Thickened bones	Osteopetrosis and other rare syndromes	
	Achondroplasia, basilar impression	Short limbs or abnormal skull base	Communicating or noncommunicating hydrocephalus

*Hypomelanosis of Ito is a neurocutaneous condition in which characteristic whorls of skin depigmentation provide a clue to associated cerebral malformation.
CSF, cerebrospinal fluid; ERG, electroretinogram; IV, intravenous; IVH, intraventricular haemorrhage; MCAP, megalencephaly-capillary malformation syndrome; MRI, magnetic resonance imaging; NF1, neurofibromatosis; PTEN, phosphatase and tensin homologue.

MEGALENCEPHALY

Definition

This is excessive brain size, not precisely defined, and most cases without neurological impairment are familial with a male preponderance. Head growth is determined by brain growth in a typically developing child so megalencephaly leads to macrocephaly (or macrocrania). Although brain size more than three standard deviations above the mean is associated with an increased relative risk of some intellectual impairment, this would be found in only a small percentage of individuals with megalencephaly. There is need, therefore, for thorough consideration of other causes of developmental impairment as in a child with normal brain size, as well as consideration of genetic causes of megalencephaly with developmental impairment, such as the *PTEN* cancer predisposition gene that produces the phosphatase and tensin homologue protein or *PIK3CA* mutation. This PI3K-AKT-mTOR pathway is essential for the typical development of many parts of the body, including the brain.

HYDROCEPHALUS

Definition and terminology

Hydrocephalus is here used to mean ventricular expansion due to elevated cerebrospinal fluid (CSF) pressure, which implies 'obstruction' to the flow of CSF. Much confusion surrounds this term because of the broader definition of hydrocephalus to mean simply excess CSF fluid in the head, of which one cause is atrophy of the cerebral parenchyma, for example after severe asphyxia. In such cases in infancy, the key clinical feature is absence of excessive head growth. This is sometimes referred to as *hydrocephalus ex vacuo*, which is not included within the narrower definition of hydrocephalus used in this book.

The longstanding division of hydrocephalus into 'communicating' and 'non-communicating' refers to communication between the CSF spaces within the brain and those on the outside of the brain and spinal cord. This is useful in that cases of non-communicating hydrocephalus are likely to have a pressure gradient between the head and spine. It is, therefore, because of risk of brain herniation, relatively less safe to perform lumbar puncture (for diagnosis or treatment) in these patients than in those with communicating hydrocephalus. Compared with later infancy, these risks are smaller in the early months because of the tendency for intracranial volume to increase with intracranial pressure, and thus reduce any pressure gradient. In general, such risks are greatest with rapid changes in pressure, such as rare instances of cerebral arterial haemorrhage in the posterior fossa, acute cerebellitis, or fulminant bacterial meningitis.

Note that 'obstructive' is *not* identical in meaning to non-communicating since obstructive hydrocephalus can be either non-communicating (e.g. obstruction at the foramen of Monro, or at the aqueduct – with a small fourth ventricle, or at the outflow from the fourth ventricle – with a large fourth ventricle), or communicating (e.g. with obstruction at the level of the arachnoid villi by blood products after IVH or meningitis).

Obstructive hydrocephalus may lead to an increase in intracranial pressure. Reference ranges for CSF pressure in infancy, as a proxy for intracranial pressure, are very scant. Mean CSF pressure of neonates was found in one study to be around 3cm of CSF (Whitelaw and Aquilina, 2012) and a pressure above 5cm is probably abnormal at this age.

Signs additional to excessive head growth associated with raised intracranial pressure due to hydrocephalus

In a young infant these are

- lethargy or reduced conscious level,

- persistent and otherwise unexplained vomiting or apnoea, and

- loss of upgaze then episodes of forced downgaze (sunsetting).

A variety of nonspecific clinical features may also be seen, including irritability, poor feeding, early developmental impairment, poor head control, apnoea, and bradycardia.

At a late stage

- spasticity of limbs, and

- extensor posturing (tonic attacks; see also Chapter 21).

Porencephaly

This refers to resorption of brain parenchyma after haemorrhage or other parenchymal insult leaving a CSF-filled space. This is not hydrocephalus, although the two conditions may occur together.

Ventricular dilatation

This is not of itself an indication of raised intracranial pressure and even a progressive increase in size can be due to atrophy (e.g. after birth asphyxia).

Ventricular index

The *ventricular index* is the distance in millimetres between the medial and lateral margins of the lateral ventricle at the level of the foramen of Monro (Figure 23.1). This measurement can be made reliably and monitored over time on cranial ultrasound scans. Reference ranges (Figure 23.2) can be used to compare serial measurements of the ventricular index with the 95th centile for age and thus compare with the expected increase in diameter of the lateral ventricles with age.

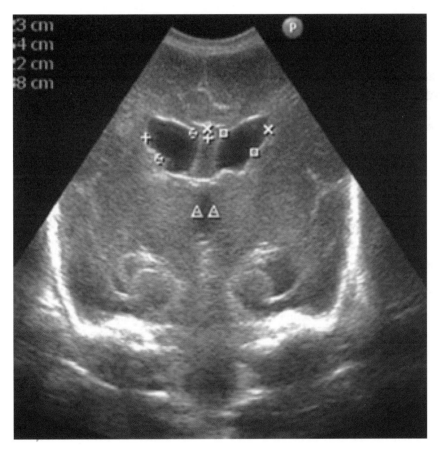

Figure 23.1 Cranial ultrasound scan showing moderate dilatation of the lateral ventricles. Coronal view with calipers showing anterior horn width (denoted by square calipers), third ventricular width (triangular calipers), and ventricular index (X and + calipers) measurements. (Reproduced from Whitelaw and Aquilina, 2012 with permission from BMJ Publishing Group Ltd.)

Monitoring of ventricular size is useful in post-haemorrhagic ventricular dilatation (PHVD; see below) and has been used as an inclusion criterion in trials of therapeutic intervention but should be combined with monitoring of head size and assessment of the coronal sutures and fontanelle to distinguish increase in ventricular index due to atrophy or porencephaly from that due to hydrocephalus. PHVD and (hereditary) porencephaly are strongly associated with mutations in the *COL4A1* or *COL4A2* genes.

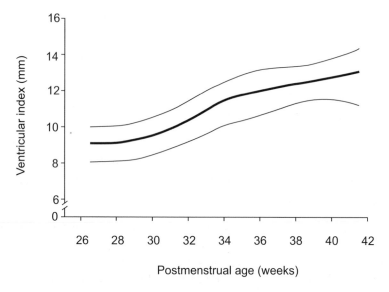

Figure 23.2 Cross-sectional chart of ventricular index against gestational age. Smoothed centiles are 3rd, 50th, and 97th centiles. (Reproduced from Levene, 1981 with permission from BMJ Publishing Group Ltd.)

Epidemiology of hydrocephalus

The incidence of hydrocephalus in the first year has been carefully tracked in Sweden over several decades (Table 23.2). In 1999 to 2002, the incidence was 0.66 per 1000 live births. Male infants outnumbered females almost 2 to 1. Infants born at more than 36 weeks' gestation accounted for 56% of all cases of hydrocephalus and there was a large increase in incidence (23 compared with 0.26 per 1000) in infants born extremely preterm, at less than 28 completed weeks of gestation, when compared with infants born at term (Persson et al. 2007). The number of cases in infants born extremely preterm was higher than in previous birth cohorts, coinciding with a decrease in their mortality. The incidence of myelomeningocele (MMC) is also higher in most countries without antenatal screening for MMC, so that the relative contribution of the different causes will show geographical variation.

PHVD

In infants born preterm most cases of hydrocephalus are secondary to haemorrhage from immature germinal matrix vessels in the subependymal layer lateral to the lateral ventricles. Such IVH is classified as grade 1 if confined to that location, grade 2 if also

Table 23.2   Incidence of hydrocephalus in the first year in Swedish infants

Hydrocephalus in first year in 1999—2002 birth cohort in western Sweden	
Hydrocephalus with myelomeningocele	0.18 per 1000
Hydrocephalus	0.48 per 1000
Malformations	49%
Intracranial haemorrhage	41%
Other	10%

(After Persson et al. 2007)

seen within the ventricle, and grade 3 if associated with PHVD. In addition to causing PHVD, haemorrhage can rupture into brain parenchyma (grade 4) with an increased risk of long-term neurological sequelae.

PHVD occurs in approximately 35% of patients with IVH and, of these, approximately 15% require shunt insertion for control of raised intracranial pressure. Severe IVH with its complications and periventricular leukomalacia remain the major determinants of brain injury in infants born preterm, and the neurodevelopmental outcome of infants with severe PHVD is extremely poor.

Surgical treatment of PHVD in the form of ventriculoperitoneal shunt insertion is effective in treating symptoms or signs of raised intracranial pressure, but has a high incidence of shunt blockage or infection in small, affected infants and carries lifelong risks associated with late infection or shunt failure. Endoscopic third ventriculostomy has been used, but is unlikely to be an effective form of treatment in the majority of cases because the extracerebral space into which fluid drains from the third ventricle is proximal to the obstruction (i.e. it is a communicating hydrocephalus).

Moderate to severe PHVD is often managed at first by intermittent removal of CSF, but randomized trials have suggested that serial removal of CSF (by ventricular taps with or without placement of a ventricular reservoir, or by lumbar puncture) does not reduce the progression to eventual shunt placement. A randomized trial of the use of acetazolamide and frusemide for PHVD and a subsequent systematic review (Whitelaw and Aquilina, 2012) showed that this treatment was both ineffective and dangerous, in that it increased the incidence of death or associated motor disability at follow-up.

Hydrocephalus due to cerebral malformation

The anatomy of cerebral malformations can usually be ascertained on CT, although MRI is preferable. The most common are those associated with MMC and aqueduct stenosis. Cystic dilation of the fourth ventricle with hypoplasia or agenesis of the vermis constitute the Dandy–Walker malformation: both features should be identified on imaging before making this diagnosis in which the long-term neurodevelopmental outcome is good in a proportion of promptly treated cases.

Hydrocephalus associated with open MMC commonly becomes clinically apparent soon after surgical closure of the MMC and requires prompt treatment to preserve the surgical closure.

Surgical treatment is the only active treatment option. Endoscopic third ventriculostomy is more physiological and has a lower complication rate than ventriculoperitoneal shunting, in which infection rates are highest in the youngest infants. However, the endoscopic method is only an option for non-communicating hydrocephalus and has a relatively lower success rate in infants than in older children.

A helpful, brief summary of the neurosurgical aspects of current management of hydrocephalus makes the important point that delayed recognition of shunt malfunction remains an important and preventable cause of death in current practice (Kandasarmy, Jenkinson, and Mallucci, 2011).

The British Antibiotic and Silver Impregnated Catheters for ventriculoperitoneal shunts multicentre randomized controlled trial (The BASICS trial) is a large trial that has recently established that antibiotic impregnated ventriculoperitoneal shunts have a significantly lower infection rate than non-impregnated ventriculoperitoneal shunts with the resulting reduction in days in hospital and other costs making this a cost-effective advance in treatment (Mallucci et al. 2019).

IDIOPATHIC (OR 'BENIGN') EXTERNAL HYDROCEPHALUS

This disorder is dominantly inherited and parental macrocephaly is a cardinal feature. Key clinical features are

- at least one parent with macrocephaly,

- OFC at birth above the mean for gestational age,

- excessive head growth deviating above and away from centiles, and

- no other neurological abnormalities in an unaffected infant.

Typically, the anterior fontanelle is large and may also be full. Some cases present with bulging of the fontanelle in a relatively unaffected infant, typically brought on by a minor viral respiratory infection. Affected infants often come to medical attention because of excessive head growth. In some cases, the trajectory of head growth is dramatically above and away from the 99th centile (Figure 23.3).

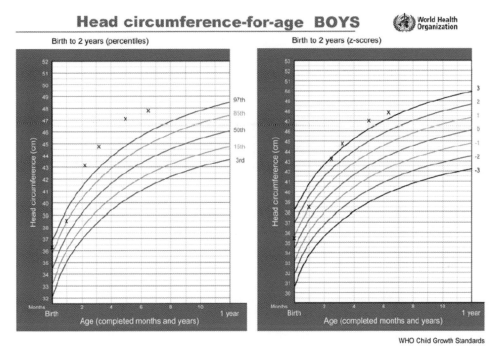

Figure 23.3 Trajectory of head growth from birth in an unaffected male infant whose father and paternal grandfather had occipitofrontal head circumferences of 60.0cm and 62.0cm. At the time of the most recent measurement he was sitting alone, passing objects from hand to hand, and babbling communicatively. The diagnosis is benign (also known as 'idiopathic') familial external hydrocephalus. The two charts are based on identical data plotted against (a) centiles and (b) z-scores. This shows how perception of the need to take action might be influenced by the specifics of chart construction. (Reprinted from WHO, 2007. Licence: CC BY-NC-SA 3.0 IGO.) A colour version of this figure can be seen in the colour plate section.

Imaging

Medical concern about head growth is often increased by cranial imaging which shows enlarged, and sometimes anteriorly very large, extracerebral CSF spaces of CSF intensity/density. On MRI, these can be difficult to distinguish from subdural collections, although complete symmetry, widened, rather than flattened, cerebral sulci, and a broad interhemispheric fissure are typical features. Visualization of the arachnoid membrane on MRI will confirm that the fluid is subarachnoid in distribution. Plump, rather than markedly expanded, lateral ventricles are also typical of benign external hydrocephalus. If MRI is not accessible, the distinction from chronic symmetrical subdural collections of blood can be even more difficult on CT scan and requires recognition of the above-mentioned typical features (Figure 23.4).

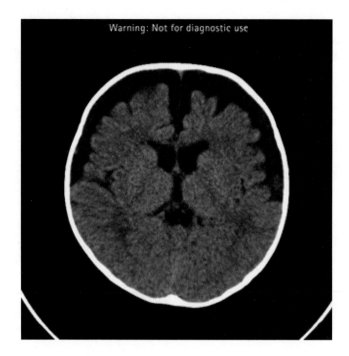

Figure 23.4 Computed tomography scan at age 7 months of the same infant whose head growth is shown in Figure 23.3. This shows plump cerebral ventricles and enlarged frontotemporal extratemporal cerebrospinal fluid spaces. Identical attenuation in these spaces with that in the cerebral ventricles, enlargement of the interhemispheric fissure, and the fact that the cerebral sulci appear enlarged rather than compressed are important features. The appearances are typical of benign enlargement of the extracerebral spaces (also known as benign external hydrocephalus). No intervention is required.

Other investigations

No other investigations are required in most cases, although consideration should be given to checking urine organic acids to exclude dominantly inherited glutaric aciduria, which can lead to both cerebral atrophy and subdural haemorrhage, but without acute presentation. Some history of neurological difficulties in the affected parent or child is likely in such cases. There is no indication to undertake lumbar puncture, but if CSF pressure is measured it may be above the reference range for infants. This is, however, 'normal' for infants with the other features described and does not require any intervention.

Management

In the absence of developmental problems other than delayed sitting, cranial imaging can often be avoided and investigation can be confined to monitoring of the child's clinical progress in the community. Developmental progress is typical except that independent sitting can be delayed. Motor milestones revert to normal once the child is able to stand independently. Medium- and long-term neurological outcome is completely typical with macrocephaly.

CRANIOSYNOSTOSIS

Definition

This refers to premature fusion of the sutures between the cranial bones while the brain is still growing and may be associated with ridging of the affected suture (see the section on signs at the beginning of this chapter). This can occur in a number of syndromic conditions with associated dysmorphism. Primary synostosis of all sutures could lead to microcephaly with normal head shape but is rare and more often leads to turricephaly (pointed or conical top of skull). Scaphocephaly (literally, keel head), due to sagittal synostosis, is the most common and is the single-suture synostosis most likely to require treatment within the first few months of life. Dolichocephaly, brachycephaly, trigonocephaly, and plagiocephaly follow from sagittal, coronal, metopic, and unilateral (coronal or lambdoid) synostosis respectively. Secondary microcephaly with sutural fusion may be symmetrical when the rate of head growth is greatly reduced secondary to cerebral atrophy, with or without reduction in CSF volume (e.g. birth asphyxia or shunt placement for PHVD, see above) with associated encephalomalacia. This is not, strictly speaking, craniosynostosis unless the brain growth is being constrained by fusion of the sutures.

Treatment

Surgical treatment of craniosynostosis is clearly indicated only in certain dysmorphic syndromes or when accompanied by raised intracranial pressure. In these cases, subspecialist craniofacial expertise is needed. Some cosmetic benefit for the more severe examples of fusion of a single suture are best considered in the light of the views of the child and parents and balanced against the risks of surgery.

ABNORMAL HEAD SHAPE WITHOUT SYNOSTOSIS

Symmetrically abnormal head shape is seen in a number of genetic syndromes. Abnormal head shape in the absence of synostosis may be postural; for example, dolichocephaly in infants born extremely preterm, brachycephaly in some cases of profound motor impairments, and plagiocephaly with chest deformity resulting from asymmetrical postural preferences in infancy. These posturally induced deformities of head shape can be corrected by increasing time in non-preferred postures. Sleeping in the supine position is, however, effective in reducing the risk of sudden infant death and should be continued in all infants. In these situations, it is important to minimize exposure to X-rays and to rely on clinical assessment, as detailed at the beginning of this chapter, as much as possible to distinguish positional plagiocephaly from synostosis (Figure 23.5).

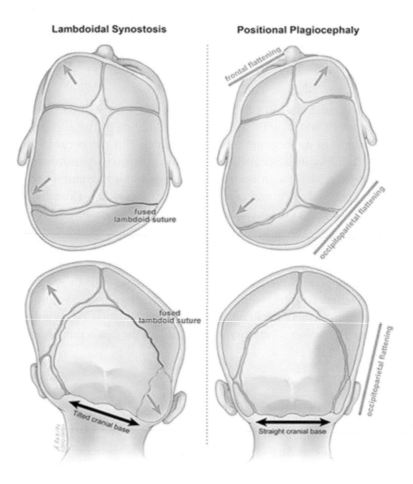

Figure 23.5 Differentiation of lambdoid synostosis from positional plagiocephaly. Clinical distinction between the two reduces the infant's exposure to potentially harmful X-rays. (Reproduced from the site of The International Society of paediatric Neurosurgery, www.ispn.guide.)

BRAIN TUMOURS

Detailed consideration of brain tumours in infancy is beyond the scope of this chapter but a recent and detailed account of this topic for neurologists is given elsewhere (Kennedy, Chakraborty, and Walker, 2018). WHO CNS 2016 replaces previous classifications of CNS tumours and uses, for the first time, molecular parameters in addition to histology (see https://braintumor.org/wp-content/assets/WHO-Central-Nervous-System-Tumor-Classification.pdf).

The overall incidence of brain tumours, including those that are benign at age 0 to 19 years, is more than 5 per 100 000 and about 10% of them present before the age of 2 years. A significant number of these are 'congenital' (presenting within 2 weeks of birth) or 'probably congenital' presenting within the first year. About 40% of these are gliomas with their biological behaviour varying widely within that group. In infants, in contrast to older children, there is a predominance of supratentorial tumours. Low grade tumours account for 40% of childhood brain tumours. Hypothalamic-chiasmatic low grade tumours most commonly present in the first 2 years of life and about 15% of these are associated with neurofibromatosis type 1. There is a trend towards younger patients presenting with larger tumours.

In infancy, brain tumours may present with symptoms or signs of increased intracranial pressure, focal neurological deficits, or epilepsy. Presentation with symptoms but no abnormal clinical signs is rare, except in the case of epilepsy. The initial symptomatology is often nonspecific and delayed acquisition of developmental milestones and behavioural disturbances are common presenting features. A systematic review of reports of the presenting features of brain tumours found that in infancy, macrocephaly is frequently a feature and, surprisingly, that a prompt diagnosis is actually more likely to be made in children aged less than 3 years than in older children (Wilne et al. 2007). Less common manifestations include intracranial haemorrhage, seizures (occasionally infantile spasms), focal neurological signs, and the diencephalic syndrome of emaciation. The UK HeadSmart Be Brain Tumour Aware campaign launched in 2011 produced a number of useful resources. These are downloadable at https://www.headsmart.org.uk/clinical/healthcare-resources/and include a quick reference guide, a medical educational poster, and pocket-sized symptoms cards listing the most common clinical features in infants.

Infants with tumours have an 80% to 90% chance of survival at 3 years with low grade gliomas, but lower survival rates with other histologies. Surgery is difficult because of the large size of many tumours and the relatively high risks of surgery associated with small circulating blood volume. Risk of the unwanted effects of radiation is highest in infancy and it is used less than previously as a consequence, excepting an increasing role for focal radiotherapy for certain brain regions (e.g. the posterior fossa) when long-term effects appear to be less burdensome. Chemotherapy is no panacea either, with high rates of disease progression at 12 to 18 months and an as yet poorly defined role in increasing the unwanted effects of radiotherapy.

Quality of life for survivors of infant brain tumours is often poor. Furthermore, the emergence of problems only appears when the surviving child reaches the age at which the function would normally be expected to occur. In addition, the decrease in scores over time on neurocognitive assessments following the diagnosis of a brain tumour in the developing brain typically reflect a failure to acquire skills at the expected rate rather than a loss of previously acquired skills; taken together these result in a tendency to 'grow into' deficits. One single-centre study in Switzerland of 27 followed-up consecutive patients diagnosed in the first year of life reported that 11 of them were survivors. Of these 11, nine had persistent neurological complications and eight had cognitive complications leading to school problems or impaired choice of occupation (Gerber et al. 2008).

Another single institution (St Judes Children's Research Hospital) study reported on 51 infants with low grade gliomas diagnosed in the first year of life. Of these, 25 had undergone cognitive assessments which covered domains of intellectual functioning, academic achievement, verbal memory, fine motor control, social-emotional functioning, attention, adaptive behavior, and executive functioning. The 25 assessed children were representative of all 51 infants, although significantly older and more likely to be simply observed initially than the 26 non-assessed infants. In assessed participants, the median number of chemotherapy regimens and tumour-directed surgical procedures was 2 and 1 respectively (range 0−5), while 11 had received focal and one had cranio-spinal radiotherapy. At a median follow-up interval of 9.7 years (range 1−17.6 years), 76% and 71% of assessed infants had scores that fell >1SD below expected mean level on intellectual and adaptive functioning respectively. Greater numbers of chemotherapy regimens and surgical procedures (but not the use of focal radiotherapy) were associated with worse outcomes. The assessed participants approached criteria for an intellectual disability with mean scores of 75.5 and 71.3 for IQ and adaptive functioning respectively (Heitzer et al. 2019). Avoidance of severe neurocognitive impairment is the predominant driver of parent treatment preferences, even over cure, in childhood cancer (Greenzang et al. 2020) so this is not a good outcome.

COMMON MYTHS ABOUT ASSESSMENT OF THE CRANIUM AND VENTRICLES

Myths about cranial imaging. One myth is that a diagnosis of hydrocephalus is possible without cranial imaging. It is not possible to diagnose hydrocephalus without establishing that there is enlargement of the cerebral ventricles and good reason to think that the enlargement is pressure-driven.

Myths about size of the third ventricle. Another myth is that diagnosis of neurological conditions can be based on the dimensions of the third ventricle. There are no reference ranges for the dimensions of the third ventricle that can usefully distinguish normal from abnormal in the absence of enlargement of the lateral ventricles. In an individual with expanded lateral ventricles, the third ventricle also dilates and serial measurements of its diameter in such an individual can sometimes be easier to com-pare with each other than lateral ventricular measurements because the dimensions of the third ventricle are less influenced by positioning of the head in the scanner.

Myths about the anterior fontanelle. Another myth is that diagnosis of neurological con-ditions can be based on anterior fontanelle dimensions. Considerable variation exists in the size and age at closure of the anterior fontanelle and, in the absence of dys-morphism, these variations do not show useful associations with neurological condi-tions and do not require investigation. Small, early-closing fontanelles may raise the question of craniosynostosis, especially if there is ridging of the sutures (see elsewhere in this Chapter and Chapter 22). Large, late-closing fontanelles are a feature of some dysmorphic syndromes (e.g. with macrocephaly in *PTEN* mutation).

Myths about a cavum septum pellucidum. Another myth is that diagnosis of neurological conditions can be suspected in the presence of a cavum septum pellucidum. The pres-ence of a cyst between the leaflets of the septum pellucidum is a normal variant and does not require intervention.

REFERENCES

Alvarez LA, Maytal J, Shinnar S (1986) Idiopathic external hydrocephalus: natural history and relationship to benign familial hydrocephalus. *Pediatrics* 77: 901–907.

Baxter P (2011) Head size: WHOse growth charts?*Dev Med Child Neurol* 53: 3–4.

Gerber NU, Zehnder D, Zuzak TJ, Poretti A, Boltshauser E, Grotzer MA. (2008) Outcome in children with brain tumour diagnosed in the first year of life: long-term complications and quality of life. *Arch Dis Child* 93: 582–89.

Greenzang KA, Al-Sayegh H, Ma C, Najafzadeh M, Wittenberg E, Mack JW (2020) Parental con-siderations regarding cure and late effects for children with cancer. *Pediatrics* 145: e20193552. https://pediatrics.aappublications.org/content/145/5/e20193552

Heitzer AM, Ashford JM, Hastings C, et al. (2019) Neuropsychological outcomes of patients with low-grade glioma diagnosed during the first year of life. *J Neurooncol* 141: 413–420.

Kandasarmy J, Jenkinson MD, Mallucci CL (2011) Contemporary management and recent advances in paediatric hydrocephalus. *BMJ* 343: 146–151.

Kennedy C, Chakraborty A, Walker D (2018) Tumours of the CNS, other space-occupying lesions and pseudotumor cerebri. In: Arzimanoglou A, ed, *Aicardi's Diseases of the Nervous System in Childhood*, 4th edn. London: Mac Keith Press, pp 729–800.

Levene MI (1981) Measurement of the growth of the lateral ventricles in preterm infants with real-time ultrasound. *Archi Dis Child* 56: 900–904.

Mallucci CL, Jenkinson MD, Conroy EJ, et al. (2019) Antibiotic or silver versus standard ventricu-loperitoneal shunts (BASICS): a multicentre, single-blinded, randomised trial and economic evaluation. *Lancet* 394: 1530–1539.

Persson EK, Anderson S, Wiklund LM, Uvebrant P (2007) Hydrocephalus in children born in 1999-2002: epidemiology, outcome and ophthalmological findings. *Child Nerv Syst* 23: 1111–1118.

Whitelaw A, Aquilina K (2012) Management of posthaemorrhagic ventricular dilatation. *Arch Dis Child Fetal Neonatal Ed* 97: doi:10.1136/adc.2010.190173

WHO (2007) The WHO Child Growth Standards. World Health Organization https://www.who. int/ childgrowth/standards/en/

Wilne S, Collier J, Kennedy C, et al. (2007) Presentation of childhood CNS tumours: a systematic review and meta-analysis. *Lancet Oncol* 8: 685—695.

Wright CM, Inskip HM, Godfrey K, Williams AF, Ong KK (2011) Monitoring head size and growth using the new UK-WHO growth standard. *Arch Dis Child Fetal Neonatal Ed* 96: 386—388.

Resources

Arzimanoglou A, ed, (2018) *Aicardi's Diseases of the Nervous System in Childhood*, 4th edn. London: Mac Keith Press.

HeadSmart (2011) Resources relating to clinical presentation of brain tumours in infants and children. Downloadable at: https://www.headsmart.org.uk/clinical/healthcare-resources/

Levene MI, Chervenak FA, eds, (2009) *Fetal and Neonatal Neurology and Neurosurgery*, 4th edn. London: Churchill Livingstone.

Louis DN, Perry A, Reifenberg G, et al. (2016) The 2016 World Organization classification of tumors of the central nervous system. *Acta Neuropathol* 6: 803—830. Available at: https://braintumor.org/wp-content/assets/WHO-Central-Nervous-System-Tumor-Classification.pdf

CHAPTER 24

The floppy infant

Helgi Hjartarson and Thomas Sejersen

Key messages

- The floppy infant is essentially a constellation of clinical features that has an extensive list of potential differential diagnoses.
- Central causes account for 60% to 80% of cases and hypoxic-ischaemic encephalopathy, sepsis, intracerebral haemorrhage, and congenital heart disease are more common than all other causes combined.
- A key feature of peripheral and central causes is the presence or absence of weakness.
- A thorough history and examination is essential in localizing the origin of hypotonia and reduces the list of differential diagnoses.
- Clinical evaluation of critically ill neonates and infants is difficult even for experienced experts. Practice is the only way of becoming proficient at it.

Common errors

- The belief that floppiness in an infant is synonymous with an inherent neuromuscular disorder.
- The belief that the term 'floppy infant' pertains only to infants that are symptomatic at birth.
- The prejudice that neuromuscular disorders are never treatable.

When to worry

- Delays in acquiring, and especially loss of motor skills, is particularly worrisome and should lead swiftly to investigation.

DEFINITION

The floppy infant is a descriptive term that denotes infants presenting with severe generalized muscular hypotonia (hereafter referred to as hypotonia). Hypotonia is a common symptom in the newborn period, in infants born preterm as well as at term, although gestational age is relevant. Before the 28th gestational week, flaccid arm extension and a frog-like leg posture are physiological (i.e. normal) phenomena. This gradually changes after the 32nd week and the infant's limbs are typically flexed at term equivalent age in both infants born preterm and infants born at term.

The term 'floppy infant' is used in two distinct clinical situations:

1. Severe hypotonia in a newborn infant, and

2. delayed motor development in an older infant, typically 3 to 4 months old, either from birth or initial typical development followed by stagnation.

The clinical picture in infant hypotonia is not very variable despite the many possible aetiologies (Box 24.1).

Box 24.1 Objective clinical manifestations
☑ Floppy ('rag-doll' or 'frog-like') appearance
☑ Poor head control
☑ Scarcity of spontaneous movements
☑ Delayed motor development
☑ Hypermobile joints common
☑ Feeding difficulties
(Adapted from Hjartarson, 2017 with permission from Studentlitteratur AB)

Normal muscle tone requires both an intact nervous system and healthy muscles. Hence, hypotonia is a common clinical sign in neurological disorders, resulting in an extensive differential diagnosis. Hypoxic-ischaemic encephalopathy (HIE), sepsis, and congenital heart diseases are important causes in neonates. Most of the remaining conditions have a genetic aetiology (Box 24.2).

Neuromuscular disorders may manifest at any age. In neonates this often manifests as floppiness and in older infants as hypotonia of a varying degree, in combination with delayed motor development. Distinguishing between hypotonia and weakness is important. Weakness pertains to a muscle's reduced maximal voluntary force, while hypotonia is defined as a skeletal muscle's reduced resistance to passive movement.

Box 24.2   Examples of genetic causes in neonatal hypotonia

Genetic causes in neonatal hypotonia

- ☑ Congenital muscular dystrophies
- ☑ Congenital myasthenic syndromes
- ☑ Congenital myopathies
- ☑ Congenital myotonic dystrophy type 1
- ☑ Pelizaeus—Merzbacher disease
- ☑ Pompe disease
- ☑ Prader—Willi syndrome
- ☑ Spinal muscular atrophy type 1
- ☑ Trisomy 13
- ☑ Trisomy 18
- ☑ Trisomy 21 (Down syndrome)
- ☑ Zellweger syndrome

(Adapted from Hjartarson, 2017 with permission from Studentlitteratur AB)

ORIGIN OF HYPOTONIA

It is helpful to think of hypotonia in terms of its origin being in the central or peripheral nervous system. The former accounts for 60% to 80% of cases and the single most common cause in neonates is HIE. Certain conditions may affect both locations, for example, metabolic disorders and certain congenital muscular dystrophies. An underlying disorder causing severe hypotonia may also predispose a child to perinatal complications, which in turn may cause HIE.

Central hypotonia

Central hypotonia can arise anywhere in the central nervous system (CNS) in the neural pathway, above the spinal cord anterior horn cells or cranial nerve motor nuclei (Table 24.1). The history may support this suspicion, as in perinatal asphyxia. Neonates with central hypotonia often display CNS symptoms, e.g. obtundation, seizures, brisk deep tendon reflexes or clonus, and an *absence of weakness*. As they get older, hypotonia may be replaced by hypertonia and delays in other modalities may become apparent.

Table 24.1   Central hypotonia of the newborn infant

Examples	
Systemic disease*	HIE*
	Sepsis*
	Intracerebral hemorrhage*
	Congenital heart disease*
	Inborn errors of metabolism
Syndromes	Trisomies (13, 18, 21)
	Angelman syndrome
	Prader—Willi syndrome
	Smith—Lemli—Opitz syndrome
	Other deletion syndromes
Other	CNS malformation on brain MRI
	TORCH
	Delayed myelination
	Spinal cord injury

*More common than all other central and peripheral causes combined.
CNS, central nervous system; HIE, hypoxic-ischaemic encephalopathy; MRI, magnetic resonance imaging; TORCH, toxoplasmosis, other, rubella, cytomegalovirus, herpes simplex. (Adapted from Hjartarson, 2017 with permission from Studentlitteratur AB)

Peripheral hypotonia — motor unit

Peripheral hypotonia (Table 24.2) indicates a neuromuscular disorder, i.e. a disorder affecting the motor unit. The most common peripheral causes in infants are spinal muscular atrophy (SMA), congenital myotonic dystrophy type 1 (DM1), and the congenital myopathies. Affected infants are generally vital, albeit weak, with ambiguous or absent deep tendon reflexes. They show no sign of irritability and have a normal circadian rhythm. Typically, weakness is significant and in certain conditions there is substantial underdevelopment or atrophy of musculature. Concomitant congenital birth defects are less common, apart from joint problems, as are dysmorphic features, except for micrognathia, myopathic face, and ptosis. Males may have cryptorchidism. Difficulties eating and breathing are not unusual. Cognitive development is more often typical.

Table 24.2 Peripheral hypotonia in the newborn infant

Examples	
Anterior horn	Spinal muscular atrophy*
Nerve	Hereditary motor and sensory neuropathies
Synapse	Transient neonatal myasthenia
	Botulism
	Congenital myasthenic syndromes
Muscle	Congenital myopathies
	Congenital muscular dystrophies
	Congenital DM1

* The single most common cause of peripheral neonatal hypotonia. DM1, myotonic dystrophy.

(Adapted from Hjartarson, 2017 with permission from Studentlitteratur AB)

CLINICAL APPROACH

In the history

- Consanguinity increases the likelihood of autosomal recessive (AR) disorders and recurrent miscarriages suggest a multisystem disorder or syndrome.

- Polyhydramnios implies bulbar weakness with difficulties swallowing.

- Low Apgar score may support suspicion of asphyxia.

- Onset of symptom within the first 24 hours may imply sepsis or an inborn error of metabolism, as does rapid progression of neurological symptoms.

- Upper motor neuron signs (see Chapter 6) suggest CNS damage.

Box 24.3 highlights a few important points from the medical history.

On examination

- Does the clinical picture fit a recognizable syndrome?

- Are there dysmorphic features? Primary, as part of syndrome or secondary, e.g. pectus excavatum resulting from weak respiratory muscles, or plagiocephaly caused by excessive lying supine?

- Is there muscle atrophy?

- What is the head circumference?

> **Box 24.3**   Medical history
>
> ☑   Family history: Affected relatives? Consanguinity? Stillbirths?
>
> ☑   Maternal illness: Myasthenia gravis? Myotonic dystrophy? Advanced maternal age?
>
> ☑   Pregnancy: Drug exposure? Infections? Polyhydramnios? Paucity of fetal movements?
>
> ☑   Perinatal history: Apgar scores? Hypoxic-ischaemic encephalopathy?
>
> ☑   Age at onset?
>
> ☑   Symptoms?
>
> ☑   Course: Static? Progressive? Fluctuations?

Evaluating a critically ill newborn infant in a neonatal intensive care (NICU) setting is difficult for obvious practical reasons, and the physical examination may be limited to inspection. The key difference between central and peripheral hypotonia is the presence or absence of weakness. Assessing muscle tone and strength is difficult and highly subjective in the youngest group. Weak infants are typically hypotonic, but hypotonia may exist without weakness.

Examples of clinical signs and manoeuvres — taking into account the child's age:

- Pull-to-sit (Figure 24.1a): Holding the infant's hands, slowly pull to the sitting position. Head-lag should be minimal in a term infant by postnatal age of 2 to 3 months.

- Vertical suspension (Figure 24.1b): Place your hands under the infant's axillae and lift to a vertical position. A hypotonic child slips through the examiner's hands.

- Frog-like leg posture (Figure 24.1c): Hips externally rotated, knees touching the ground.

- Ventral suspension (Figure 24.1d): With the infant in the prone position, place one hand under the torso and lift. Typically developing neonates born at term flex their extremities and can briefly hold their head at nearly 180 degrees.

- Scarf-sign: Pull the supine infant's one arm across the torso until you meet resistance. The test is considered positive if the elbow can cross the midline.

Observe the child's movements and movement patterns. Facial expression, breathing, and crying are relevant when assessing strength. Fetal akinesia may result in arthrogryposis multiplex congenita. Fasciculations denotes denervation, most easily detectable in the tongue, strongly suggesting SMA. Deep tendon reflexes are difficult to interpret

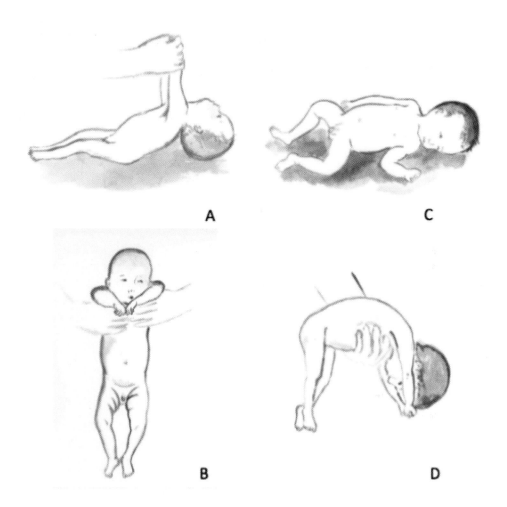

Figure 24.1 Illustration of floppy infant. Head lag is noted during traction in lying position (a), lack of axial control and lack of resistance in shoulders in 'shoulder suspension test' (b), 'frog-legged' posture (c), and inability to lift head and limbs against gravity in the 'ventral suspension' test (d). (Illustration by Rebecka Lagercrantz.)

in the neonate, but should be evaluated in older infants, where areflexia or hyporeflexia (i.e. absent or diminished deep tendon reflexes) indicate a peripheral cause. Ophthalmological examination may reveal signs of congenital infection or of genetic disorders that also involve the eye.

Table 24.3 shows associations between clinical features and underlying pathology in different parts of the nervous and muscular systems.

Table 24.3 Clinical signs and symptoms in hypotonia causes by disorder at different levels

	Tone	Strength	Reflexes	Vitality	Fascicu-lation	Muscle mass
CNS damage	↓ then ↑	0 / ↓	0 / ↑	↓	No	0 / ↓
CNS syndrome	↓	0 / ↓	0	0	No	0 / ↓
α-motor neuron	↓	↓	↓↓	0	Yes	↓↓ (proximal)
Nerve	↓	↓	↓	0	No	↓ (distal)
Motor endplate	0 / ↓	↓	0 / ↓	0	No	0 / ↓
Muscle	↓	↓	↓↓	0	No	↓ (proximal)

↑ = increase, ↓ = decreased, 0 = normal.

(Adapted from Hjartarson, 2017 with permission from Studentlitteratur AB)

INVESTIGATIONS

Some of the investigations at your disposal are invasive and painful. Use these judiciously! Figure 24.2 suggests an approach to investigating neonatal hypotonia.

Laboratory evaluation

In the newborn infant, initial blood testing aims to detect an eventual infection and to look for evidence of asphyxia. Subsequently, testing is broadened based on the specific clinical picture (Box 24.4, and below). Consider congenital infections – TORCH (toxoplasmosis, other, rubella, cytomegalovirus, herpes simplex). There are no specific blood tests that screen for inherent muscle disorders, but creatine kinase (CK) is a marker for muscle damage and comes closest to this. CK is sensitive to trauma and blood concentrations of CK may be elevated in neonates and greatly elevated in asphyxia.

Genetics

Consider karyotyping. Order targeted genetic tests when appropriate, e.g. in case of specific syndromes, DM1 or SMA.

Whole genome sequencing has recently become a tool available to clinicians even in the work-up of seriously affected infants. Bioinformatics is simplified by specifically

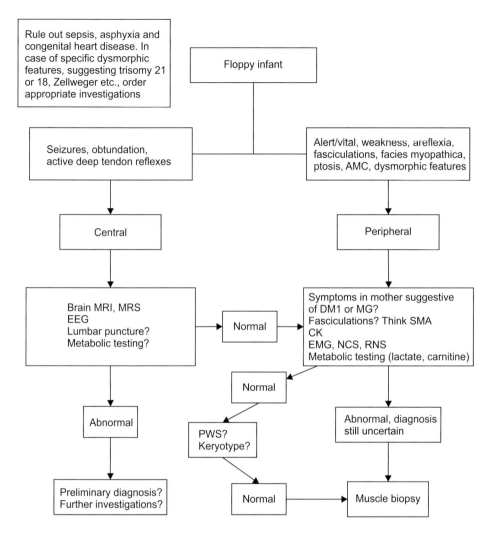

Figure 24.2 Schematic illustration showing approach to investigating hypotonia in the newborn infant. AMC, arthrogryposis multiplex congenita; CK, creatine kinase; DM1, myotonic dystrophy type 1; EEG, electroencephalograpy; EMG, electromyography; MG, myasthenia gravis; MRI, magnetic resonance imaging; MRS, magnetic resonance spectroscopy; NCS, nerve conduction studies; PWS, Prader–Willi syndrome; RNS, repetitive nerve stimulation; SMA, spinal muscular atrophy. (Adapted from Hjartarson, 2017 with permission from Studentlitteratur AB.)

examining certain genes (e.g. known neuromuscular or neurometabolic disease genes). The clinical examination, along with a thorough phenotypic description, is nonetheless very important, even when used in conjunction with advanced genetic methods.

> **Box 24.4** First-tier laboratory testing in the hypotonic newborn infant
>
> ☑ Complete blood count, blood gas
>
> ☑ Creatine kinase (CK)
>
> ☑ C-reactive protein (CRP)
>
> ☑ Cultures — blood, urine, cerebrospinal fluid (CSF)
>
> ☑ CSF analysis
>
> ☑ Electrolytes, including calcium and magnesium
>
> ☑ Glucose
>
> ☑ Liver function tests
>
> ☑ Consider congenital infection (TORCH)
>
> ☑ Consider testing for metabolic disorders — lactate, ammonia, transferrin isoelectric focusing, urine organic acids, and plasma amino acids

Neurophysiology

Electromyography (EMG), nerve conduction studies (NCS), and repetitive nerve stimulation (RNS) are useful investigations in suspected peripheral hypotonia. They may be used in combination and their aim is to localize the pathology to the anterior horn, axon, motor endplate, or muscle, thereby guiding further investigations. EMG is painful and all three of these investigations may be difficult to interpret in the newborn infant.

Muscle biopsy

Muscle biopsy is still the criterion standard in suspected myopathies. Further genetic studies are frequently guided by its results. Whichever affected muscle may be biopsied, it is prudent to consult the muscle pathologist beforehand, and a discussion with metabolic experts is advisable when a mitochondrial disorder is part of the differential diagnosis.

Imaging

Brain imaging is recommended in suspected central hypotonia. Ultrasound may be appropriate in the newborn infant, but otherwise MRI is supreme. In certain congenital muscular dystrophies, MRI may reveal specific CNS abnormalities. Magnetic resonance spectroscopy has added diagnostic value in metabolic disorders. In older infants, the MRI appearance of specific muscles may provide important diagnostic information and thereby guide further investigation. Cardiac ultrasound is essential if cardiac involvement is suspected

TREATMENT

With the exception of antibiotics in sepsis, enzyme replacement therapy (ERT) in Pompe disease, intrathecal Spinraza injections, and gene therapy with Zolgensma in SMA, treatment is generally supportive, irrespective of the cause. For children with chronic conditions, the emphasis is on habilitative measures, with the help of, among others, physiotherapists, occupational therapists, speech therapists, and specialists in rehabilitation. Nutrition is often a long-term issue that may necessitate placement of a gastrostomy tube. The child may need ventilatory support (see also section on SMA type 1). Secondary skeletal deformities are common and may be difficult to prevent even with aggressive bracing and other orthopaedic measures.

PROGNOSIS

Prognosis is entirely dependent upon the individual aetiology. The terms 'benign developmental delay' and 'benign congenital hypotonia' have been used for children with delayed gross motor development, especially delayed walking, without any demonstrable disorder. Some have displayed neonatal symptoms so pronounced as to warrant the term 'floppy'. Allegedly, their outcome appears to be favourable.

SPECIFIC CONDITIONS

SMA type 1 (Werdnig-Hoffmann disease)

SMA is an autosomal recessive disorder affecting 1 in 11 000 neonates, 60% of whom have type 1, the most common genetic cause of infant mortality. SMA is caused by mutations in the SMN1 gene, leading to progressive degeneration of α-motor neurons in the spinal cord and brainstem, with subsequent muscle weakness. The main dictator of the phenotype is the SMN2 gene copy number. SMA type 1 is the commonest SMA type and these patients almost always have two copies of the SMN2 gene, consistent with this being most common also in the general population. Patients with milder types 2 or 3 usually have a higher number of SMN2 copies. Diagnosis is confirmed by genetic analysis.

SMA type 1 manifests before 6 months of age, with symmetrical hypotonia and weakness accompanied by progressive muscle atrophy. Heart and extraocular muscles are spared, as is the diaphragm, although other respiratory muscles are weak causing paradoxical breathing and a bell-shaped thorax. Reflexes are reduced or impossible to elicit. Tongue fasciculations are almost universal. Sensory modalities are normal and so is intellectual development.

Affected children do not achieve independent sitting and the most seriously affected have difficulties feeding and swallowing. Failure to thrive is common. Treatment of SMA type 1 has until recently been entirely symptomatic. Mortality has been approximately 95% by age 18 months, with most patients succumbing to an infection in combination with chronic respiratory failure. International recommendation guidelines for SMA, published in 2017, advocates the use of non-invasive positive pressure (NIV) in symptomatic infants with SMA type 1, partly as a means of palliation. Tracheotomy ventilation, on the other hand, is a much more ethically difficult decision where it is imperative to weigh carefully the expected long-term benefits as well as burden of an invasive medical treatment. This is optimally done in a multidisciplinary setting. We have traditionally advised against this in the case of infants with progressive diseases, including SMA type 1.

In December 2016, the US Food & Drug Administration (FDA) approved Spinraza as the first drug for the treatment of SMA. The European Medicines Agency (EMA) followed suit 6 months later. Spinraza has been shown to be effective in SMA types 1 and 2. It modulates alternate splicing of mRNA from the mostly non-functional SMN2 gene, increasing the production of a functional SMN protein. The drug is administered intrathecally, initially as four loading doses over a 2-month period, and thereafter as maintenance doses every 4 months. Risdiplam is an orally administered drug with similar mode of action, that shows promising results in clinical SMA trials and it is currently under FDA consideration.

In May 2019, Zolgensma was approved by the FDA for use in patients with SMA under the age of two years. It is approved in Japan since March 2020 and in May 2020 the EMA granted conditional approval for its use in SMA type 1, as well as in an SMA patient who has three SMN2 gene copies, with a weight of up to 21kg. The drug is an adeno-associated virus vector-based gene therapy which delivers a fully functional copy of the human SMN1 gene into the child's motor neuron cells. It is the first approved gene therapy for treating a neuromuscular disorder and is administered as a one-time intravenous infusion.

Further studies are on-going, but as of June 2020, no long-term data are available. Furthermore extreme cost has already proven to be an issue, with many countries unable to afford Spinraza. No doubt, the same will apply to the following novel drugs e.g. Zolgensma, with a price tag of $2 million for the needed single dose. This raises important ethical issues as the consequences undoubtedly will be a fundamentally different prognosis for children with the same disease in different - and sometimes neighbouring - countries. For symptomatic children, neither Spinraza nor Zolgensma offers a cure, as already vanished neurons cannot be replaced. Instead, they potentially transform a fatal condition to a chronic one. The sooner the treatment is initiated the better, which in turn has implications for newborn screening programs. These new treatments will change the standards of care for SMA in the years to come and the positive is obviously that the therapeutic landscape for this devastating disorder seems to be radically changing.

Congenital DM1

This is a multiorgan disorder with an autosomal dominant inheritance. It is caused by a trinucleotide sequence (CTG) expansion in the DMPK gene on the long arm of chromosome 19. In DM1 the copy number is increased, with severity and disease onset correlating with the copy number. In the context of floppiness, only the congenital form is relevant, affecting approximately 1 in 20 000 live births. These children have >800 copies, many times greater than the normal 5 to 34 copies. A genetic analysis confirms the diagnosis.

In people with 35 to 60 copies, the repeat count increases in the germ line, especially in the mother. This phenomenon of parent-to-child amplification is called anticipation. A child with the serious congenital form practically always has a symptomatic mother.

The onset is prenatal with decreased fetal movements. Polyhydramnios is present in approximately 50% of cases. The newborn infant is hypotonic and weak, with myopathic facies and a tented upper lip. Congenital contractures are common. Myotonia is not displayed in the first few years. Respiratory failure as well as bulbar weakness often necessitates immediate need for both respiratory and nutritional support in an NICU setting.

Motor function improves in those who survive the neonatal period, with most children acquiring independent walking. Intellectual disability is universal. Treatment is purely symptomatic. Regular follow-ups are important, with the intervals depending on patient's age and disease severity. An important aspect is an annual electrocardiogram (ECG).

Prader—Willi syndrome

This is a complex genetic condition characterized by muscular hypotonia, initial feeding difficulties followed by excessive appetite and obesity, short stature, and intellectual deficit. A decrease in fetal movement is common. The neonate may display symptoms requiring a nasogastric tube for weeks.

Children with Prader—Willi syndrome often display certain dysmorphic features that hint at the diagnosis, e.g. small hands and feet, almond-shaped eyes, a narrow forehead, and a thin upper lip. A genetic test is required to confirm the diagnosis.

Infantile Pompe disease (glycogenosis type II)

Deficiency in acid maltase results in an inability to break down glycogen which subsequently accumulates in tissues, including muscle. This disorder has traditionally been classified in to three groups. The only one relevant in the context of floppiness is the classic infantile form.

Pompe disease is caused by different mutations in the GAA gene on the long arm of chromosome 17, and inheritance is AR. It manifests on average at 1 to 2 months of age, with severe generalized hypotonia and weakness, feeding difficulties, and poor weight gain. Heart failure usually manifests somewhat later. Macroglossia, hepatomegaly, and hearing loss are common. Deep tendon reflexes may be reduced. CK is usually elevated. Oligosaccharide concentrations in urine may hint at the diagnosis. ECG is abnormal and muscle biopsy may reveal a vacuolar myopathy.

Upon suspicion, acid maltase activity is determined in muscle cells, white blood cells, or fibroblasts. In the classic infantile form, enzyme activity is <1%. Genetic testing confirms the diagnosis.

Muscle weakness and cardiac failure are progressive and, without specific therapy, lead to death on average at 6 to 7 months of age.

Intravenous ERT has been available since 2006 and should be initiated as soon as possible. ERT is not curative but it is life saving as it reverses the otherwise fatal hypertrophic cardiomyopathy in the majority of patients with the infantile form. Long-term effects of ERT are being elucidated continually, as the oldest treated patients with the infantile form have reached adulthood. Sadly, ERT does not have the same dramatic effect on striated skeletal muscle and most patients have significant residual hypotonia and weakness, and progressive muscle weakness has been described in patients who initially responded well to treatment.

Congenital myopathies

This is a heterogeneous group of disorders with at present 32 known disease genes and a wide variation in severity, even within subgroups. Generalized weakness and hypotonia at birth are typical and the clinical course is most often static or slowly progressive.

Congenital myopathies are typically caused by mutations in genes that code for proteins important for sarcomere function or for the influx of calcium, resulting in ineffective contraction. There may be structural abnormalities within the myofibrils, sometimes with accumulation of aberrant proteins (inclusions). EMG may confirm the presence of a myopathy. There is no dystrophic process visible on histopathological examination and CK is most often normal.

The group contains several different disorders with different types of inclusions. Making a definite diagnosis can be challenging as the different disorders have overlapping phenotypes.

Myotubular myopathy is a serious X-linked form of centronuclear myopathy, caused by mutations in the MTM1 gene. There is a history of polyhydramnios and decreased fetal movements. Affected males display pronounced weakness and hypotonia requiring respiratory support. Facial weakness and ophthalmoplegia are common as is cryptorchidism. Fingers and toes are long, and length and head circumference may be above the 90th centile. Of the most seriously affected, almost 40% die within the first year and most survivors are respirator dependent around the clock.

Congenital muscular dystrophies

This is also a heterogeneous group where the children often are symptomatic at birth, with severe weakness and hypotonia. Depending on the subtype, there may be cardiac, CNS, eye, and connective tissue involvement. There is variable involvement of respiratory and bulbar muscles. CK is typically elevated and the muscle biopsy is most often consistent with a dystrophic process. The course is often relatively static with regards to muscle strength.

Classification is based on the clinical picture, biochemical testing, and genetic finding. As with congenital myopathies, there is considerable overlap between phenotypes. Inheritance is usually AR, with, at present, 32 known disease genes. The relative incidence of different types varies in different populations.

Transient neonatal myasthenia

This disorder occurs in 12% of infants whose mothers have autoimmune myasthenia gravis. The cause is a passive placental transfer of antibodies to the fetus. Affected neonates present in the first few days with generalized hypotonia, a weak cry, and feeding difficulties. Fatigable weakness is typical.

Neurophysiological studies are pathological and affected neonates are often positive for autoantibodies. Children of myaesthenic mothers should be observed in hospital for at least 7 days. Recovery is complete, most often within the first month. A small subset of infants with transient neonatal myasthenia may require treatment with acetylcholinesterase (AChE) inhibitors.

Congenital myasthenic syndromes (CMS)

This is a group of disorders resulting from failure in neuromuscular signal transmission. Unlike transient neonatal myasthenia, CMS are genetic disorders and testing for autoantibodies is negative. Except for slow-channel syndrome, heredity is AR.

CMS are caused by mutations in genes important for (1) acetylcholine (ACh) production, (2) production of the enzyme AChE, and (3) making of the acetylcholine receptor (AChR). The resulting impairment in neuromuscular transmission is presynaptic in 10%, synaptic in 15%, and postsynaptic in 75%. The onset may be prenatal, neonatal, or infantile. In the neonate, respiratory failure, feeding difficulties, ptosis, and a weak cry are common. Symptom fluctuation is typical as is fatigability. CK is normal. Decrement is seen on repetitive nerve stimulation.

Treatment is symptomatic and it needs to be tailored to the exact type. Immunosuppressive therapy is ineffective. AChE inhibitors are effective in the majority but may worsen symptoms in slow-channel syndrome. Other possible therapies include 3,4-diaminopyridine, ephedrine, fluoxetine, and quinidine.

Infant botulism

This is a condition caused by a neurotoxin produced by the bacterium Clostridium botulinum, a spore-forming bacterium whose spores may be found in soil and certain foods (e.g. honey). The spores are resilient but are usually destroyed in heat-sterilized and canned products. The neurotoxin itself is heat-sensitive and does not survive boiling.

Transmission of spores is oral. They germinate into bacteria that colonize the gut where they produce the neurotoxin, which then prevents the release of ACh. 95% of cases occur in children between 3 weeks and 6 months of age, often coinciding with the introduction of regular foods. The clinical picture is myasthenia-like, and the spectrum varies from a relatively mild to fulminant fatal disease. There is usually a period of 1 to 4 days with lethargy, feeding difficulties, and constipation, followed by deterioration with loss of head control, symmetrical weakness, and facial weakness. Eye contact is normal. Deep tendon reflexes are initially normal, but later reduced. Finally, paralysis and respiratory failure ensues. Clinical suspicion is supported by history of introduction of honey into the diet, neurophysiological studies and confirmed aetiologically through detection of C botulinum in faeces or food, or by demonstrating the presence of toxin in blood, faeces, or food.

Treatment consists of rapid administration of an antitoxin, which shortens the disease course. Treatment is otherwise symptomatic, and recovery takes approximately 3 weeks. Antibiotics are not recommended.

Hereditary motor and sensory neuropathies (HMSNs)

This is a large and heterogeneous group of disorders seldom affecting infants and extremely rarely neonates. The genetics are complex with a large number of known disease genes and a number or inheritance patterns. The distribution of weakness is for distal muscles to be more affected than proximal muscles, in contrast to all the aforementioned conditions. Congenital hypomyelinating neuropathy is an extremely severe type with prenatal onset. Manifestations are severe generalized hypotonia, weakness, and areflexia. Respiratory and swallowing difficulties are common, as is congenital arthrogryposis. Nerve conduction velocities are extremely low or absent, affecting both motor and sensory fibers. Dejerine–Sottas disease (HMSN type III or CMT3) is a similar but distinct disorder with overlapping phenotype, which may manifest in an infant with hypotonia, weakness, and delayed motor milestones.

REFERENCES

Hjartarson HT (2017) Floppy infant-syndrome. In: Jägervall M, Lundgren J, editors, *Barnneurologi*. Lund: Studentlitteratur AB, pp 277–289.

Resources

Bodensteiner JB (2008) The evaluation of the hypotonic infant. *Semin Pediatr Neurol* 15: 10–20.

Bonne G, Rivier F Genetable of neuromuscular disorders. An online gene table database concerning neuromuscular disorders. Updated regularly. User-friendly and linked to various other databases. Available from: http://www.musclegenetable.fr/(Accessed 8th November 2018)

Finkel RS, Mercuri E, Meyer OH et al. (2017). Diagnosis and management of spinal muscular atrophy: Part 2: Pulmonary and acute care; medications, supplements and immunizations; other organ systems; and ethics. *Neuromuscul Disord* 28: 197-207

Hahn A, Schanzer A. (2019). Long-term outcome and unmet needs in infantile-onset Pompe disease. *Ann Transl Med*, 7: 283.

Igarashi M (2004) Floppy infant syndrome. *J Clin Neuromuscul Dis* 6: 69–90.

Laugel V, Cossée M, Matis J, et al. (2008) Diagnostic approach to neonatal hypotonia: retrospective study on 144 neonates. *Eur J Pediatr* 167: 517–23.

Mercuri E, Finkel RS, Muntoni F, et al. (2017) Diagnosis and management of spinal muscular atrophy: Part 1: Recommendations for diagnosis, rehabilitation, orthopedic and nutritional care. *Neuromuscul Disord* 28: 103-115

Nimmo GA, Cohn RD (2018) The Floppy Infant. In: Swaiman KF, Ashwal S, Ferriero DM, et al. (eds) *Swaiman's Pediatric Neurology*. Edinburgh: Elsevier, pp e2351–2364.

Peredo DE, Hannibal MC (2009) The floppy infant: evaluation of hypotonia. *Pediatr Rev* 3: e66–76.

Prasad AN, Prasad C (2011) Genetic evaluation of the floppy infant. *Semin Fetal Neonatal Med* 16: 99–108.

Schorling DC, Kirschner J, Bönnemann CG (2017) Congenital Muscular Dystrophies and Myopathies: An Overview and Update. *Neuropediatrics* 48: 247–261.

CHAPTER 25

Infant sleep and behaviour

Outi Saarenpää-Heikkilä, E Juulia Paavonen, and Kaija Puura

Key messages

- Parental concern about an infant's sleep is very common.
- Fragmented sleep is usually normal during infancy.
- Sleep disturbances during infancy are very common though mostly benign.
- Behavioural sleep interventions should be used to treat sleep disturbances.
- Breathing difficulties during sleep in infancy are the most serious sleep disorder in infancy.

Common errors

- Not knowing the dynamic process of sleep development in infancy.
- Trying to treat normative sleep behaviours in infancy.
- Not recommending behavioural treatments for an infant's insomnia.
- Ignoring breathing problems during sleep.

When to worry

- Parental report of continuous snoring, mouth breathing, and breathing difficulties in sleep.
- Frequent (>2 times per night) night awakenings after 8 months of age.
- Restlessness and otherwise unexplained daytime irritability (sleep debt?).
- Approaching half of total sleep occurring in daytime after 3 to 4 months of age.
- Co-occurring problems with two or three of: sleep, feeding, and excessive crying — especially if parent–child interaction is also problematic.

TEMPERAMENT

There are differences among infants in how well or poorly they can regulate their emotions and behaviour which we tend to describe as different temperament types (fussy, adaptable, slow to warm up), but they are not disorders or even problems in themselves.

SLEEP REGULATION

About 30% of infants suffer from single or multiple regulatory problems in their first year of life (Schmid et al. 2010), although prevalence rates vary depending on the definition and methodological approaches applied. Key symptoms include excessive crying, sleeping problems, and feeding problems, which may be challenging for the infant and the family.

The symptoms can occur separately or in any combination. Co-occurring feeding problems plus excessive crying, or feeding problems plus sleeping problems are reported in about 7% of infants born at term; excessive crying plus sleeping problems co-occur in only 2%; and co-occurrence of all three regulatory problems in a further 2% of infants (Martini et al. 2017).

Although regulatory problems constitute transient problems in many cases, they persist in some infants (Schmid et al. 2010; Winsper and Wolke 2014). There is also increasing evidence that infant regulatory problems are associated with increased childhood behaviour problems such as externalizing problems (i.e. attention-deficit/hyperactivity disorder, oppositional defiant disorder, and conduct disorder; Hemmi, Wolke, and Schneider, 2011). The co-occurrence of more than one regulatory problem has greater predictive power for longer-term problems than a single regulatory problem occurring in isolation (Wake et al. 2006; Hemmi, Wolke, and Schneider, 2011).

RISK FACTORS

Regulatory problems in infancy may arise

- as a consequence of neurodevelopmental vulnerabilities of the infant and/or of problems in parent—infant interaction;

- in infants born very preterm (<32 weeks' gestation) who are at risk of disruptions in brainstem development upon which regulatory functions are dependent. The early signs of this disturbance include excessive crying and difficulties with sleeping and feeding. The early effects of prematurity on brain development may thus manifest themselves as comorbid regulatory problems (Bilgin and Wolke, 2017);

- if there is a dysfunctional parent—infant interaction pattern, which can lead to, aggravate, or maintain early regulatory problems (Laucht, Esser, and Schmidt, 2002). Risk factors include anxiety difficulties or depression in the parent and parental personal experience (Field et al. 2007; van der Wal, van Eijsden, Bonsel, 2007; Petzoldt at al. 2016; Martini et al. 2017);

- as a result of maternal depression which has been associated with infant sleeping problems. This may be due to shared genetic factors as well as dysfunctional parent—infant interaction (Field et al. 2007; Martini et al. 2017) although other researchers found no significant relation between the quality of parenting and infant regulatory problems (Dale et al. 2011).

MANAGEMENT

Parents of infants with regulatory problems should be offered

- information on the nature of the problems, which includes explaining the probable neurodevelopmental vulnerability and exploring whether the parents feel anxiety or lowered mood in their parental role. Clinicians should reassure parents that regulatory problems might occur despite nurturing parenting;

- careful monitoring of crying, sleeping, and feeding behaviours of infants who were born preterm. Interventions should be considered in those infants with comorbid regulatory problems (Douglas and Hill 2013); and

- intervention and support when infant problems seem to be associated with problematic parent—infant interaction. If the parent or parents are suffering from anxiety or depression, adequate care for their own condition may be also be needed.

THE DEVELOPMENT OF INFANT SLEEP

Sleep structure is described according to electrophysiological changes in the brain (measured by electroencephalogram [EEG]), cardiorespiratory and muscle functions, and temperature regulation (Olini and Huber, 2014; Bathory and Tomopoulos, 2017).

There are five different stages of sleep that are differentiated using EEG. In the mature brain, each sleep cycle moves out of wakefulness (W) into light sleep (N1, N2) followed by deep sleep (N3) with rapid eye movement (REM) sleep (R) occurring at the end of the cycle. Arousals and awakenings usually occur between the cycles. One sleep cycle is circa 50 to 60 minutes in infancy but within a few years it reaches 90 minutes, which is typical for older children and adults. Nocturnal sleep consists of several sleep cycles, in an adult usually five to six cycles.

Different stages of sleep are typified by changes in heart rate, respiratory rate, and muscle tone. Heart rate and respiration slow down while falling asleep, being slowest during deep sleep. In REM sleep, they accelerate again becoming irregular resembling the function while awake. Muscle atonia is also a typical feature of REM sleep. For this reason, no motor movement is seen during this sleep phase. This atonia affects the auxiliary respiratory muscles during REM sleep and breathing is, therefore, especially prone to disturbances in this sleep phase. The extraocular muscles and diaphragm are, however, not atonic and continue to function.

During the neonatal period these phases are still immature and cannot be differentiated. However, it is possible to use EEG to define quiet sleep – which is considered to be the precursor of deep sleep; active sleep – which is the precursor of REM sleep and intermediate sleep – which is characterized by features typical of both quiet and active sleep. Intermediate sleep disappears during the first 6 months of life as sleep neurophysiology matures.

There are many differences in the infant sleep EEG compared to the mature sleep EEG. First, the brain waves are more disorganized and wavelengths are slower than in more mature brains. Second, a period of infant sleep may begin with REM sleep, which is pathological later in life. Third, the distribution of sleep phases is different in infants to that in older children and adults. In infants, more than half of total sleep consists of REM sleep, but its percentage decreases rapidly during the first year of life being only 20% in toddlerhood and later in life. Accordingly, the percentage of deep sleep increases gradually reaching 30% by toddlerhood with further decreases to around 20% in adolescence.

Body temperature and the secretion of melatonin and cortisol display circadian variation that is evident from the age of 1 to 2 months. Melatonin is secreted from the pineal gland at the beginning of nighttime, stimulated by a fall in light, and levels fall at dawn. It has no cyclical secretion until 3 months of age (Mirmiran, Maas, and Ariagno, 2003). Cortisol secretion increases during sleep, reaching the peak value in the morning. It is not dependent on the sleep–wake cycle but dark-light circadian variation. Its secretion also matures during the first months. The maturation of temperature regulation (with a decrease in core body temperature after falling asleep) has a similar timetable, although it is possible to accelerate the process by enhancing the natural light and dark variation in the infant's environment.

The neonate has no day-to-night rhythmicity in sleep: the sleep and wake periods are distributed randomly throughout the 24 hours. With the maturation of circadian rhythms, the longest sleep periods start to occur during the nighttime in many infants as early as 5 weeks of age, but at the latest at the age of 3 months. One core feature in the maturation process is the rising percentage of nighttime sleep while daytime sleep shortens, particularly after 6 months of age. By the end of the first year, the majority of total sleep appears at night. Usually infants have one to two naps during the day until the age of 2 years after which children have one nap until the age of 3 to 4 years, some even until 6 to 7 years. However, if the child is sleeping too much during the daytime, the quality or duration of nighttime sleep can worsen.

Several developmental features make infants prone to night awakenings. First, immaturity in the sleep structure predisposes infants to night awakenings because the arousal threshold is lower during REM sleep than during deep sleep. Moreover, shorter sleep cycles typical of infancy cause sleep to lighten more frequently. The immaturity of the circadian rhythm also affects the continuity of sleep; sleep periods at night are relatively short even though the total amount of sleep is high.

Sleep requirements during 24 hours average 16 hours in neonates and 12 to 14 hours at the age of 1 year, but it is important to know that the variation of this in typically developing infants is extremely large (Galland et al. 2012). The best way to estimate the sufficiency of sleep is to assess infant's behaviour during the daytime, because lack of sleep is related to daytime symptoms, such as irritability, restlessness, or tiredness. Conversely, if the child seems to be in good health during the daytime, sleep deprivation is unlikely.

EVALUATION OF INFANT SLEEP

Because of the immaturity of sleep development during the first 3 months of life not much regularity can be expected in this early period. Parents who are worried about sleep at this age need to be given advice and information about normative sleep—wake development and practices that are beneficial in the long run, such as encouraging regular daytime rhythms, providing appropriate lighting conditions (reduced evening light), and regular bedtime routines. Beyond the age of 6 months, sleeping problems need to be evaluated systematically. The first objective of the evaluation is to decide whether or not there is a deviation from normative development. Sometimes the parents are worried about sleep phenomena that are normal for infants (such as frequent night awakenings). Even when there are no sleep disturbances, it is valuable to support the parents and to give them advice and preventive sleep education on how to help the infant improve his/her sleep quality.

To evaluate infant's sleep problems first evaluate the quality and the quantity of achieved sleep via parent interviews and completed sleep questionnaires.

- Parents should be given a sleep diary to follow the infant's sleep prospectively. It is a useful tool to gather information about sleep duration and quality, as well as the sleep—wake rhythm (Figure 25.1).

- The actual sleep quantity and the sleep—wake rhythm are then evaluated from the sleep diary. The average sleep duration is calculated and its range is documented and compared to the reference values for the age group. The achieved sleep duration should not fluctuate by more than 2 hours from day to day.

Next, the infant's sleep—wake rhythm is evaluated.

- At about the age of 3 to 4 months infants' circadian rhythms have started to mature towards a regular sleep—wake rhythm.

- Appropriate sleep—wake rhythm is quite stable after 4 to 6 months of age and daytime sleep starts to decrease so that the percentage decreases from about 50% at birth to around 25% at the age of 8 months and 15% at the age of 24 months. However, individual differences are quite large.

Finally, sleep disorders are assessed by interviewing the parents on the following:

- An evaluation of bedtime routines in the family, parental behaviours at bedtime, regularity of the sleep habits in the family.

- Sleeping environment and potential disturbing factors (such as excessive noise or lighting, insufficient space, inadequate or excessive temperature, insufficient food at night).

- Symptoms of sleep disordered breathing and somatic symptoms that may impair the infant's sleep quality (such as acute infections, eczema, allergies, gastro-oesophageal reflux, pain).

- Night awakenings, other sleep disorders, and daytime events should also be marked in the diary.

BEHAVIOURAL INSOMNIA OF CHILDHOOD

Difficulty with falling asleep and night awakenings are very common in infants. They are usually not indicative of sleep disturbances (i.e. deviation from typical development) because a few awakenings (1—2) are still quite common at the age of 1 to 2 years (Galland et al. 2012). If sleep onset difficulties or night awakenings are more severe than average, a diagnosis of behavioural insomnia of childhood should be considered. According to the International Classification of Sleep Disorders (ICSD), two subtypes of behavioural insomnia in childhood have been defined: sleep-association type and limit-setting type (Vriend and Corkum, 2011).

SLEEP DISORDERS

Sleep disorders are classified according to the ICSD (Sateia, 2014). The main categories of sleep disorders in childhood in this classification are insomnia, circadian rhythm sleep wake disorders, sleep related breathing disorders, parasomnias, hypersomnolence (not seen in infants), and movement disorders (Table 25.1).

Instructions for completion

Symbols to add each day

1. Moments with
   – tiredness   ○
   – short nap   ●

2. Sleeping time also scheduled naps

3. Time of going to bed   ↓

4. Time of waking up   ↑

5. Short awakenings at night   ↕

6. Meal times   **S**

7. Column for 'Sleep quality' assessed on a scale of 1 to 10 (worst t best)

8. Column for 'Medication or other' with numbers ①, ②, ③, etc to indicate either medication use or additional clinical features.
   Description to be given underneath, as shown beneath two day excerpt.

Two day excerpt of a completed diary (normally one page per week)

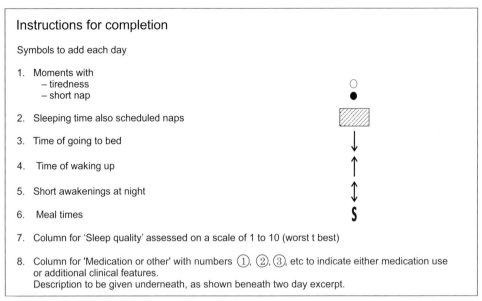

Additional symptoms, description
① Crying for an hour
② Flu symptoms disturbing sleep

Figure 25.1   Sleep diary. The example above indicates, on the date 17/4, asleep between 0.00–6.00 hrs and woke at 6.15. Tiredness between 9.30–10 hrs. Slept between 13.15–14.15 hrs and 16.30–17.30 hrs. Put to bed at 20.45 and fell asleep at 21.00. Several short awakenings through the night. Woke up on 18/4 at 5.15 and picked up at 6.15. Short nap between 6.45–7.05 hrs. Cried between 9–10 hrs. Slept between 14.00–16.00 hrs. Tiredness between 20.00–21.00 hrs and at 21.00 put to bed and fell asleep quickly. A short awakening at 22.10. The first night's sleep quality good (8pts) and the second night's bad (3pts). Flu on the second day. Meal times marked with S.

Sleep-association type insomnia

Sleep-association insomnia is a subtype of behavioural insomnia of childhood that results from negative sleep associations which lead to increased night awakenings (Vriend and Corkum, 2011). A sleep association is any factor that is related to the ability to fall asleep. Infants with negative sleep associations are unable to fall asleep without a certain practice or behaviour at bedtime. Typically, the infant is settled to sleep by the parents through behaviours such as breastfeeding. In older children, sleep-onset can be associated with the parent being present or falling asleep in the parents' bed. If the

Table 25.1 Main categories and subtypes of infant sleep disorders according to the International Classification of Sleep Disorders

Sleep disorder classification in infants	
Insomnia	Sleep association disorder
	Limit setting disorder
Circadian rhythm disorders	Advanced sleep—wake rhythm disorder
	Delayed sleep—wake rhythm disorder
	Irregular sleep—wake rhythm disorder
	Non-24-hours sleep—wake rhythm disorder
Breathing disorders	Central apnoea of prematurity/infancy
	Congenital central alveolar hypoventilation syndrome
	Obstructive sleep apnoea, paediatric
Parasomnias	Pavor nocturnus (night terrors)
Movement disorders	Sleep-related rhythmic movement disorder
	Benign myoclonus during sleep

infant is unable to self-soothe, the child will also need parental help at night to be able to fall asleep after night awakenings between the sleep cycles. In the worst case, the child may wake up after every sleep-cycle (i.e. every hour). Typically, infants with a sleep-association problem start to cry when they wake up at night and calm down very quickly when breastfeeding starts again. Some parents adopt all kinds of other habits intended to help the infant to fall asleep: rocking, tapping, or even travelling in the car have been used to get the infant to fall asleep. The diagnosis can be based on parental interview, as the parents typically report frequent night awakenings along with use of a specific bedtime habit to help the infant to fall asleep.

Some somatic diseases should be borne in mind as alternative causes for disturbance of the infant's sleep: circadian sleep—wake disorders, gastro-oesophageal reflux, food allergy, acute infections, ear infections, and sleep breathing disorders can all cause night awakenings and restless sleep. However, it is important to note that, in contrast to sleep association insomnia, somatic disease is not usually associated with ease in settling the infant back to sleep.

The key element in the behavioural treatment of sleep association disorder is to support the infant in learning to fall asleep on her/his own (Honaker and Meltzer, 2014). It is treated behaviourally by supporting the child gradually to learn new sleeping habits. Treatment should not be initiated until the infant is at least 5 to 6 months old as only at that age is the infant mature enough to learn new habits. The basic principle in treating this condition is to support the infant to learn little by little to fall asleep without parental interaction, while nevertheless avoiding excessive crying which increases the infant's arousal level and makes it more difficult for them to fall asleep. There are several different variations on the treatment of sleep association disorder, but they all aim to reduce interaction between the child and the parent when the child is falling asleep at bedtime. Learning to fall asleep independently is a basic developmental milestone and reflects improving self-regulation. It is usually acquired during the first year, although some infants need more support from the parents to be able to learn independent sleeping.

Limit-setting type

Another type of behavioural insomnia of childhood is defined by problems in limit-setting at bedtime (Vriend and Corkum, 2011). These children are reluctant to go to sleep at bedtime and they can use a variety of strategies to avoid bedtime. They have already learned how to express their will and resist going to bed, thus testing the limits parents try to set. This is typical for children aged 2 years or older.

The treatment of this condition is based on behavioural intervention to strengthen appropriate behaviours at bedtime. The intervention might comprise various elements such as regular routines, developing positive sleep associations, and implementing relaxation skills. Bedtime routines need to be clear, consistent, and positively supported: good behaviours are encouraged by positive feedback to the child while negative behaviours should be ignored. Protests can be repeatedly ignored (Honaker and Meltzer, 2014). Sometimes it is useful to temporarily delay the bedtime to make it easier for the child to fall asleep. When this delayed bedtime runs smoothly, the bedtime can be advanced gradually to the desired time (e.g. 15 minutes every 3 days).

Circadian rhythm disorders

There are several types of circadian rhythm disturbances that may occur after the age of 6 months. The infant's main sleep period may be delayed or advanced or sleep—wake rhythms can be irregular. Typically, sleep quality is relatively good in circadian rhythm disorders and there are no abnormal awakenings. Advanced rhythms can be treated by delaying the bedtime gradually when the time of rising in the morning is also delayed. Delayed rhythm is treated by keeping the time of rising early enough and taking care that the infant does not sleep too much during the daytime. Positive routines may also help to get the infant to go to bed in a happy mood making it gradually easier to advance the bedtime. In fact, delayed rhythm is often associated with behavioural insomnia of childhood. Bright light therapy is a very effective tool for treating circadian rhythm disorders. It is given in the early morning in delayed sleep phase disorder and in the early evening in advanced sleep phase disorder.

Children with autism are particularly prone to both insomnia and circadian rhythm disorders which may be challenging to treat behaviourally (Souders et al. 2009). Orally administered melatonin treatment at bedtime may help the infant to fall asleep or, in some cases, slow-release melatonin may also have an effect on early awakening (Schroder, Bataillard, and Bourgin, 2014). Circadian sleep disturbances are very common in intellectual impairment, especially in patients with Angelman or Smith-Magenis syndrome (De Leersnyder, 2013). The worst disturbance is irregular sleep—wake rhythm disorder which may be seen in autistic and severely intellectually impaired patients. In blind infants, non-24-hour sleep—wake rhythm disorder may be seen, with the rhythm gradually becoming increasingly delayed because the synchronizing effect of light on the brain is lacking. The treatment of these last two disorders is difficult: good sleep hygiene alone is not effective and medication is often also needed, melatonin being the most commonly used.

BREATHING DISORDERS

Central apnoea of prematurity/infancy

Infants born preterm are very prone to central apnoeas or periodic breathing due to immature function of respiratory centre in the brainstem (Sateia, 2014). In 0.5% to 2% of infants born at term, central apnoeas are still seen. If the apnoeas last more than 20 seconds or the infant has one or more oxygen desaturations, a decrease in heart rate, pallor, cyanosis, or floppiness, the problem requires hospital admission to determine whether it could be life-threatening. Apnoea may be diagnosed using either a sleep study with polysomnography or oxygen saturation monitoring with simultaneous respiratory recording. The American Academy of Sleep Medicine criteria for respiratory events in infants are helpful for the evaluation of apnoea in these infants (Berry et al. 2012). Gastro-oesophageal reflux and epilepsy are possible underlying aetiologies and should also be considered whenever evaluating infant apnoeas. Short apnoeas are also seen as a normal phenomenon during infant sleep but do not cause significant disturbance of gas exchange or heart rate (Evans et al. 2018). In severe cases of central apnoea, respiratory stimulants (caffeine, theophylline) are used as treatment for a few months. Maturation is usually reached by the age of 6 months and medication can be stopped.

Congenital central alveolar hypoventilation (CCH) syndrome

CCH (also called Ondine's curse) is a life-threatening disorder in respiratory regulation. The patient's respiration diminishes during deep sleep causing severe gas exchange problems. The disorder can be life-threatening and it causes, as a minimum, developmental harm and cor pulmonale if untreated. It is caused by mutation of the *PHOX2* gene. These infants may also have Hirschsprung disease, autonomic dysfunction, neural tumours, swallowing dysfunction, and ocular abnormalities. Ventilatory support is needed during sleep as a treatment; some patients may also need it during the daytime (Weese-Mayer et al. 2017).

Obstructive sleep apnoea and sleep disordered breathing (SDB)

Obstructive sleep disordered breathing is a relatively common disorder even as early as infancy (Kaditis et al. 2017). Snoring is the major symptom but sometimes only very strict breathing without any noise is seen. In sleep, respiration may seem to require more effort than normal and the patient may be a mouth breather with the neck hyperextended (i.e. the head thrown back). There may also be excessive sweating. During the daytime, the infant may be tired and irritable despite apparently sufficient sleep and may also be a mouth breather when awake. The causes of the disorder in infancy are predominantly craniofacial structure (e.g. midface hypoplasia, Crouzon syndrome, mandibular hypoplasia [Pierre Robin sequence], laryngomalacia, macroglossia – Down syndrome), abnormal tone (e.g. cerebral palsy), and respiratory infections. All these conditions are associated with a reduced diameter of the airways and, thus, compromised airflow. There is some evidence that breastfeeding protects against SDB (Ponce-Garcia et al. 2017).

When the infant's obstructive breathing disorder is in doubt, polysomnography is needed but is not available widely. Polysomnography includes recording of EEG, electrooculogram (EOG), chin electromyography (EMG), electrocardiogram, oxygen saturation, respiratory chest movement sensors, thermistor, nasal pressure cannula, and capnography (sometimes transcutaneous CO_2-recording). A microphone to record snoring and video are also used. Cardiorespiratory studies (excluding EEG, EOG, and EMG to stage sleep) are an acceptable alternative (Kaditis et al. 2017).

True apnoeas are quite rare in infants, but hypopneas and partial obstruction are more common. If respiratory gas exchange is disturbed and/or sleep structure is disturbed by arousals and awakenings due to obstruction, clinically relevant obstructive breathing disorder can be diagnosed. In fact, obstructive apnoea-hypopnoea index >1 (more than one obstructive apnoea or hypopnea per hour in polysomnography) is considered pathological in infants.

During infancy, adenoidectomy is the treatment of choice. Rarely, tonsillotomy (preferred to tonsillectomy during infancy because it is safer) may also be needed in more severe cases. When there are congenital facial or respiratory tract anomalies, ventilatory support is needed because the effect of surgery may be too slow to resolve the acute respiratory problem (Kaditis et al. 2017).

PARASOMNIAS

Parasomnias are behavioural phenomena during sleep, which usually do not disturb the children's sleep even though they may concern parents. The brain is not mature enough to produce these parasomnias during the first year and parasomnias are rare during the first two years of life. Only pavor nocturnus (sleep terrors) can manifest approximately from the age of 18 months. Pavor nocturnus occurs during the first half of the night, most often after the first sleep cycle. The infant suddenly sits up and starts to scream or cry loudly. He/she has tachycardia and tachypnoea and hyperhydrosis may also be apparent. The infant is not aware of the parents and parental calming is not effective. This usually lasts 5 to 15 minutes and often disappears as suddenly as it started.

The background of the phenomenon is that deep sleep does not lighten up evenly across the brain: the frontal zone of the brain is still in deep sleep while the motor area is 'awake'. Pavor nocturnus and the related phenomena of confusional arousal and sleep walking are called arousal parasomnias (Provini et al. 2011). Commonly, the child will have confusional arousals or sleepwalking later in childhood having had pavor nocturnus when younger. If the infant has a lot of pavor-like symptoms and if these occur during the second half of the night, the differential diagnoses of sleep association and, more rarely, epilepsy should be considered.

There are predisposing factors for arousal parasomnias: genetic factors, fever, sleep debt, other sleeping difficulties, and stress. In most cases no treatment is needed, at least during infancy. If the parasomnias occur very frequently and are prolonged, it is useful to reduce stress factors. In pavor nocturnus, avoidance of sleep debt and reduction of fever are important. Generally, parental reassurance is all that is required.

MOVEMENT DISORDERS

Sleep-related rhythmic movement disorder (SRMD)

SRMD (body rocking and/or head banging) in infancy has been reported to be observable at some point in almost half of all infants (Gwyther, Walters, and Hill, 2017), but a recent study using objective methods did not support this view, and found, on the contrary, that it affected only 0.34% to 2.78% of typically developing infants (Gogo et al. 2019). It disappears during toddlerhood but some cases may even continue into adulthood. Rocking side to side movement of the body and/or head and/or head banging targeted at the wall or the bedside are the main patterns of the disorder. Sometimes intense vocalization also occurs. The symptoms usually appear when the infant is falling asleep, sometimes also during light sleep. If the symptoms occur at every sleep–wake transition during the night, it may fragment infant's sleep and be very disturbing to the other family members. Injuries are rare, but occasionally dermal bruises and scarring, retinal detachment, and cataract and bone skull injury may occur. Differential diagnosis can rarely include epileptic seizures. Padding or a collar may be used to protect the skull. No drug treatment studies exist but the use of clonazepam and tricyclic antidepressants has been reported in single cases. Usually, SRMD is easy to diagnose based simply on the description provided by parents. Home videos recorded on a mobile phone are also very informative. Sometimes a sleep study in hospital is needed if the symptoms are very severe. Other varieties of sleep movement disorders (bruxism, periodic leg movement disorder, restless legs) are not usually seen or diagnosed in infancy.

Benign myoclonus during sleep

During the first months of life, the infant can have myoclonic twitches during sleep which disappear immediately when the infant wakes up. The phenomenon is totally benign and has nothing to do with epilepsy. No epileptic activity is seen during EEG recorded during the episode. It disappears with maturation, usually by age 6 months.

REFERENCES

Bathory E, Tomopoulos S (2017) Sleep regulation, physiology, and development, sleep duration and patterns, and sleep hygiene in infants, toddlers and pre-school age children. *Curr Probl Pediatr Adolesc Health Care* 47: 29—42.

Berry RB, Budhiraja R, Gottlieb DJ, et al. (2012) Rules for scoring respiratory events in sleep: update of the 2007 AASM Manual for the Scoring of Sleep and Associated Events. Deliberations of the Sleep Apnea Definitions Task Force of the American Academy of Sleep Medicine. *J Clin Sleep Med* 8: 597—619.

Bilgin A, Wolke D (2017) Development of comorbid crying, sleeping, feeding problems across infancy: Neurodevelopmental vulnerability and parenting. *Early Hum Dev* 109: 37—43.

Dale LP, O'Hara EA, Keen J, Porges SW (2011) Infant regulatory disorders: Temperamental, physiological, and behavioural features. *J Dev Behav Pediatr* 32: 216—224.

De Leersnyder H (2013) Smith-Magenis syndrome. *Handb Clin Neurol* 111: 295—296.

Douglas PS, Hill PS (2013) Behavioural sleep interventions in the first six months of life do not improve outcomes for mothers or infants: a systematic review. *J Dev Behav Pediatr* 34: 497—507.

Evans HJ, Karunatilleke AS, Grantham-Hill S, Gavlak JC (2018) A cohort study reporting normal oximetry values in healthy infants under 4 months of age using Masimo technology. *Arch Dis Child* 103: 868—872.

Field T, Diego M, Hernandez-Reif M, Figueiredo B, Schanberg S, Kuhn C (2007) Sleep disturbances in depressed pregnant women and their newborns. *Infant Behav Dev* 30: 127—133.

Galland B, Taylor B, Elder D, Herbison P (2012) Normal sleep patterns in infants and children: a systematic review of observational studies. *Sleep Med Rev* 16: 213—222.

Gogo E, van Sluijs RM, Cheung T, et al. (2019) Objectively confirmed prevalence of sleep-related rhythmic movement disorder in pre-school children. *Sleep Med* 53: 16—21.

Gwyther A, Walters A, Hill CM (2017) Rhythmic movement disorder in childhood: an integrative review. *Sleep Med Rev* 35: 62—75.

Honaker SM, Meltzer LJ (2014) Bedtime problems and night wakings in young children: an update of the evidence. *Ped Resp Rev* 15: 333—339.

Kaditis AG, Alonso Alvarez ML, Boudewyns A, et al. (2017) ERS statement on obstructive sleep disordered breathing in 1- to 23-month-old children. *Eur Respir J* 50: 1700985.

Hemmi MH, Wolke D, Schneider S (2011) Associations between problems with crying, sleeping and/or feeding in infancy and long-term behavioural outcomes in childhood: a meta-analysis. *Arch Dis Child* 96: 622—629.

Laucht M, Esser G, Schmidt MH (2002) Vulnerability and resilience in the development of children at risk: The role of early mother—child interaction. *Revista de Psiquiatria Clínica* 29: 20—27.

Martini J, Petzoldt J, Knappe S, Garthus-Niegel S, Asselmann E, Wittchen HU (2017) Infant, maternal, and familial predictors and correlates of regulatory problems in early infancy: The differential role of infant temperament and maternal anxiety and depression. *Early Hum Dev* 115: 23—31.

Mirmiran M, Maas YG, Ariagno RL (2003) Development of fetal and neonatal sleep and circadian rhythms. *Sleep Med Rev* 7: 321—334.

Olini N, Huber R (2014) Ageing and sleep: sleep in all stages of human development. In: Bassetti C, Đogaš Z, Peigneux P, eds, *Sleep Medicine Textbook* 1st edn. Regensburg, Germany: ESRS, pp 73—82.

Petzoldt J, Wittchen H-U, Einsle F, Martini J (2016) Maternal anxiety versus depressive disorders: specific relations to infants' crying, feeding and sleeping problems. *Child Care Health Dev* 42: 231—245.

Ponce-Garcia C, Hernandez IA, Major P, Flores-Mir C (2017) Association between breast feeding and paediatric sleep disordered breathing: a systematic review. *Paediatr Perinat Epidemiol* 231: 348—362.

Provini F, Tinuper P, Bisulli F, Lugaresi E (2011) Arousal disorders. *Sleep Med* 12: S22—S26.

Sateia M, ed (2014) *International Classification of Sleep Disorders*, 3rd edn. Darien, IL: American Association of Sleep Medicine.

Schroder C, Bataillard M, Bourgin P (2014) Circadian rhythm sleep disorders / Comorbidities and special population /autism spectrum disorder. In: Bassetti C, Đogaš Z, Peigneux P, eds, *Sleep Medicine Textbook*, 1st edn. Regensburg, Germany: ESRS, pp 348—350.

Souders M, Mason T, Valladares O, et al. (2009) Sleep behaviors and sleep quality in children with autism spectrum disorders. *Sleep* 32: 1566—1578.

Schmid G, Schreier A, Meyer R, Wolke D (2010) A prospective study on the persistence of infant crying, sleeping and feeding problems and preschool behaviour. *Acta Paediatr* 99: 286—290.

van der Wal MF, van Eijsden M, Bonsel GJ (2007) Stress and emotional problems during pregnancy and excessive infant crying. *J Dev Behav Pediatrics* 28: 431—437.

Vriend J, Corkum P (2011) Clinical management of behavioral insomnia of childhood. *Psychol Res Behav Manag* 4: 69—79.

Wake M, Morton-Allen E, Poulakis Z, Hiscock H, Gallagher S, Oberklaid F (2006) Prevalence, stability, and outcomes of cry-fuss and sleep problems in the first 2 years of life: prospective community-based study.*Pediatrics* 117: 836—842.

Weese-Mayer D, Rand C, Zhou A, Carroll M, Hunt C (2017) Congenital central hypoventilation syndrome: a bedside-to-bench success story for advancing early diagnosis and treatment and improved survival and quality of life. *Pediatric Res* 81: 192—201.

Winsper C, Wolke D (2014) Infant and toddler crying, sleeping and feeding problems and trajectories of dysregulated behaviour across childhood. *J Abnorm Child Psychol* 42: 831—843.

CHAPTER 26

Early developmental impairment and neurological abnormalities at birth

Richard W Newton, Ilona Autti-Rämö, and Audrone Prasauskiene

Key messages

- The first consultation with parents to discuss significant neurodevelopmental impairment in their infant child is a major life event for them: see them together, if possible, and choose your words with care.
- Negative attitudes and exclusion by society are major contributors to disability and inability to participate in everyday life and social activities.
- All children need love, opportunity, setting of limits regarding what constitutes acceptable behaviour, and encouragement.
- There is no safety limit for drinking during pregnancy. Binge drinking should be avoided if becoming pregnant is possible. Maternal biomarkers may aid diagnosis.
- Alcohol consumption during pregnancy can lead to a large variety of adverse outcomes ranging from a severely malformed infant with typical facial features to a child with a normal phenotype but a specific learning disorder.
- Open spinal defects in myelomeningocele should be closed within 24 hours of birth.
- Progressive hydrocephalus must be treated by ventriculoperitoneal shunting, not by prescribing acetazolamide (Diacarb) or any other diuretics.

Common errors

- Failing to recognize that most children with early developmental impairment do have a long-term future with positive aspects.
- Failing to consider alcohol exposure as an aetiological factor and thus failure to recognize fetal alcohol spectrum disorder.
- Not performing spinal X-ray or magnetic resonance imaging to define the level of the lesion in spina bifida (very important for management and prognosis).
- Not initiating clean intermittent catheterization in spina bifida.

Common myths

- *Early assessment or imaging accurately predicts future development*
  For many children a diagnostic label is associated with a wide range of potential. The passing of time allows a more accurate assessment of potential to emerge. The best indication of how a child will make progress in future is how they are making progress at present, rather than what imaging shows. Ultimately, many young people with a developmental impairment may achieve some degree of independence as adults if given the right opportunity and encouragement.
- *Intensive intervention alters outcome*
  Instead emphasize love, opportunity, and encouragement (which all children need to reach their potential). Concentrate on treating the treatable (see above), help parents to identify realistic goals and what activities to include in their play with the child to encourage the next developmental step.
- *Brain stimulants/megavitamins/sicca-cell injections/stem cells alter outcome*
  There is no evidence base for any of these (see also Chapter 13) but there are cases of reported harm being done to children treated with them

When to worry

- In general, when there is a deterioration in development.
- In fetal alcohol syndrome, when alcohol consumption within the family is not moderated, there is risk of maltreatment and neglect of the child.
- In myelomeningocele, when irritability or sleepiness, bulging or pulsing fontanelle, vomiting, or poor feeding is observed.

> **Box 26.1** Terminology derived from the International Classification of Functioning, Disability and Health: Child and Youth Version
>
> In the context of health:
>
> ☑ Bodily functions are the physiological functions of body systems (including psychological functions).
>
> ☑ Body structures are anatomical parts of the body such as organs, limbs, and their components.
>
> ☑ Impairments are deviations from the norm or loss of body function or structure.
>
> ☑ Activity is the execution of a task or action by an individual.
>
> ☑ Participation is involvement in a life situation.
>
> ☑ Activity limitations are difficulties an individual may have in executing activities.
>
> ☑ Participation restrictions are problems an individual may experience in involvement in life situations.
>
> ☑ Environmental factors make up the physical, social, and attitudinal environment in which people live and conduct their lives.
>
> (WHO, 2007)

As indicated in Box 26.1, the International Classification of Functioning, Disability and Health: Child and Youth Version (ICF-CY) has two *parts*, each with two *components*.

Part 1. Functioning and Disability

a. Body functions and structures.

b. Activities and participation.

Part 2. Contextual Factors

c. Environmental factors.

d. Personal factors.

Each component can be expressed in both positive and negative terms.

DEFINITIONS

The terms disorder, impairment, disability, and disadvantage (handicap) have precise meanings that should be used in a consistent way by professionals. Between 1980, when the World Health Organization (WHO) first published an 'International Classification of Impairments, Disabilities, and Handicaps' (WHO, 1998), and the present time, the emphasis has shifted away from a purely medical view and towards a social model for disability. The ICF-CY (WHO, 2007; Box 26.1) provides a common language for those who help young people with body impairments which limit activity and compromise potential. It also provides concepts and terms which describe the functional daily living consequences of body impairments and activity limitations. It describes levels of functionality, identifies strengths and weaknesses, and encodes them. The tool is culturally adaptable, helping clinicians target interventions based on individual performance in each developmental domain, i.e. motor abilities, communication, cognition, social skills, emotional regulation/behavior, and self-care skills/adaptive functioning. The ICF-CY was merged with the ICF between 2012 and 2015 (https://www.who.int/classifications/icf/en/).

This social model allows an interdisciplinary perspective on disability that reflects the views of many professionals and, more importantly, the views of disabled people themselves. It proposes that barriers, negative attitudes, and exclusion by society (purposefully or inadvertently) are the things which define who is disabled within a particular society. It recognizes that many people with a physical or intellectual impairment may be disadvantaged in specific situations unless society takes steps to minimize these disadvantages. This model does not deny the existence of individual limitations or impairments but instead emphasizes that these should not be the cause of individuals being excluded. The disadvantage of a particular impairment is situationally specific and many people are disabled not by the impairment but rather by the lack of help the society in which they live (including their doctors) feels able to offer.

Thus, the extent to which a disorder, impairment, or disability imposes a disadvantage on an individual depends not only on its severity but also on:

- the attitudes and ambitions of the child and family,

- the financial resources of the family,

- secondary problems created by professionals, including doctors,

- the prejudices of the society in which the person lives,

- adaptations of the physical environment, and

- legislation in support of the disabled.

Nonfatal disabling conditions are among the main causes of children receiving intervention and interdisciplinary habilitation services. To maintain quality, such services need to use the ICF-CY 2007 terminology and framework that is shared by all professionals involved. Goals for intervention and rehabilitation have become less focused on body impairments and typical development (activity) and more focused on a child functioning within context (i.e. participation). This requires involvement of family members and other persons in a child's natural environment in deciding upon and implementing interventions. Traditionally, habilitation teams have carried out assessments, written reports, and filed them, and thus, the disabled person's world does not change. The ICF-CY encourages team members to contact other significant people in the young disabled person's life, to explain the nature of the condition, to take away fear, to answer questions, and to pave the way for greater inclusion. In this way the young person's world will change.

The term 'early developmental impairment' (Francoeur et al. 2010) should now replace 'global developmental delay'. The latter term is misleading to parents (it implies their child will 'catch up') and is often inaccurate as many children have difficulties in only a few areas of development and are not 'globally' affected.

The challenge for the clinician is:

- to understand the underlying biology (i.e. cause),

- to explain this to parents,

- to use it to generate a probability statement to predict future outcome,

- to establish, regardless of cause, the developmental strengths and limitations of the individual child, and

- to create, with the help of allied professionals (e.g. remedial therapists and teachers), family-focused love, opportunity, and encouragement to allow children to reach their potential and to enable participation.

EPIDEMIOLOGY

Definition and incidence of developmental impairment

Developmental impairment is defined as a developmental/intelligence quotient (DQ/IQ) of <70, a visual acuity of <6/60, a hearing loss of $\geq$90 decibels, or severe non-ambulant cerebral palsy. International classifications identify ranges of function based on standard scores of DQ/IQ.

Assessment is based not only on DQ/IQ scores, but also takes into consideration a young person's adaptive functioning so that attainment is not measured rigidly. For example, it must be acknowledged that a person with developmental cognitive impairment may function well socially or in certain work settings.

Most DQ/IQ standard scoring systems identify the bottom 2% of the population (i.e. more than 2 standard deviations from the mean) as being in the impaired group. In practical terms we should regard children as having early developmental impairment when they show significant limitations in two or more domains of development before the age of 5 years, in cases where those difficulties are not better explained by another developmental disorder (e.g. autism spectrum disorder, cerebral palsy).

CAUSES OF DEVELOPMENTAL IMPAIRMENT

- Genetic disorders.

- Acquired brain injury — pre-, peri-, or postnatal:

    o Infection.

    o Vascular disease (e.g. arterial ischaemic stroke).

    o Hypoxia-ischaemia.

    o Maternal drug abuse (e.g. alcohol).

- Social deprivation (e.g. poor diet or health care, or physical abuse).

RED FLAG FACTORS OF POTENTIAL CONCERN

Antenatal

- Poor growth.

- Oligo- or polyhydramnios.

- Reduced fetal movement.

- Breech or other malpresentation.

Neonatal

- Low Apgar scores, but quick response to resuscitation.

- Unusual appearance at birth:

    o Dysmorphism.

- Obvious congenital abnormalities:

    o Neural tube defects.

    o Synostosis (see Chapters 22 and 23).

o   Micro- and macrocephaly (see Chapters 22 and 23).

o   Limb defects.

Unusual neonatal behaviour

- Sleepiness.

- Failure to wake for feeds.

- Poor suck: often difficulty with breast, but not bottle, feeds.

- Poor cry.

- Irritability, presence of withdrawal symptoms.

Obvious neurological abnormalities

- Hypotonia – early developmental impairment is an important cause of floppy infant syndrome (see Chapter 24).

- Hypertonia.

- Unusual patterns of tone (e.g. increased extensor tone, arching).

- Unusual patterns of movement (e.g. jerky, dystonic).

- Seizures.

Later detection

- All the above.

- Poor visual function.

- Poor hearing function.

- Delay in achieving developmental milestones.

- Irritability, inconsolable when upset.

- Disturbed behaviour and/or social behavior.

- Obvious dysmorphism.

Additional points in the history:

- Family/genetic history?

- Consanguinity?

CLINICAL APPROACH

History

Seek more information on all the above points.

Examination

Use the clinical method (see Chapters 5 and 6).

Investigations

In blood, full blood count, chromosomal karyotype (if single chromosome abnormality is suspected, e.g. Down syndrome, otherwise array comparative genomic hybridization), amino acids, thyroid function tests, possibly lactate. In urine, mucopolysaccharides, organic acids. Additional investigations should be tailored to the specific clinical features. Some investigations will not be available in all centres.

Neonatal screening programmes (see Chapter 7)

Apart from screening for cystic fibrosis, sickle-cell disease, and thalassaemia, the UK programme includes screening for conditions associated with intellectual disability: hypothyroidism; phenylketonuria (PKU); medium-chain acyl-CoA dehydrogenase deficiency (MCADD); maple syrup urine disease (MSUD); isovaleric acidaemia (IVA); glutaric aciduria type 1 (GA1); homocystinuria; pyridoxine-unresponsive; hearing loss.

PRINCIPLES OF MANAGEMENT

What to tell the parents: giving the news of developmental impairment

Parents want news about diagnosis

- together,

- as soon as possible,

- sympathetically and in private, and

- with accuracy and honesty.

They also want

- help with how to pass on the news to family and friends, and

- to have the infant/child present.

Language to use and language to avoid is outlined below.

- Remember parents will take note of every word.

- Do not be too negative about future predictions if deterioration is not evident.

- Do not provide information or advice that you are not confident about. It is better to say that you or perhaps nobody knows an answer to a particular question than give false 'expert' opinions.

- Compare: 'I am very sorry, but I have some very bad news for you. Your child has Down syndrome' with 'I have some news you were not expecting. Your child has a condition known as Down syndrome. This may be something you have heard of but know little about. I shall do the best I can to explain something about it to you and then explain how we can help'.

- Do not be too positive.

- Present a balanced view on therapies.

- Parents may believe that remedial therapy may 'heal'. Rather, explain that therapy maximizes developmental potential and limits secondary complications.

- Warn them of the unproven, and at times harmful, effect of alternative therapies (see below).

Remember the following:

- Parents are going through a major life event in receiving advice about their infant. Consequently, they will recall little of this first consultation and may misunderstand some of what they do remember.

- Always try to see both parents together at important interviews.

- See if an advocate is available to attend with them (health visitor, social worker, ward nurse, or a friend they know well).

- See them again soon to answer any questions they may have.

- Help them understand their own feelings.

- Many parents show features of bereavement after the birth of a child with a developmental impairment. Tell them that the intensity of this grief will decrease with time.

- The family will learn to find a way to find happiness and joy, and to laugh again.

- Mothers and fathers may work through their grief at a different pace. Help them understand each other's feelings.

What to tell the parents: how to deal with uncertainty

- Uncertainty is stressful; parents want to know what the future holds for the child as soon as possible. However, this may not be possible. Tell them they will need to be brave and patient.

- A diagnostic label is no more than a probability statement; for example, the range of ability in Down syndrome is broad, from profound to borderline developmental impairment.

- It is not unusual to have to wait until the infant is 10 or more months old before a preliminary estimate of future developmental performance can be made, although this depends on the type and degree of impairment.

TREATMENT AND THERAPY

What to tell the parents: give them a plan

- What they can do and who can help.

- Disabled children need what all children need: love, opportunity, setting of limits regarding what constitutes acceptable behaviour, and encouragement.

- Encourage parents to have confidence as their child's main carers, teachers, and therapists.

- Remedial therapists/community workers will explain how to maximize learning opportunity by teaching positioning, postures, interactive play, and the provision of seating or toys.

- Therapists will assess and explain how parents can help and advise them on specific interventions.

- Encourage liaison between parents, carers, teachers, and out-of-school activity groups (e.g. scouts/guides, church groups, youth clubs, sports clubs, riding for the disabled) in order to help people see a child's real potential and create opportunity for participation.

Specific diagnoses

In the remainder of this chapter we will consider in turn epilepsy, neural tube defects, fetal alcohol spectrum disorders, Down syndrome, and finally other specific genetic syndromes. In the newborn period poor feeding, failure to wake for feeding, a weak cry, and ultimately failure to thrive are common. Delayed milestones then become more evident over the subsequent months. For each condition recognizable features, presentation and a guide to future health surveillance will be reviewed.

Remember that all these syndromes may present with a history of reduced fetal movement, malpresentation, or polyhydramnios.

The child with epilepsy

Manage as for all the epilepsies as follows:

- confirm it is an epilepsy (history, electroencephalography),

- identify/classify the epilepsy if possible,

- explain the biology to the family,

- teach first aid,

- use an antiepileptic drug, in most cases, if epilepsy is confirmed.

The child with a metabolic disorder

- Investigate and treat the treatable, for example, pyridoxine dependency, the biotin- or folinic acid-responsive disorders (see Chapter 15).

The child with a surgically treatable disorder

- Developmental disability should not be regarded as a contraindication to appropriate treatment (e.g. in neural tube defects: see below);

- hydrocephalus and spina bifida;

- recognized comorbidities; for example, cardiac defects in Down syndrome; tracheo-oesophageal fistulae; anal atresia.

NEURAL TUBE DEFECTS

Incidence

There is marked geographical variation: fetal incidence of neural tube defect is 17 per 10 000 pregnancies; live birth incidence is 5.7 to 6.7 per 10 000 live births. The difference in these figures is due to termination of pregnancy and deaths in utero, particularly in cases with severe defects.

Cause

Multifactorial

- *Genetic*: risk of recurrence for non-syndromic sibling of proband: from 3% to 5%; 0.7% with preconceptional folate supplementation.

  - Folate-dependent metabolic pathway gene polymorphisms (e.g. *PCMT1*, *MTHFR*, methionine synthase, and methionine synthase reductase).

  - Folate-independent pathways (lipomyelomeningoceles are folate-resistant).

  - Syndromes such as 22q11 microdeletion, X-linked, and autosomal dominant Mendelian disorders (e.g. Currarino triad: sacral, anal and urological anomalies).

- Folic acid deficit: dietary.

- Maternal factors: obesity, diabetes with hyperinsulinaemia, first-trimester fever, antiepileptic drugs: valproate, phenytoin, carbamazepine, polytherapy; retinoins.

Presentation

- *Antenatal*: combined test (ultrasound with maternal alpha-fetoprotein) gives 99% sensitivity (see under Down syndrome below).

- Fetal ultrasonography (18–20 weeks of pregnancy):

- Head:

  - concavity of the frontal bones (the 'lemon sign'); present in 50% from 16 to 24 weeks' gestation;

  - ventriculomegaly (moderate to severe), present in 70% from late second trimester and up to 90% by term;

- Chiari II malformation: from 16 weeks' gestation the 'banana sign' reflecting abnormal anterior cerebellum with obliteration of cisterna magna; very few false positives.

- Spine:

  - C- or U-shaped vertebrae in sagittal views.

There is raised maternal alpha-fetoprotein (AFP) at 16 to 20 weeks of pregnancy in 70% to 75% of cases of open spina bifida. If AFP is raised, acetylcholinesterase will be raised in amniotic fluid. Serial fetal ultrasound monitors growth and development.

Prenatal management

What to tell the parents: Unlike many conditions considered below, the presence and potential impact of this condition will be immediately obvious to the doctor. The immediate situation needs handling with skill. Parents need a calming and reassuring statement, such as 'We can see from the results that your baby has some underdevelopment of part of the backbone. We need to discuss this with some other specialists, perhaps do some more tests, and then we will be able to work out how best to help'. Following these steps an explanation of the management plan can follow. It is important for all staff concerned to be calm, positive, and reassuring. In due course they can be counselled on the immediate, medium-, and long-term care plan. Parents will, over time, need information on the primary and secondary complications of the condition (see below) and the recurrence risk for future children and prenatal diagnostics.

Fetal surgery: The Management of Myelomeningocele Study (MOMS) (Farmer et al. 2018) demonstrated that fetal surgery has acceptable maternal and fetal risks in experienced centres. The anesthetic and maternal requirements for successful fetal surgery demand careful attention to uterine tone in particular. In time, an endoscopic approach may prove equally successful.

Mode of delivery: When, as is usual, myelomeningocele is diagnosed antenatally, birth should be by Caesarean section. The paediatric team should be present at the delivery.

Management at birth

What to tell the parents

In this situation too, always be mindful of the parental need for information. Choose words carefully and be positive (see above, antenatal diagnosis, for the key information points).

Clinical and radiological assessment

May need to involve a neurosurgeon, a renal or urological specialist, and/or spinal orthopaedic surgeon. The lesion may be obvious or subtle. After birth, position the infant either on its side, or prone. In the routine examination of the back look for:

- an open lesion and its configuration,

- large midline lipoma, preventing positioning or care in the supine position,

- asymmetrical natal cleft,

- dermal sinus above the natal cleft (distinguish from benign sacral dimple in the coccygeal region),

- midline naevus, for example, hair patch (a subtle dermal sinus may also be present),

- kyphosis or scoliosis,

- talipes equinovarus (may be asymmetrical).

Any of these may be present, signifying an open or occult neural tube defect. Then, identify the level of the spinal lesion, the major determinant of morbidity:

- *Radiological level:* use X-ray or magnetic resonance imaging (MRI) of the spine; MRI has no known risks related to exposure to the magnetic fields and is preferable to computed tomography in infants, who are at higher risk than older children of long-term risks associated with exposure to radiation.

- *Neurological level:* often higher than the anatomical level and determines future disability. Assess muscle bulk, spontaneous antigravity movements, spinal reflexes, abnormal spread of reflexes, and sacral sensation (see Table 26.1).

Also note the following:

- Associated central nervous system (CNS) malformations.

- Measure head circumference serially.

- Bone or joint deformities; for example, congenital hip dislocation (20%), kyphosis, and talipes equinovarus. Refer to specialist orthopaedic team.

- Dermal sinus tract. Leads to risk of CNS infection. Often associated with underlying spinal malformation defined by ultrasound scan/MRI. Refer to neurosurgeon.

- Non-neurological anomalies (e.g. check anus, heart).

- Bowel dysfunction. Assess anal tone. Neurogenic constipation often present (also effects of concurrent anorectal anomalies).

- Bladder dysfunction: often incomplete bladder emptying against outflow resistance, leading to secondary reflux nephropathy. Check for a good urinary stream — measure urine output by weighing nappies — seek an urgent urology/nephrology opinion if poor.

Table 26.1 Clinical signs related to level of lesion

Site of lesion	Clinical view	Functional prognosis
Thoracic lesion	Innervation of the upper limb and neck musculature and variable function of trunk musculature are present with no volitional lower limb movements. Patients with thoracic malformations tend to have more involvement of the CNS and associated cognitive deficits. Sensation is disordered below hips.	Wheelchair is used for mobility from early childhood.
Upper lumbar lesion (L1—L2—L3)	Variable hip flexor and hip adductor strength is characteristic, some sensation below hip joint, and absence of hip extensors, hip abductors, and all knee and ankle movements are noted.	Long orthosis (knee-ankle-foot orthosis) and crutches for ambulation. For longer distances use a wheelchair.
Lower lumbar lesion (L4—L5)	Hip flexor, adductor, medial hamstring, and quadriceps strength is present; strength of the lateral hamstrings, hip abductors, and ankle dorsiflexors is variable; and strength of the ankle plantar flexors is absent. This means that voluntary knee flexion movements and foot dorsiflexion and eversion (turning outwards) movements are possible.	For independent walking usually needs ankle-foot orthosis and, in some cases, crutches or sticks. In later childhood, may use wheelchair for mobility.
Sacral lesion	The power in foot flexors and/or hip extensors (gluteus maximus) may be moderately reduced.	Usually walks independently. Sometimes may need foot orthosis.

Care of open lesions

Recommended presurgical care for open lesions:

- Cover wound with sterile gauze, wash daily with normal saline, change dressing when soiled; maintain a sterile, latex-free environment.

- Give ampicillin 200mg/kg/day in two divided doses, gentamycin 5mg/kg/day in two doses (monitoring drug levels to avoid oto- or nephro-toxicity) with or without cloxacillin 100mg/kg/day in two doses until wound is clean and dry. Antibiotic protocols may vary between regions.

- Treat for meningitis if fever and/or seizures and/or depressed conscious level.

The lesion should be closed as soon as possible and always within 24 hours. The surgical site should be inspected every day for any signs of infection and cerebrospinal fluid leak. Where there was a prenatal repair and the operative site is well-healed, no special medical care is needed acutely.

Longer-term sequelae

Part of longer-term sequelae goes beyond infancy and so is outside the scope of this handbook. Nevertheless, the information given here should be very helpful for planning long-term goals and a treatment/habilitation scheme.

The child needs to be monitored closely for the development of secondary complications. This is the role of the general paediatrician, involving community-based medical services (general practitioners or neurodevelopmental paediatricians) working alongside the habilitation team or specialist services (neurosurgery, orthopaedics, nephrology, or urology) as necessary.

- *Hydrocephalus:* occurs in 80% of myelomeningocele cases, often precipitated by surgical closure of the back lesion. It requires ventriculoperitoneal (VP) shunting, often with some urgency because of rapid progression. It is uncommon in other variants. Monitor head circumference weekly for the first month, then monthly; assess pressure symptoms, irritability or sleepiness, bulging or pulsing fontanelle, vomiting, poor feeding. Serial cranial ultrasound should be performed at 2 weeks and 6 weeks and 4 months.

- *Chiari type II malformation:* occurs in 80% to 100% of cases, and is the main cause of hydrocephalus. Symptoms relate to brainstem compression and lower cranial nerves dysfunction: dysphagia, repetitive vomiting, impaired suction, impaired gag reflex, dizziness, characteristic weak or squeaky cry, or stridor caused by vocal cord palsy, apnoeic episodes, nystagmus, bradycardic episodes, and repeated aspirations leading to pneumonia. Torticollis, opisthotonus, facial weakness, and motor disorders may occur (5–10%). They may become apparent only after lesion closure and may be associated with increasing ventriculomegaly.

- *Cord-tethering syndrome:* back pain, mixed upper and lower motor neuron signs, enlarging area of sensory disturbance and incontinence. Symptoms may start appearing at any age, especially during periods of rapid growth.

- *Syringomyelia:* caused by subarachnoid obstruction to cerebrospinal fluid flow (11–77%). Signs and symptoms are similar to those of Chiari type II malformation, tethered cord, or VP shunt malfunction. Syringomyelia and tethered cord are treated surgically.

- *Bladder and bowel dysfunction:* affects 97% of cases. The neurogenic bladder leads to overflow and urge incontinence, bladder dyssynergia, and vesicoureteral reflux with a risk of urinary tract infections, upper tract dilatation, and chronic renal insufficiency. Manage with continence advice, regular catheterizations, medication (pro- or anticholinergics), and surgical procedures (intravesical botulinum toxin injections; vesicostomy; bladder augmentation and bladder neck procedures).

  Regular renal/urology team follow-up should include:

  - renal function tests, blood pressure measurement, and urine culture 3-monthly;

  - pre- and post-micturition ultrasound scan of the urogenital tract 3- to 6-monthly, as a measure of residual urine;

  - antibiotic prophylaxis is indicated;

  - bladder catheterization is discussed;

  - examination for cryptorchidism with referral for surgical treatment if necessary;

  - assessment and treatment of bowel movement disorders;

  - management of bowel dysfunction; constipation with overflow soiling; faecal impaction may worsen urinary dysfunction. Managed with continence advice, diet, laxatives, and enemas. Refer to paediatric surgeons. Conduit procedures for anterograde colonic washouts may be required.

- *Orthopaedic problems:* kyphoscoliosis (20–40%) with secondary cardiorespiratory complications, hip dislocation, knee contractures, pathological fractures from bone demineralization, internal and external tibial torsion, foot deformities (clubfoot, equinovalgus, cavus, calcaneovarus, calcaneovalgus) are common.

Orthopaedic assessment is recommended for each of the above at 3 months, 6 months, and 12 months. Treatments include bracing, rigid orthoses, spasticity management, physiotherapy, and surgery.

- *Latex allergy:* the risk increases with age and is minimized by avoiding latex articles, educating parents, and using silicone or vinyl as a substitute. Up to 70% of affected children have latex allergy. Allergy symptoms include tearing of the eyes and runny nose, sneezing, wheeziness, skin rashes, urticaria, itching, or swelling at the site of contact; in severe cases there are respiratory disorders and, rarely, anaphylactic shock.

- *Trophic skin lesions:* poorly healing, pressure ulcers on pelvic ischia and feet in the area of sensory deficit. The risk is minimized by frequent inspection (by parents or the child) of at-risk areas; noting redness of 45 minutes duration or more; keeping skin clean and dry; wearing footwear inside and outside; care with choice of clothing and footwear; care with braces and orthoses; maintaining weight symmetry while lying or sitting in a wheelchair, with frequent position changes, nursing care to affected areas.

- *Growth disorders:* short stature seen in 50% to 60% of patients. Usually related to skeletal deformity and hypothalamic-pituitary dysfunction, which can predetermine premature puberty and lack of growth hormone. Shortage of growth hormone is diagnosed in 10% to 20% patients with myelomeningocele. Either inadequate nutrition or obesity may occur.

- *Tumours:* teratoma and benign dermoid cysts may present late with paraparesis.

- *Dental hygiene:* arrange dental care with advice to parents on diet, teeth-cleaning.

- *Seizure control:* seizures occur in 10% to 30% and are related to associated brain malformations or may be a sign of shunt malfunction or infection.

Note that deterioration of neurological status, rapid progression of a scoliosis, disparity between the myelomeningocele level and neurological level, emergence of asymmetry of neurological signs, and a suspicion of Chiari type II malformation, should each lead to an urgent MRI of the spinal cord/head with neurosurgical referral as appropriate.

Outlook

- *Ambulation:* lesion level predicts ambulatory ability. Cognitive, perceptual, and coordination impairments, spasticity and bone deformities may also limit activity. Ankle dorsiflexion (L5) strength predicts community ambulation: outdoors walking and independent transfers. Use ankle orthoses and foot care only. Knee extension (L3–L4) strength predicts household ambulation: standing for transfers, walking short distances with hip-knee-ankle-foot orthoses, rigid gait orthoses, and wheelchair for longer distances. Poor trunk stability and hip flexion (T6–L2) predicts impaired ambulation: therapeutic weight bearing with orthoses. Wheelchair indoors for mobility. Ambulation may deteriorate in later childhood.

- *Cognition:* the majority of children with myelomeningocele do not have overt developmental impairment. Mean IQ is lower than average, about 90. Performance IQ is typically below Verbal IQ. Recurrent VP shunt infections predict lower IQ. Monitor head circumference monthly; assess pressure symptoms, irritability or sleepiness, bulging or pulsing fontanelle, vomiting, poor feeding; serial cranial ultrasound at 2 weeks, 6 weeks, 13 weeks, and 5 months. Urgent referral is needed for VP shunt if hydrocephalus is confirmed.

- *Vision and hearing:* test as a routine, as for all children with a developmental impairment.

- *Psychosocial issues:* puberty and sex education, poor self-image, educational and occupational exclusion all may need to be addressed.

- *Mortality and morbidity:* increased risk of death in infancy with high spinal lesions, open lesions, and multiple malformations. Causes of increased mortality: decompensated hydrocephalus, VP shunt infection; renal failure; perioperative (particularly scoliosis surgery). Most children can expect to survive well into adulthood: 30% of adults continue to require daily additional help. Quality of life affected by sequelae and functional limitations rather than level of lesion per se.

Creating opportunity and encouragement for the child

This is best achieved by helping parents adjust to their child's condition. Remedial therapists will help minimize the disadvantages attendant on the child's impairment (it is important to emphasize that they do not 'put the problem right') by the provision of aids and advice to parents and teachers on how to create opportunities for improved function. Excellent communication between home, hospital, and school is required. All professionals involved should direct parents to information specific to their child's condition (associations, websites, etc.). A suggested approach to habilitation is given in Table 26.2.

Table 26.2   A suggested approach to habilitation in spina bifida and contributions from individual team members

	Issues concerned	Tests	Therapy
Physiotherapist	Muscle strength and range of joint movement of lower limbs, correct body posture, selection of compensatory aids, and orthoses	Assessment of muscle strength with the help of manual muscle testing. Assessment of range of motion in the joints of lower limbs with the help of goniometry. Assessment of senses with the help of ASIA sensory topographic scheme. Follow-up of skin status (trophic ulceration)	Passive movements and muscle strengthening of lower limbs, muscle stretching exercises, position, training of head control, trunk control, sitting balance. Advice to family on care of infant with myelomeningocele. Posture for routine activities. Selection and adaptation of aids (sitting chair, standing frame) and orthoses
Occupational therapist	Fine motor and self-care skills	Clinical follow-up (fine motor skills as infant moves or plays). Focus should be given to child's posture, coordination, transferring movements (e.g. from bed to chair). Use clinical observation, PEDI. Assess joint mobility, muscle function and strength, tone, and coordination.	Hand function and hand—eye coordination is encouraged through play. Special seating is adapted for feeding and playing. Special feeding aids are selected, if necessary
Speech and language therapist	Assess nonverbal and then verbal communication		Games and nursery rhymes which encourage the child to attribute meaning to signs (language) and the rhythms of speech; helped by Portage, a UK-based home-visiting early education service with equivalents in many European countries

Table 26.2 (continued)   A suggested approach to habilitation in spina bifida and contributions from individual team members

	Issues concerned	Tests	Therapy
Psychologist	Identifying developmental and educational strengths and weaknesses	Cognition Use age appropriate Wechsler, Leiter, KABC, or any other nationally adapted and validated test	Counselling parents, teachers and habilitation team members; helping adjustment to level of ability, setting realistic educational goals. Intervening to improve self-image and confidence
Social worker	Identifying social need according to ability		To share experiences of parents who have overcome any attendant difficulties; and provide information on the benefit system

ASIA, American Spinal Injury Association; KABC, Kaufman Assessment Battery for Children; PEDI, Pediatric Evaluation of Disability Inventory.

FETAL ALCOHOL SPECTRUM DISORDERS (FASD)

Marked geographical variation occurs in the prevalence of fetal alcohol spectrum disorders (FASD) within and between countries. Estimated worldwide prevalence is 9 in 1000 live births, but the latest study from the United States gives a conservative estimate of 1.1% to 5% among 7-year-old children, and a less conservative approach gives an estimate of 3% to 10%.

Alcohol is a teratogen. In early pregnancy, binge drinking (five or more units on one occasion) can lead to severe organ malformation or be lethal; and in later pregnancy it is especially detrimental to growth and CNS development. No universal safety limit (time, kind, or amount) has been identified. The longer the mother drinks the poorer the outcome; every day without alcohol benefits the child. There is biological variability (genetic, nutrition, socioeconomic) and each woman and fetus are different, but there is no way to foresee the limit for a harmful dose in individual cases. The evidence of harm is clearer the more the mother drinks per occasion and/or per week; binge drinking is especially detrimental. One unit is 330ml of beer, 120ml of wine, or 40ml of spirits (be aware that strengths vary), and the only safe advice is *do not drink when pregnant or planning pregnancy.*

A specific pattern of prenatal growth deficiency, developmental impairment, and craniofacial abnormality caused by prenatal alcohol exposure originally confined to fetal alcohol syndrome (FAS), is now viewed as a spectrum of disorders (FASD) including FAS, partial FAS, alcohol-related neurodevelopmental disorder, and alcohol-related birth defects (see Table 26.3).

Table 26.3 Clinically relevant features of the fetal alcohol spectrum disorder (FASD) subgroups

	Fetal alcohol syndrome (FAS)	Partial fetal alcohol syndrome (PFAS)	Alcohol-related neurobehavioral disorder (ARND)	Alcohol-related birth defect (ARBD)	Comments
Required features (vary between guidelines)	1, 2, 3	1 and 3b (depending on guideline)	3b	4	Phenotype identifies FAS and PFAS. ARND and ARBD need historical information
1. Facial features	Short palpebral fissure Smooth philtrum Thin upper lip	Short palpebral fissure Smooth philtrum Thin upper lip	No identifiable facial features of FAS	Required for IOM criteria	Either 2 or all 3 features must be fulfilled (varies by guideline)
2. Growth deficiency	Pre- and/or postnatal height or weight ≤10th centile for ethnicity	Pre- and/or postnatal height or weight ≤10th centile for ethnicity	Postnatal growth may fall short of genetic target		In FAS and PFAS, males remain thin into adulthood; females' weight often normalizes after puberty
3a. Brain structure (optional in some guidelines)	Any of microcephaly, structural abnormalities, epilepsy	May have microcephaly, structural abnormalities, epilepsy	Occasional structural abnormalities on MRI		OFC ≤3rd or 10th centile, varying by guideline. Head growth often slow in FAS

Table 26.3 (continued)   Clinically relevant features of the fetal alcohol spectrum disorder (FASD) subgroups

	FAS	PFAS	ARND	ARBD	Comments
3b. Brain function	Usually dysfunction in ≥3 domains of brain function, often also behavioral difficulties	Usually dysfunction in ≥3 domains of brain functions, often also behavioral difficulties	Typically therapy-resistant cognitive and behavioral difficulties		Function <−1.5 or −2SD, varying by guideline. Distinguish from behavioural difficulties secondary to adverse postnatal events
4. Organ malformations, hearing, and vision defects	Need to be screened	Need to be screened	Screening recommended especially if unplanned pregnancy and possibility of binge drinking in early pregnancy	Cardiac, skeletal, and renal malformations	Organ malformations are specific for the timing of binge drinking. All organs can be affected.
5. Alcohol exposure during pregnancy	Drinking every week and binge drinking	Usually ≥2 drinks/occasion. Also bingeing, especially in first trimester	Usually occasional binge-ing or social consumption (1–2 drinks)	Binge drinking in early pregnancy (e.g. unplanned)	Level of exposure and need for confirmation of this varies by guideline

Various existing guidelines differ in specific criteria. The proportion between the subgroups differs between countries. In western countries the proportion of FAS and PFAS together is 10% to 20% and ARND covers the rest. In South Africa the proportion of FAS and PFAS is much higher. IOM, Institute of Medicine; MRI, magnetic resonance imaging; OFC, occipitofrontal head circumference.

Diagnostic criteria for a diagnosis of FASD

Currently three sets of diagnostic criteria for FASD are mostly in use: the updated Institute of Medicine criteria (Hoyme et al. 2016), the 4-digit diagnostic code (Astley, 2004) and the Canadian guidelines criteria (Clarren, Lutke, and Sherbuck, 2011). The main differences between these diagnostic systems are (1) the required number of characteristic facial features, (2) the definition of central nervous dysfunction, and (3) the definition of the amount/level of prenatal alcohol exposure (Astley Hemingway et al. 2019).

Diagnosis may be difficult, especially if alcohol consumption is concealed. Prenatal alcohol exposure has traditionally been assessed by maternal self-reporting with questions directed at consumption before and during pregnancy and how it changed once pregnancy was confirmed (reliable answers requiring confidentiality and trust). The applicability of biomarkers as an adjunct to this is currently being assessed. These include fatty acid ethyl esters (FAEEs), and ethyl glucuronide (EtG) in meconium and phosphatidylethanol (Peth) in blood. It is likely that either in combination with self-reporting or independently they will prove to be more sensitive and specific for prenatal alcohol exposure.

Presentation

A high percentage of children with FASD do not carry characteristic dysmorphism. If FASD is suspected, screen heart and kidney for associated abnormalities and vision and hearing for impairment. Affected infants are at high risk of secondary developmental problems due to adverse life events (maltreatment, multiple placements, neglect of care) and delayed diagnosis or misdiagnosis.

Neonatal presentations: There may be microcephaly already at birth and the rate of post-natal head growth is often slower than normal. Feeding and weight-gain are often poor. The infant may be very irritable and tremulous, with a marked startle reflex, and require sedation. Further feeding problems and constipation may follow. Dysmorphism may include small palpebral fissures, smooth philtrum, and a thin upper lip (see http://depts.washington.edu/fasdpn/htmls/lip-philtrum-guides.htm). Some children exposed to binge drinking in early pregnancy have organ malformations, especially renal or cardiac abnormalities.

Long-term health surveillance: Later presentation is also common with developmental impairment, specific learning disorder, or behavioural difficulties first observed at pre-school/school age. Developmental and, in some cases, behavioural difficulties may not be evident in infancy but emerge through childhood.

DOWN SYNDROME

Incidence is about 1 in every 700 live births. Causes include trisomy 21, 21 translocation, or mosaicism.

Diagnostic

Prenatally by amniocentesis or chorionic villus biopsy following maternal AFP screen linked to maternal age. Recommendations from the Serum Urine and Ultrasound

Screening Study (SURUSS) and National Institute for Clinical Excellence (NICE) guidelines currently recommend the following:

- Combined test: nuchal translucency scanning plus serum measurement of free beta-human chorionic gonadotrophin (hCG) and pregnancy-associated plasma protein A (PAPP-A) should be offered to females at between 11 weeks and 13 weeks + 6 days of gestation.

- The quadruple test: this measures free beta-hCG, AFP, inhibin-A, and uE3 and is the best to offer for females presenting in the second trimester(see Table 7.1).

- New technology now allows cell-free fetal DNA to be analysed from 10 weeks' gestation onwards (>98% for 0.2% false positive rate; test failure rate is about 4%). To complement this analysis of the allelic ratios of polymorphisms present within the methylated promoter of a DNA sequence on chromosomes 13, 18, and 21 is also available. These modern tests allow maternal blood tests to replace the invasive chorionic villus biopsy and amniocentesis methods.

- Postnatally, through distinctive dysmorphism: microcephaly, brachycephaly, eyes slanting downward medially and narrow palpebral fissures, single palmar crease, wide space between great and second toe, small ears, macroglossia.

- Hypotonia: Down syndrome is an important cause of the floppy infant.

Issues for early infancy

Poor feeding and congenital heart disease are common; ideally screen with echocardiogram (usually atrioventricular canal defects); may need urgent treatment. Transient myeloproliferative disease; duodenal atresia, Hirschprung disease, severe respiratory syncytial virus bronchiolitis.

Long-term health surveillance issues

Long-term cardiovascular surveillance; atlanto-axial instability (usually after infancy). Intellectual disability. Hearing and vision problems are common, arrange screening. Screen for hypothyroidism.

Other common associations

Overexpression of more than 50 genes in the Down syndrome critical region on chromosome 21 along with epigenetic mechanisms lead to many disease susceptibilities. Clinicians should be aware of an enhanced risk of disordered autoimmunity: celiac disease; hypothyroidism, often associated with thyroiditis; inflammatory arthritis, diabetes; enhanced risk of acute myeloid leukaemia (more than 50-fold increased risk compared to the general population); testicular tumours; immunodeficiency, impaired cellular immunity predisposes to bacterial or fungal infections; dry skin may require oilatum emollient in the bath and moisturizing creams (later psoriasis and eczema is more common); and at end of a shortened life, Alzheimer disease. For management guidance and detail see Newton et al. (2015).

CONGENITAL HYPOTHYROIDISM

Incidence of severe deficiency is 1 in 4000 births. Worldwide iodine deficiency is the most common cause; elsewhere it is due to gland underdevelopment or genetically determined inborn error of thyroxine or triiodothyronine production). If untreated it leads to growth failure and intellectual disability. Thyroxine treatment is effective and inexpensive.

Prevention: effective neonatal screening programmes. Without screening less than 50% with severe deficiency are diagnosed.

Suspect: when there is excessive sleepiness, poor feeding, low muscle tone, a hoarse cry, constipation, prolonged physiological jaundice, and low body temperature. Occasionally, severe prenatal onset in athyreosis with large anterior fontanelle, persistent posterior fontanelle, umbilical hernia, and macroglossia occur.

SPECIFIC GENETIC SYNDROMES OTHER THAN DOWN SYNDROME

If the clinical phenotype refers to a specific genetic syndrome, the clinical geneticist should be consulted about further investigations. Defer labelling a condition as a specific syndrome until definite evidence from further investigations, if potentially available, supports the diagnosis.

Prader—Willi syndrome

Incidence is 1 in 12 000 to 15 000 live births. The cause is chromosome 15p deletion (paternal) or uniparental disomy (maternal).

Presentation: marked hypotonia with feeding problems and poor weight gain in infancy (often requiring tube-feeding). Often happy, placid infants with short stature, small hands and feet, and fair skin.

Dysmorphism: distinctive facial features: narrow face, almond shape eyes, small mouth with thin upper lip and downturned corners.

Long-term health surveillance: severe obesity (often between 1 year and 6 years) due to obsessive overeating with associated diabetes, hypertension, chronic venous insufficiency, cellulitis, and hypoventilation. Hypogonadism, undescended testicles, small

penis,
delayed puberty. Also, strabismus, scoliosis, osteoporosis (with childhood fractures in some cases), disturbed sleep and sleep apneoa, enuresis, dental problems, including soft tooth enamel, thick saliva, poor oral hygiene, bruxism (teeth grinding).

Behaviour problems may include temper tantrums, violent outbursts, obsessive/compulsive or oppositional defiant behaviour.

Phenylketonuria

There is marked geographical variation. Incidence is 1 in 15 000 live births. The cause is an inborn error of metabolism: phenylalanine hydroxylase deficiency (autosomal recessive).

Phenylketonuria is normally detected through neonatal screening at 6 to 14 days after birth. If undetected it may present with seizures, albinism, and a 'musty odour' to the infant's sweat and urine. Strict diet can prevent progression of the disease. Untreated children are developmentally typical at birth but then present with an evolving developmental impairment and acquired microcephaly. Seizures are common.

Rett syndrome

Incidence is 1 in 10 000 to 22 000 live births. The cause is mutations in the *MECP2* or, more rarely, the *CDKL5* or *FOXG1* genes and is seen almost exclusively in females.

Development is typically normal until the age of 6 months or so, then development slows, purposeful hand use is lost and there is a deceleration of head growth. Hand stereotypies appear such as wringing and/or repeatedly putting hands into the mouth and holding the shoulders abducted with the hands at the level of the mouth.

Plateauing and then regression of development follows with the long-term emergence of a dystonia, avoidance of eye contact, lack of social skills, a loss of communication skills and, in the adolescent years, scoliosis. Seizures are common.

Neurocutaneous syndromes

The incidence of neurofibromatosis type 1 (NF1) is 1 in 3000 to 4000 live births; that of tuberous sclerosis is 10 to 16 per 100 000 live births.

Causes are:

- NF1: mutation of chromosome 17q11.2 encoding neurofibromin.

- NF2: mutation of chromosome 22q12 encoding NF2 (Merlin).

- Tuberous sclerosis: autosomal dominant pattern with variable penetrance. Two-thirds result from new sporadic genetic mutations. Mapped to two genetic loci,

TSC1 and *TSC2*. *TSC1* encodes for the protein hamartin and is located on chromosome 9q34; *TSC2* encodes for the protein tuberin and is located on chromosome 16p13.3.

The café-au-lait patches associated with neurofibromatosis or depigmented patches associated with tuberous sclerosis may be evident in the newborn period requiring further clinical assessment followed by special investigation, as necessary.

Apart from nonspecific features such as evolving developmental impairment throughout infancy, it would a be unusual for the neurocutaneous syndromes to present with medical problems in infancy. The one exception is in the context of the epileptic spasms and hypsarrhythmia of West syndrome, of which tuberous sclerosis is a common cause.

The velocardiofacial syndrome

Incidence is 1 in 4000 live births. The cause is a deletion in chromosome 22q11.2.

Presentation and signs: may present in the newborn period with cyanosis related to an associated congenital heart disease, craniofacial dysmorphism with a round face, prominent parietal bones, and a bulbous nasal tip. The face appears long and hypotonic with narrow palpebral fissures, puffy upper eyelids, a squared nasal root, and a narrow alar base with thin alae nasi. There may be cleft palate, hypospadias, and long tapering fingers.

Other features: nasal regurgitation, hypocalcaemia, poor feeding.

Long-term health surveillance: check for cardiac abnormalities and disorders of calcium metabolism. Monitor growth and development (short stature seen in about 30%).

Angelman syndrome

The incidence is 1 in 12 000 to 20 000 live births. The cause is 15q11–13 deletion (maternal) or uniparental disomy (paternal).

Angelman syndrome is often not diagnosed in the newborn period.

Presentation: as infancy progresses, developmental impairment becomes more obvious. The behavioural phenotype is one of a happy demeanour. Spontaneous laughter is a characteristic but inconstant feature. Children often have jerky arm movements due to cortical myoclonus hand flapping movements, are restless with a short attention span, and may have episodes of overbreathing or hyperventilation.

There is evolving microcephaly, seizures may develop in infancy (usually by 3 years of age) associated with large-amplitude posterior slow waves and spikes on the electroencephalogram.

Characteristic facial appearance includes a broad jaw. A wide-based stiff-legged ataxic and apraxic gait evolves.

Long-term health surveillance: classification management of seizures.

Klinefelter syndrome

The incidence is 1 in 500 to 1000 males. The cause is karyotype 47, XXY.

Presentation in the newborn period or early infancy is rare. Developmental impairment emerges in the second half of infancy with an emphasis on low tone and delayed motor development. Later in childhood, language impairment emerges in 25% to 85%, as reported in published studies.

Long-term health surveillance: hypogonadism with the effects emerging at puberty.

Turner syndrome

The incidence is 1 in 2500 females. The cause is karyotype 45, X.

Presentation and signs: may be identified antenatally with a heart or renal abnormality, cystic hygroma, or ascites.

Dysmorphism: symmetrical growth restriction, lymphoedema of hands and feet, shield like chest with wide-spaced nipples, low hairline, low-set ears, small fingernails.

Health surveillance: visual impairment from scleral or corneal abnormalities or glaucoma; screen for heart abnormalities.

Developmental impairment emerges throughout infancy.

Triple X syndrome

The incidence is 1 in 1000 live births in females. The cause is karyotype 47, XXX.

Does not usually present in the newborn period or infancy. Indeed, may not present throughout life. Associated with hypotonia and delayed development in some. The clue to the diagnosis is often disorders of menstruation after puberty.

Williams syndrome

The incidence is 1 in 20 000 live births. The cause is a deletion on chromosome 7 which may include several genes to give a varying phenotype: *CLIP2*, *ELN* (connective tissue abnormalities and cardiovascular disease, specifically supravalvular aortic stenosis), *GTF2I*, *GTF2IRD1* (facial features), and *LIMK1*.

Newborn period and presentation: dysmorphism: an elfin facial appearance with a low nasal bridge. There may be failure to thrive and low muscle tone. Presentation often occurs after infancy with developmental impairment, good verbal skills but poor understanding.

Health surveillance issues: cardiac abnormalities including supravalvular aortic stenosis and transient hypercalcaemia.

Fragile X syndrome

The incidence is 1 in 4000 males; 1 in 8000 females. The cause is mutations in the FMR1 gene encoding fragile X intellectual disability 1 protein, which probably has a role in synapse development. CGG triplet repeats are expanded in the *FMR1* gene and ability relates to the size of the expansion.

Presentation: even though this is an X-linked disorder both males and females can be affected. Recognizable dysmorphism becomes more evident with impairment; but features are very variable. Look for prominent ears, macrocephaly with a prominent forehead, flexible finger joints, high palate, pes planus. Pubertal enlargement of testicles and a long face. Impairment ranges from mild learning disabilities to severe intellectual disability. There is developmental impairment, especially speech and language (most often in males). Later in childhood, attention-deficit/hyperactivity disorder or poor attention span, or autism and autistic behaviours, such as hand flapping, hand biting, and chewing on clothes, may be identified.

Long-term health surveillance: much related to behaviour. Social and emotional problems, such as aggression in males or shyness in females with frequent tantrums; may get anxious, but often have a good sense of humour.

In common with many children with developmental impairments, they may be very sensitive to stimuli such as sound.

REFERENCES

Astley SJ (2004) *Diagnostic Guide for Fetal Alcohol Spectrum Disorders.* The 4-digit code, 3rd edn. Seattle: University of Washington.

Astley Hemingway SJ, Bledsoe JM, Brooks A, et al. (2019) Comparison of the 4-Digit Code, Canadian 2015, Australian 2016 and Hoyme 2016 fetal alcohol spectrum disorder diagnostic guidelines. *Adv Pediatr Res* 6: 31.

Clarren SK, Lutke J, Sherbuck M (2011) The Canadian guidelines and the interdisciplinary clinical capacity of Canada to diagnose fetal alcohol spectrum disorder. *J Popul Ther Clin Pharmacol* 18: e494—e499.

Farmer DL, Thom EA, Brock JW, et al. (2018) The Management of Myelomeningocele Study: full cohort 30-month pediatric outcomes. *Amer J Obstet Gynecol* 218: e1—e256. https://doi.org/10.1016/j.ajog.2017.12.001

Francoeur E, Ghosh S, Reynolds K, Robins R (2010) An international journey in search of diagnostic clarity: early developmental impairment. *J Dev Behav Pediatr* 4: 338—340.

Hoyme HE, Kalberg WO, Elliott AJ, et al. (2016) Updated clinical guidelines for diagnosing fetal alcohol spectrum disorders. *Pediatrics* 138: pii: e20154256.

Newton RW, Puri S, Marder L, eds (2015) *Down Syndrome: Current Perspectives.* London: Mac Keith Press.

WHO (2007) *International Classification of Functioning, Disability and Health—Child and Youth Version.* Geneva: WHO.

WHO (1998) *International Classification of Impairments, Disabilities and Disadvantages (Handicaps).* Geneva: WHO.

Resources

Björck-Åkesson E, Wilder J, Granlund M, et al. (2010) The ICF-CY as a tool in child habilitation/early childhood intervention — feasibility and usefulness as a common language and frame of reference for practice. *Disabil Rehab* 32: S125—S138.

WHO (2014) Guidelines for the identification and management of substance use and substance use disorders in pregnancy. Geneva: WHO. Available at: https://www.who.int/substance_abuse/publications/pregnancy_guidelines/en/

CHAPTER 27

Cerebral palsy

Florian Heinen and Peter Baxter

Key messages

- Cerebral palsy (CP) can be diagnosed in the first year(s) of life.
- It has no cure but does have appropriate interdisciplinary and multimodal management, especially functional therapy (e.g. physiotherapy, postural management, orthosis). Physiotherapy is necessary but lacks specificity.
- Good communication with parents regarding diagnosis and realistic expectations is key.
- Diagnosis of CP has three key aspects:
  - **clinical type** (spastic > dystonic > ataxic) and pattern (bilateral vs unilateral) per Surveillance of Cerebral Palsy in Europe,
  - **severity** according to Gross Motor Function Classification System,
  - **aetiology** (history, anatomical distribution, timing of lesion) per brain magnetic resonance imaging (MRI)
- Essentials for development: evaluation and treatment of comorbidities, bonding, family involvement, and educating parents supportively.

Common errors

- False positive: misdiagnosing transitory neurological phenomena or a single missed milestone at a single timepoint as 'early or likely CP', or misinterpreting the early signs of dopa-responsive-dystonia as dystonic CP.
- False negative: diagnosis is not confirmed within the first year of life.

- Misleading communication: pressure, not support: 'you must do this to avoid that'.
- Therapeutic misconceptions, or 'the-more-you-give-the-more-you-get medication', or 'if-we-do-not-do-everything-we-will-miss-something' (vitamins, minerals, 'cognitive enhancers', 'complementary medicine' etc.).

When to worry

Risk factors

- Birth <32 weeks gestational age or birthweight <1500g.
- Neonatal seizures, encephalopathy, hyperbilirubinaemia, or hypoglycaemia.
- Abnormal cranial ultrasonography and/or brain MRI (e.g. periventricular leukomalacia, infarction, thalamic lesions).

Possible signs

- Reduced spontaneous motor behaviour, including poor sucking and feeding.
- Abnormal muscle tone; initial hypotonia, poor head control. Later, hypertonia with scissoring, or fisting (thumb in palm).
- Motor milestones delayed beyond stated limit (but see also 'Common errors' above): head control 4 months; rolling over 5 months; sitting unsupported 9 months; standing with assistance 14 months; walking alone 18 months.
- Characteristic 'catch' on fast passive movement at the ankle, suggesting spasticity.
- Pathologically brisk deep-tendon reflexes together with other upper motor neuron signs.
- Persistent primitive and neonatal reflexes: Moro, asymmetric tonic neck reflexes, etc.

DEFINITION

Owing to the complexity of the biological systems involved (cortico-subcortico-spino-muscular), no single definition is available that covers all aspects of cerebral palsy (CP). The following three suggestions for definition of terms have good practical use.

CP

CP describes a group of permanent disorders of the development of movement and posture and limiting activity that are attributed to nonprogressive disturbances arising in the developing fetal or infant brain. The motor disorders of CP are often accompanied by disturbances of sensation, visual perception, cognition, communication or behaviour, epilepsy, and/or secondary musculoskeletal problems.

This definition highlights, on the one hand, the priority of the motor system disorder and on the other, the important comorbidities. Within the first year of life the motor system is the easiest developmental ability to observe and examine (AACPDM, 2007).

Spasticity (hypertonia)

The US Pediatric Motor Disorder Task Force proposed the following definition of spasticity (as distinct from dystonia or rigidity). Hypertonia is used as an umbrella term. 'Spasticity' is defined as hypertonia in which one or both of the following signs are present: (1) resistance to externally imposed movement increases with increasing speed of stretch and varies with the direction of joint movement and/or (2) resistance to externally imposed movement, above a threshold speed or joint angle, rises rapidly.

'Dystonia' is defined as a movement disorder in which involuntary sustained or intermittent muscle contractions cause twisting and repetitive movements, abnormal postures, or both (Sanger et al. 2003). Dystonia is not very velocity-dependent.

Upper motor neuron syndrome

Damage to the motor areas and/or pathways of the central nervous system (CNS) may give rise to a specific type of movement disorder arising rostral to (i.e. above) the level of the lower motor neuron and, therefore by definition, being an upper motor neuron syndrome (UMNS). In the context of this syndrome, an easily triggered muscle stretch reflex and a velocity-dependent increase of muscle tone upon passive stretching (pathological tonic stretch reflex) of affected motor segments are considered the most important clinical criteria for the presence of spasticity.

Classic descriptions of UMNS differentiate between clinically negative and clinically positive symptoms. Clinically negative symptoms include paresis, reduced selective motor control, impaired coordination, and impaired control of movement together with easy fatigability of the limb(s). Positive symptoms include spasticity, abnormal posture (spastic dystonia), and changes over time in the mechanical properties of muscles with a tendency to develop contractures, which are initially dynamic and later fixed. Extensor plantar responses may be seen in typically developing infants age <12 months but are otherwise usually due to a lesion in the efferent motor pathway between the cerebral cortex and the motor neuron, loss of the reflex righting, and orienting limb response to cutaneous stimulation (positive Babinski sign), and are a feature of spastic CP. In dystonic CP, the plantars may be flexor or may be extensor due to an abnormal reflex righting and orienting limb response to cutaneous stimulation (pseudo-Babinski sign).

CLINICAL APPROACH

While taking the history (especially guided by the 'When to worry' points above), observe the infant's spontaneous motor behaviour, eye contact, and visual behaviour ('go by the eyes'), interaction with their parents and adaptive motor behaviour, for example, undressing.

With the child on a stable warm surface, offer objects that are suitable for the first year of life and observe visual interest, reaching, grasping, etc. Then perform a flexible and adaptable neurological examination including (1) cranial nerves, (2) muscle stretch (i.e. deep-tendon) reflexes, (3) motor reactions, and (4) milestones. Use the formalized help of the Basic Neurological Examination to differentiate typical from atypical neurological development (Novak et al. 2017; and see Tables 27.1–27.5, below).

Make special note of the head size, response to visual and auditory stimuli, head control, pronator and thumb adductor tone, hip joint mobility (especially abduction), slow (range of motion) and fast (modified Tardieu test) ankle dorsiflexion (known in some countries as 'flexion'), presence or absence and symmetry of the Moro response, asymmetric tonic neck and righting reflexes, and response to visual threat defensive responses.

Obtain these data at two assessments separated in time by a minimum of several weeks to ensure that the findings are consistent, i.e. neither transient nor progressively worsening, to decide whether this is or is not a CP, or whether a more prolonged period of monitoring is needed to decide.

If the findings are consistent, decide on the type of CP according to the Surveillance of Cerebral Palsy in Europe (SCPE) classification (Cans et al. 2007).

More specifically, decide whether it is:

- bilateral or unilateral,

- spastic, dyskinetic (i.e. dystonic or choreo-athethoid), or ataxic.

Note: within SCPE terminology 'hypotonic' CP is no longer considered a diagnostic option (see Chapter 21).

Note: it is well known that mixed types of CP exist. Use the predominant one in diagnosis. If you or your team are not familiar with the SCPE system, details are available on an educational DVD at www.scpenetwork.eu.

Note: hypertonia or spasticity are rarely present in the neonatal period or in the first 3 months of life.

In unilateral CP (e.g. after neonatal stroke), even when there is a demonstrated cause such as a porencephalic cyst, an infant may not show any features at all until after 3 months. It may then be noted that the affected arm is not being moved or used as much as the other side, and there is a tendency to hold it pronated and fisted (with the thumb adducted across the palm). Neglect of a limb can be an early feature.

In bilateral CP, truncal hypotonia and poor head control are the main signs in the first few months of life and may be difficult to differentiate from other causes of neonatal hypotonia (see also Chapter 21). Some can also show asymmetric axial tone with head lag when being pulled to sit, but reasonable head control when held prone. Bottom shuffling can be a later presenting feature – but also remember that most bottom shufflers will simply be following a known normal motor developmental variant. Many with severe early-onset problems can be unsettled infants who cry a lot – but also be mindful that most unsettled infants do not have a CP.

Decide the severity using the GMFCS levels (before the age of 2 years)

Table 27.1   Gross Motor Function Classification System (GMFCS)

GMFCS level	Features
Level I	Infants move in and out of sitting and floor sit with both hands free to manipulate objects. Infants crawl on hands and knees, pull to stand, and take steps holding on to furniture. Infants walk between 18 months and 2 years of age without the need for any assistive mobility device.
Level II	Infants maintain floor sitting but may need to use their hands for support to maintain balance. Infants creep on their stomach or crawl on hands and knees. Infants may pull to stand and take steps holding on to furniture.
Level III	Infants maintain floor sitting when the low back is supported. Infants roll and creep forward on their stomachs.
Level IV	Infants have head control but trunk support is required for floor sitting. Infants can roll to supine and may roll to prone. Children may achieve self-mobility using a manual or powered wheelchair.*
Level V	Physical impairments limit voluntary control of movement. Infants are unable to maintain antigravity head and trunk postures in prone and sitting. Infants require adult assistance to roll. Some children achieve self-mobility using a powered wheelchair with extensive adaptations.*

* See Hielkema et al. (2017).

See Table 27.1. Within the second half of the first year you will be able to use the Gross Motor Function Classification System (GMFCS) to get an idea of severity of the CP. The GMFCS is a very good tool, but when it is used before the age of 2 years, the GMFCS level may change at a later stage. Explain this to the parents and re-evaluate every time you see the child.

Communicate your estimated GMFCS level to the parents, therapists, and carers and — if you like — use the GMFCS treatment curves to communicate an idea about the perspective of the developmental curve of the child beyond the first year of life (see Resources and Figure a) (Heinen et al., 2010).

Aetiology and epidemiology

Known aetiology plays a crucial role for any planning and the communication of concepts. Aetiology (if available) is based on neuroimaging (ultrasound, computed tomography, and especially magnetic resonance imaging [MRI]), from which the nature and, thus, probable timing of the lesion can be decided (see Table 27.2).

Table 27.2 Timing of pathogenetic lesions

Probable time of insult	Approximate gestational age	Radiological or pathological findings
First and second trimester	Before 24 weeks	Malformations
Early third trimester and neonatal	25–34 weeks	Predominantly white matter disorders such as periventricular leukomalacia, intraventricular haemorrhage
Late third trimester	35 weeks to 28 days postterm	Cortical-subcortical and deep grey-matter lesions, basal ganglia lesions
Postneonatal	28 days postterm to 2 years	Traumatic, ischaemic, vascular, or infectious lesions

In general, about 1 to 2 per 1000 liveborn children are diagnosed with CP by the age of 3 to 5 years. In those born before 32 weeks' gestation or with birthweights <1500g, the prevalence rises to 80 to 100 per 1000 live births. Postneonatal causes account for approximately 5% of children with CP. The most common clinical pattern overall is bilateral spastic CP and the second most common is unilateral spastic CP, which occurs more often in infants born at term than in infants born preterm.

Clinico-radiological correlates (Krägeloh-Mann and Horber, 2007) are listed in Table 27.3.

Table 27.3 Correlation of clinical and neuroradiological findings

Type of CP	MRI positive %	
Bilateral spastic	90%	60% periventricular leukomalacia (90% if born preterm) 15% cortical or subcortical/basal ganglia/thalamus lesions (4% if born preterm) 10% malformations (1.5% if born preterm) 3% unclassified
Unilateral spastic	90%	35% periventricular leukomalacia (85% if born preterm) 30% infarction 20% malformations 5% unclassified
Dyskinetic	60—70%	50% basal ganglia/thalamus lesions 15% periventricular leukomalacia Rare: basal ganglia lesions ('kernicterus')

(Reprinted from Krägeloh-Mann and Horber, 2007)

Figure 27.1 (overleaf) Types of treatment for children with bilateral spastic cerebral palsy (CP) by age and severity of impairment. Figure 27.1a plots motor performance on the y-axis against age in years on x-axis. The five curves correspond to the five levels (I—V) of the Gross Motor Function Classification System (GMFCS; Russell et al. 2003; Palisano et al. 2008). A careful history and repeated clinical assessments provide the basis for estimating the likely trajectory and brain imaging within the first two years will provide additional information. The graph provides parents, caregivers, and the multidisciplinary team with a vehicle for discussion of management options for the individual child and a means of visualizing the projected future course of the child's motor development. The basal green curve represents therapist input to which orthoses/aids (bright green), oral medication (yellow), botulinum toxin (orange), intrathecal baclofen (red), and orthopaedic surgery (blue) can be added as necessary. The thickness of the lines A to D indicates an approximation to the percentage (0—25%, 25—50%, 50—75%, 75—100% respectively) of patients having the need for each type of therapy with a broken line indicating an intermittent requirement. Bear in mind, however, that (1) the GMFCS level calculated before the age of 2 years may subsequently change, especially in milder cases, and (2) that the phenotype of cerebral palsies in infants born preterm became less severe between 1990 and 2005 (van Haastert et al. 2011) and may well be continuing to change.

Figure 27.1b gives the indications, principles, and summary of limitations of the different treatment options indicated by the different coloured lines in Figure 27.1a, illustrated by examples. Indications for selective dorsal rhizotomy are not shown. For each treatment, the potential benefit has to be weighed against the limitations. These figures can be downloaded from Heinen et al. 2010, supplementary data. BSCP, bilateral spastic cerebral palsy.

(Reprinted from Heinen et al. 2010 with permission from Elsevier. A colour version of this figure can be seen in the colour plate section.)

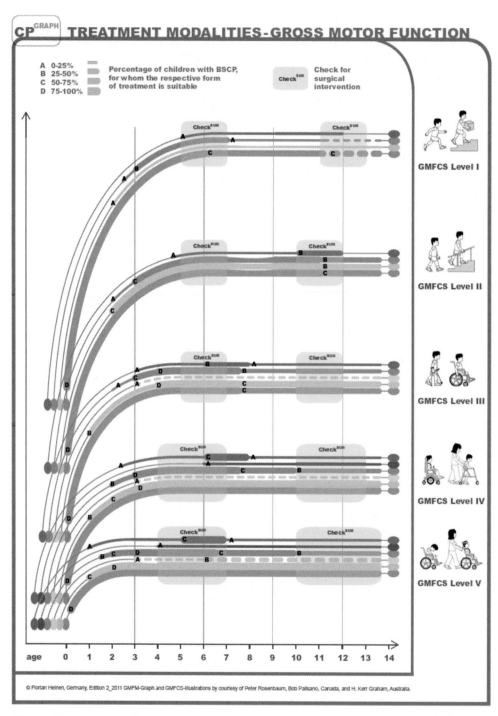

Figure 27.1a Types of treatment for children with bilateral spastic cerebral palsy (CP) by age and severity of impairment

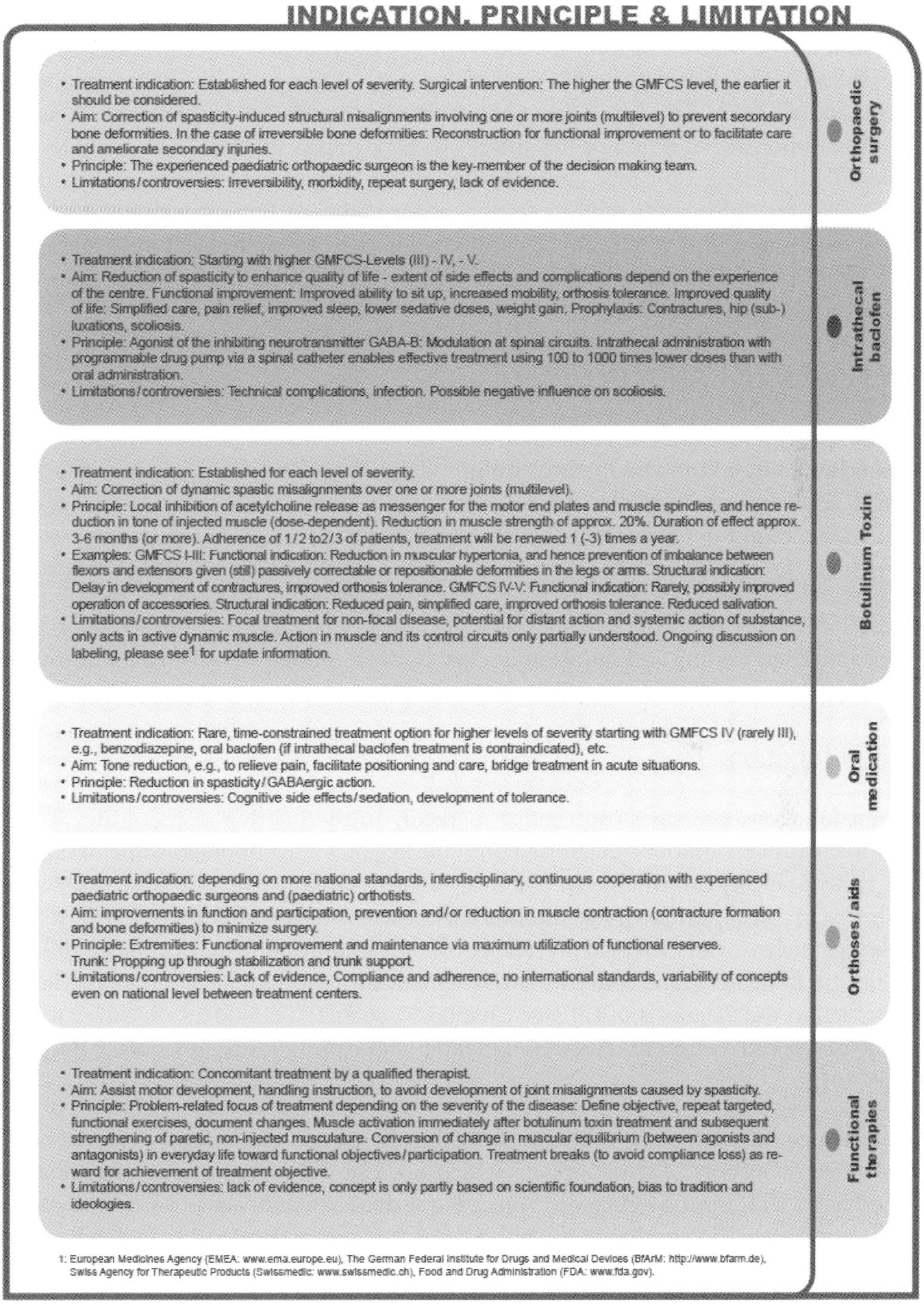

INDICATION, PRINCIPLE & LIMITATION

- Treatment indication: Established for each level of severity. Surgical intervention: The higher the GMFCS level, the earlier it should be considered.
- Aim: Correction of spasticity-induced structural misalignments involving one or more joints (multilevel) to prevent secondary bone deformities. In the case of irreversible bone deformities: Reconstruction for functional improvement or to facilitate care and ameliorate secondary injuries.
- Principle: The experienced paediatric orthopaedic surgeon is the key-member of the decision making team.
- Limitations/controversies: Irreversibility, morbidity, repeat surgery, lack of evidence.

Orthopaedic surgery

- Treatment indication: Starting with higher GMFCS-Levels (III) - IV, - V.
- Aim: Reduction of spasticity to enhance quality of life - extent of side effects and complications depend on the experience of the centre. Functional improvement: Improved ability to sit up, increased mobility, orthosis tolerance. Improved quality of life: Simplified care, pain relief, improved sleep, lower sedative doses, weight gain. Prophylaxis: Contractures, hip (sub-) luxations, scoliosis.
- Principle: Agonist of the inhibiting neurotransmitter GABA-B: Modulation at spinal circuits. Intrathecal administration with programmable drug pump via a spinal catheter enables effective treatment using 100 to 1000 times lower doses than with oral administration.
- Limitations/controversies: Technical complications, infection. Possible negative influence on scoliosis.

Intrathecal baclofen

- Treatment indication: Established for each level of severity.
- Aim: Correction of dynamic spastic misalignments over one or more joints (multilevel).
- Principle: Local inhibition of acetylcholine release as messenger for the motor end plates and muscle spindles, and hence reduction in tone of injected muscle (dose-dependent). Reduction in muscle strength of approx. 20%. Duration of effect approx. 3-6 months (or more). Adherence of 1/2 to2/3 of patients, treatment will be renewed 1 (-3) times a year.
- Examples: GMFCS I-III: Functional indication: Reduction in muscular hypertonia, and hence prevention of imbalance between flexors and extensors given (still) passively correctable or repositionable deformities in the legs or arms. Structural indication: Delay in development of contractures, improved orthosis tolerance. GMFCS IV-V: Functional indication: Rarely, possibly improved operation of accessories. Structural indication: Reduced pain, simplified care, improved orthosis tolerance. Reduced salivation.
- Limitations/controversies: Focal treatment for non-focal disease, potential for distant action and systemic action of substance, only acts in active dynamic muscle. Action in muscle and its control circuits only partially understood. Ongoing discussion on labeling, please see[1] for update information.

Botulinum Toxin

- Treatment indication: Rare, time-constrained treatment option for higher levels of severity starting with GMFCS IV (rarely III), e.g., benzodiazepine, oral baclofen (if intrathecal baclofen treatment is contraindicated), etc.
- Aim: Tone reduction, e.g., to relieve pain, facilitate positioning and care, bridge treatment in acute situations.
- Principle: Reduction in spasticity/GABAergic action.
- Limitations/controversies: Cognitive side effects/sedation, development of tolerance.

Oral medication

- Treatment indication: depending on more national standards, interdisciplinary, continuous cooperation with experienced paediatric orthopaedic surgeons and (paediatric) orthotists.
- Aim: improvements in function and participation, prevention and/or reduction in muscle contraction (contracture formation and bone deformities) to minimize surgery.
- Principle: Extremities: Functional improvement and maintenance via maximum utilization of functional reserves. Trunk: Propping up through stabilization and trunk support.
- Limitations/controversies: Lack of evidence, Compliance and adherence, no international standards, variability of concepts even on national level between treatment centers.

Orthoses/aids

- Treatment indication: Concomitant treatment by a qualified therapist.
- Aim: Assist motor development, handling instruction, to avoid development of joint misalignments caused by spasticity.
- Principle: Problem-related focus of treatment depending on the severity of the disease: Define objective, repeat targeted, functional exercises, document changes. Muscle activation immediately after botulinum toxin treatment and subsequent strengthening of paretic, non-injected musculature. Conversion of change in muscular equilibrium (between agonists and antagonists) in everyday life toward functional objectives/participation. Treatment breaks (to avoid compliance loss) as reward for achievement of treatment objective.
- Limitations/controversies: lack of evidence, concept is only partly based on scientific foundation, bias to tradition and ideologies.

Functional therapies

1: European Medicines Agency (EMEA: www.ema.europe.eu), The German Federal Institute for Drugs and Medical Devices (BfArM: http://www.bfarm.de), Swiss Agency for Therapeutic Products (Swissmedic: www.swissmedic.ch), Food and Drug Administration (FDA: www.fda.gov).

Figure 27.1b

In the early 2000s, approximately 16% of children with CP were reported to have normal findings on MRI (Krägeloh-Mann and Horber 2007; Reid et al. 2014) but this percentage is likely to have fallen with the development of more sensitive MRI sequences. In the unusual case without imaging abnormalities, conditions mimicking CP, such as dopa-responsive dystonia or hereditary spastic paraparesis, should be considered, especially if there is a positive family history. If the diagnosis by history and clinical course is CP, additional metabolic testing is not indicated but a metabolic disorder being misdiagnosed as CP should be considered if there are clinical features suggestive of a neurometabolic disease (e.g. progression, involvement of organs other than the CNS, episodes of worsening/crises).

MANAGEMENT AND FOLLOW-UP

Management relies on close collaboration between parents and professionals. This is best achieved by an interdisciplinary multimodality team who meet together with parents to report progress and plan interventions. It is important to understand the beliefs and resources of the parents and their motivation for 'do's and don'ts' (Heinen et al. 2010).

Provision for the child's non-neurological health needs is beyond the scope of this book, but their feeding and nutrition is a key element of their well-being and must be given specific consideration (see Sullivan, 2009).

Motor function

Motor functions and signs can change markedly in the first few years of life. Some children with CP cannot be diagnosed until the age of 3 years or older, while in others the type or severity can change. In one study of at-risk infants, 50% of those suspected to have CP at 12 months of age did not have it when reviewed at the age of 7 years, although there was an increased prevalence of comorbidities such as learning disability, behaviour difficulties, and epilepsy. The systematic use of tools that take a standardized approach to the diagnosis of CP (see Chapter 5) enables a confident diagnosis to be made earlier and reduces the chances of making a false positive diagnosis of CP (Novak et al. 2017).

Management of the motor problems primarily relies on physiotherapy. There are several different 'schools' of physiotherapy which advocate different methods (e.g. Bobath, Conductive Education, Montessori, Vojta). None of these have been proved to be superior to the others. 'Do no harm' is a watchword that should be strictly observed, especially when it comes to painful procedures.

In the first 2 years of life other interventions such as muscle relaxants (baclofen, diazepam, etc.), botulinum toxin, orthoses, and orthopaedic surgery are not usually yet indicated. However, severe hypertonicity interfering with functional motor development like walking/mobility can improve with botulinum toxin, oral baclofen, and positioning (slight flexion of the neck). Other forms of spasticity reduction, such as intrathecal (i.e. into lumbar cerebrospinal fluid using an implanted infusion pump) baclofen or selective dorsal rhizotomy, are impractical in this age group.

Complementary medications and interventions are widely used but there are no data to prove or disprove any benefits, and they can be costly.

On follow-up, predict the motor development over the next 3 to 6 months — this is best done together with the physiotherapist — and communicate to the parents realistic developmental and therapeutic goals. A written Goal Attainment Scale (Table 27.4) can help in monitoring progress. It will need to be assessed and updated at each visit. You can define specific goals for different domains of the World Health Organization International Classification of Functioning, Disability and Health, Child and Youth version (ICF-CY) levels (body structure and function, activity and participation, environmental, and personal factors). The ICF-CY was merged with the ICF between 2012 and 2015 (https://www.who.int/classifications/icf/en/). Videos at home and in the standardized clinical setting (e.g. from mobile phones) are also useful when documenting progress.

Table 27.4 Goal Attainment Scale

Goal Attainment Scale	Level of attainment
−2	Much less than expected
−1	Somewhat less than expected
0	Expected level of outcome
+1	Somewhat more than expected
+2	Much more than expected

The GMFCS levels should also be reviewed at each visit. These measures can be used to build motor development curves (Palisano et al. 2008).

Consider hip assessment at each visit; this is best done with hip ultrasound in the first year and thereafter by radiographic imaging. The method of choice to detect inadequate positioning of the head of the femur is measuring the Reimers Migration Index (MI), standardized radiographic imaging of the pelvis in patients *older than 1 year of age*. An MI <10% right/left is normal in typically developing children. Different definitions for subluxation and luxation of the hip joint exist, but in general a 'hip at risk' in children with CP is defined as a MI ≥30% (with additional information gained using GMFCS levels or Ashworth scores; see Table 27.6). Always involve a paediatric orthopaedic surgeon for hip management. Hip surveillance programmes can prevent hips from (sub-) luxation over time when started early enough (Hägglund et al. 2005).

In a child under the age of 1 year, neither specialist wheelchairs nor adaptations to the home are required but early planning for these is important and the child may benefit from specialist seating. Table 27.5 and Table 27.6 show the measures that may be used to evaluate and classify body structure and function and activity.

Table 27.5   Classification systems used in the evaluation of cerebral palsy

Instrument	What is addressed?	ICF dimension	Target age	Clinical value	Literature
Gross Motor Function Classification System (GMFCS)	Classification of motor abilities, oriented to mobility, corresponding to age	Activity	<2, 2—4, 4—6, 6—12, 12—18 years	+ + +	www.canchild.ca; Palisano et al. (1997, 2000, 2006, 2008); Russell et al. (2003)
Manual Ability Classification System (MACS)	Classification of manual abilities for children with CP, oriented to activities of daily living	Activity	4—18 years	+ + +	www.macs.nu; Eliasson et al. (2006)
Communication Function Classification System (CFCS)	Classification of communication abilities for individuals with CP. Oriented towards everyday communication performance	Activity Participation	2—18 years	+ + +	https://cparf.org/what-is-cerebral-palsy/severity-of-cerebral-palsy/communication-function-classification-system/

+, helpful; + +, very helpful; + + +, excellent

Table 27.6 Classification systems used in the evaluation of cerebral palsy

Instrument	What is addressed?	ICF dimension	Target age	Psycho-metric criteria	Clin-ical value	Literature
Goal Attainment Scaling (GAS)	Standardized therapy goal setting (in five levels) and determination of which level has been reached	According to indi-vidual ther-apy goal: function, activity, participa-tion	All ages	+ +	+ +	Maloney et al. (1978); Maloney (1993); Palisano (1993); Cusick et al. (2006)
Range of Motion (ROM)	Passive assess-ment of joint mobility with neutral-0-method (goniometry)	Body func-tion/ struc-ture	All ages	+ +	+	McDowell et al. (2000); Allington et al. (2002); Fosang et al. (2003)
Modified Tardieu Scale	'Fast' assess-ment of joint mobility. Differentiates dynamic from fixed limitation of muscles	Body func-tion/ struc-ture	All ages	+ Upper extremity + + Lower extremity	+ + +	Boyd and Gra-ham (1999); Fosang et al. (2003); Mackey et al. (2003); Scholtes et al. (2006)
Modified Ashworth Scale	'Fast' assess-ment of joint mobility. Differentiates dynamic from fixed limitation of muscles	Body func-tion/ struc-ture	All ages	+ + For knee flexors and elbow + For all other muscles	+ +	Bohannon and Smith (1987); Fosang et al. (2003); Clopton et al. (2005); Scholtes et al. (2006)

Table 27.6 (continued)   Classification systems used in the evaluation of cerebral palsy

Instrument	What is addressed?	ICF dimension	Target age	Psycho-metric criteria	Clin-ical value	Literature
Video doc-umentation	Standardized documenta-tion of baseline and follow-up examinations to evaluate therapy progress	Activity	All ages	+ +	+ + +	Mackey et al. (2003); Maathuis et al. (2005)
Canadian Occupa-tional Per-formance Measure (COPM)	Measures changes of self-evaluated function and performance during a period of time	Function activity par-ticipation	From about 8 years (need for self evalu-ation)	+ + +	+ +	www.thecopm.ca; Carswell et al. (2004); Cusick et al. (2006)
Gross Motor Function Measure (GMFM 88 or 66)	Evaluation of quantitative changes of motor functions within defined time periods; 66 is a shortened version of 88	Activity	0.5—16 years	+ + +	+ + +	Russell et al. (2003)
Assist-ing Hand Assessment (AHA)	Evaluation of bimanual skills of children with unilateral CP	Activity	1.5—15 years	+ + +	+ + +	Eliasson et al. (2006)
Pediatric Evaluation of Disability Inventory (PEDI)	Standardized questionnaire for parents to assess the amount of functional defi-cits of everyday activities	Activity and participa-tion	0.5—7.5 years	+ + +	+ + +	www.sralab.org/ rehabilitation-measures/ pediatric-evaluation-disability-inventory

+, helpful; + +, very helpful; + + +, excellent

Comorbidities

As the lesions that cause CP often affect other brain functions, comorbidities affecting vision, hearing, communication, feeding, epilepsy, cognition, and family support are frequent and need to be actively identified and managed. This requires an interdisciplinary approach (see Table 27.7).

Table 27.7 Classification systems used in the evaluation of cerebral palsy

System	Specialists	Problems	Possible actions
Visual	Ophthalmologist, orthoptist	Strabismus, refractive errors, retinopathies, optic nerve hypoplasia, visual field defects, cortical visual agnosia	Spectacles, patching, strabismus surgery
Hearing	Otolaryngologist, audiometry	Conductive defects Sensorineural hearing loss	Hearing aids
Communication	Speech and language therapist	Bulbar dysfunction, central language disorders	Alternative and augmentative communication methods
Feeding	Speech and language therapist, dietician, nurse, paediatrician	Bulbar or pseudobulbar palsy, gastrooesophageal reflux (after first year)	Monitor growth, nasogastric tube or gastrostomy feeding, antireflux medication
Epilepsy	Paediatrician	Seizures	Electroencephalography, antiepileptic medication
Cognition	Paediatrician, psychologist	Learning difficulties	Early intervention, early nursery placement
Behaviour	Paediatrician, psychologist	Sleep problems, frequent crying	Behavioural techniques, assessment for pain
Family	Paediatrician, social services	Bereavement, education, multiple hospital visits, financial resources	Social support, financial support, respite provision

Some children with dystonic cerebral palsy, especially if it is severe, can develop acute persistent or repeated episodes of repetitive hypertonic spasms and postures, a condition called 'status dytonicus', which can last minutes, hours or days. Although episodes occur most frequently in later childhood or early adolescence, they may be seen at any age. Triggers include pain, most often of abdominal origin and related to feeds, such as gastro-oesophageal reflux, and intercurrent illness. During them the child is aware and in considerable pain and distress, reflected in a marked tachycardia and sweating. In severe cases muscle breakdown occurs causing a rise in the plasma creatine kinase (CK) level, which needs to be monitored together with renal function. In some children episodes can be life threatening. The clinical features are often florid and can be similar to those of raised intracranial pressure, malignant hyperthermia, narcotic withdrawal or status epilepticus. Treatment requires removal of the cause and heavy sedation, with if necessary drugs such as clonidine, gabapentin, or a midazolam infusion, and intensive care.

Some myths and related facts

- Specificity of treatment: there are no data showing that one type of physiotherapy intervention is superior to another.

- The more the better: trials of intense versus normal physiotherapy intervention have shown temporary short-term improvement but have not shown any difference in longer-term outcome.

- It is necessary to give every known medication (vitamins, minerals, cognitive enhancers, complementary medicines) in order not to miss something. First, do no harm (see Chapter 13 Evidence-based therapies).

- If the outcome is not the desired one, the treatment was wrong or not intense enough, or the method was wrong. These are not usually the reasons.

- Stem cell treatment: there is no indication, in the present state of knowledge, for any kind of therapy involving stem cell injections or implantations

SUMMARY

CP is the most common cause of hypertonic movement disorders in children. Although the cerebral lesion in CP is usually caused by a single event, CP has to be understood as a developmental disorder described over time as an individual develops. Throughout the last 20 years, intensive research in the field of CP has overcome different ideological 'schools' of (physio-)therapies and complementary medications. Using the above mentioned tools we now have evidence-based information to give the parents and caregivers a *corridor* of motor development by classifying CP with regard to (1) type, (2) severity, and (3) aetiology. It is the right of every family to be in possession of such information and is a prerequisite for family centred programmes.

Early classification of CP within the first year(s) of life provides the best starting point for a *preventive* strategy to reduce the risk of secondary complications (e.g. hip subluxation). This has been shown to be of benefit in large cohort studies during the last two decades. Nevertheless, the clinical profile of each child with CP remains unique and requires a personalized approach to maximize his/her potential functioning. The goal of interdisciplinary treatment is, however, not only to improve functional abilities, but also to increase the participation of each child with CP. This has to be the goal for all of our interventions.

REFERENCES

AACPDM (2007) The definition and classification of cerebral palsy. *Dev Med Child Neurol* 49(s109): 1–44.

Allington NJ, Leroy N, Doneux C (2002) Ankle joint range of motion measurements in spastic cerebral palsy children: intraobserver and interobserver reliability and reproducibility of goniometry and visual estimation. *J Pediatr Orthop Part B* 11: 236–239.

Bohannon RW, Smith MB (1987) Interrater reliability of a modified Ashworth scale of muscle spasticity. *Phys Ther* 67: 206–207

Boyd RN, Graham HK (1999) Objective measurement of clinical findings in the use of botulinum toxin type A for the management of children with cerebral palsy. *Eur J Neurol* 4: 23–35.

Cans, Christine, Dolk H, Platt MJ, et al. (2007) Recommendations from the SCPE collaborative group for defining and classifying cerebral palsy. *Dev Med Child Neurol Suppl* 109: 35–38.

Carswell A, McColl MA, Baptiste S, Law M, Polatajko H, Pollock N (2004) The Canadian Occupational Performance Measure: a research and clinical literature review. *Can J Occup Ther* 71: 210–222.

Clopton N, Dutton J, Featherston T, Grigsby A, Mobley J, Melvin J (2005) Interrater and intrarater reliability of the Modified Ashworth Scale in children with hypertonia. *Pediatr Phys Ther* 17: 268–274.

Cusick A, McIntyre S, Novak I, Lannin N, Lowe K (2006) A comparison of goal attainment scaling and the Canadian Occupational Performance Measure for paediatric rehabilitation research. *Pediatr Rehabil* 9:149–157.

Eliasson AC, Krumlinde-Sundholm L, Rösblad B, et al. (2006) The Manual Ability Classification System (MACS) for children with cerebral palsy: scale development and evidence of validity and reliability. *Dev Med Child Neurol* 48: 549–554.

Fosang AL, Galea MP, McCoy AT, Reddihough DS, Story I (2003) Measures of muscle and joint performance in the lower limb of children with cerebral palsy. *Dev Med Child Neurol* 45: 664–670.

Hägglund G, Andersson S, Düppe H, Lauge-Pedersen H, Nordmark E, Westbom L (2005) Prevention of dislocation of the hip in children with cerebral palsy. The first ten years of a population-based prevention programme. *J Bone Joint Surg Br* 87: 95–101.

Heinen F, Desloovere K, Schroeder AS, et al. (2010) The updated European Consensus 2009 on the use of Botulinum toxin for children with cerebral palsy. *Eur J Paediatr Neurol* 14: 45—66.

Hidecker MJ, Paneth N, Rosenbaum PL, et al. (2011) Developing and validating the Communication Function Classification System for individuals with cerebral palsy. *Dev Med Child Neurol* 53: 704—710.

Hielkema T, Boxum AG, Hamer E, Geertzen, JHB, Hadders-Algra M (2017) Time to update the Gross Motor Function Classification System (GMFCS) for early age bands by incorporation of assisted mobility?*Pediatr Physical Ther* 29: 100—101.

Krägeloh-Mann I, Horber V (2007) The role of magnetic resonance imaging in elucidating the pathogenesis of cerebral palsy: a systematic review. *Dev Med Child Neurol* 49: 44—151.

Mackey AH, Lobb GL, Walt SE, Stott NS (2003) Reliability and validity of the Observational Gait Scale in children with spastic diplegia. *Dev Med Child Neurol* 45: 4—11.

Maloney FP (1993) Goal attainment scaling. *Phys Ther* 73: 123.

Maloney FP, Mirrett P, Brooks C, Johannes K (1978) Use of the Goal Attainment Scale in the treatment and ongoing evaluation of neurologically handicapped children. *Am J Occup Ther* 32: 505—510.

McDowell BC, Hewitt V, Nurse A, Weston T, Baker R (2000) The variability of goniometric measurements in ambulatory children with spastic cerebral palsy. *Gait Posture* 12: 114—121.

Novak I, Morgan C, Adde L, et al. (2017) Early, accurate diagnosis and early intervention in cerebral palsy: advances in diagnosis and treatment. *JAMA Pediatr* 171: 897—907.

Palisano RJ (1993) Validity of goal attainment scaling in infants with motor delays. *Phys Ther* 73: 651—658.

Palisano RJ (2006) A collaborative model of service delivery for children with movement disorders: a framework for evidence-based decision making. *Phys Ther* 86: 1295—1305.

Palisano R, Rosenbaum P, Walter S, Russell D, Wood E, Galuppi B (1997) Development and reliability of a system to classify gross motor function in children with cerebral palsy. *Dev Med Child Neurol* 39: 214—223.

Palisano RJ, Hanna SE, Rosenbaum PL, et al. (2000) Validation of a model of gross motor function for children with cerebral palsy. *Phys Ther* 80: 974—985.

Palisano RJ, Rosenbaum P, Bartlett D, Livingston MH (2008) Content validity of the expanded and revised Gross Motor Function Classification System. *Dev Med Child Neurol* 50: 744—750.

Reid S, Dagia CD, Ditchfield MR, et al. (2014) Population-based studies of brain imaging patterns in cerebral palsy. *Dev Med Child Neurol* 56: 222—232.

Russell DJ, Leung KM, Rosenbaum PL. (2003) Accessibility and perceived clinical utility of the GMFM-66: evaluating therapists' judgements of a computer-based scoring program. *Phys Occup Ther Pediatr* 23: 45—58.

Sanger TD, Delgado MR, Gaebler-Spira D, Hallett M, Mink JW; Task Force on Childhood Motor Disorders (2003) Classification and definition of disorders causing hypertonia in childhood. *Pediatrics* 111: e89—e97.

Scholtes VA, Becher JG, Beelen A, Lankhorst GJ (2006) Clinical assessment of spasticity in children with cerebral palsy: a critical review of available instruments. *Dev Med Child Neurol* 48: 64—73.

Sullivan PB, ed (2009) *Feeding and Nutrition in Children with Neurodevelopmental Disability*. London: Mac Keith Press.

van Haastert IC, Groenendaal F, Cuno SPM, et al. (2011) Decreasing incidence and severity of cerebral palsy in prematurely born children. *Pediatrics* 159: 86—91.

Resources

Australian Hip Surveillance Guidelines: https://www.ausacpdm.org.au/resources/australian-hip-surveillance-guidelines/

DeMatteo C, Law M, Russell D, Pollock N, Rosenbaum P, Walter S (1992) *QUEST: Quality of Upper Extremity Skills Test*. Hamilton, ON: McMaster University, Neurodevelopmental Clinical Research Unit, Gross Motor Function Classification System (GMFCS): https://www.canchild.ca/en/resources/42-gmfcs-e-r

Gross Motor Function Measure (GMFM): https://www.canchild.ca/en/resources/44-gross-motor-function-measure-gmfm

Maathuis KG, van der Schans CP, van Iperen A, Rietman HS, Geertzen JH (2005) Gait in children with cerebral palsy: observer reliability of Physician Rating Scale and Edinburgh Visual Gait Analysis Interval Testing scale. *J Pediatr Orthop* 25: 268—272.

Surveillance of Cerebral Palsy in Europe (SCPE): https://eu-rd-platform.jrc.ec.europa.eu/scpe_en

CHAPTER 28

Central nervous system disorders of movement other than cerebral palsy

Peter Baxter and Florian Heinen

Key messages

- There are many different paroxysmal or persistent movement disorders in the first year of life.
- Most can be diagnosed on clinical grounds.
- Phenomenology discriminates ataxia, athetosis, chorea, dystonia, myoclonus, stereotypies, and tremor. Ballismus, Parkinsonism, and tics are rare in this age group.
- Remember that these motor disorders are most obvious in the mature brain, but in younger people they are less easily distinguished.
- Typically developing infants can also show mild forms of 'physiological' ataxia and athetosis which are age-related.

Common errors

- Mistaking the normal variation in motor development for disease.
- Mistaking normal motor asymmetry during development for disease.
- Mistaking a paroxysmal movement disorder for epilepsy (or vice versa).
- Assuming that all chronic motor abnormalities are a form of cerebral palsy.

- Inappropriate investigations for benign conditions.
- Inappropriate treatment for normal conditions.

When to worry

- When head control does not develop.
- When sitting without support is delayed beyond 9 months corrected age.
- When new motor findings appear or old ones worsen.

DEFINITIONS

(See also Sanger et al. 2003, 2006).

Ataxia (literally 'without order')

Inability to generate a normal or expected voluntary movement trajectory that cannot be attributed to weakness or an involuntary muscle activity around the affected joints. Ataxia can result from impairment of the spatial pattern of muscle activity or from impairment of the timing of the activity, or both. It can be specified as dysmetria (undershoot or overshoot), dyssynergia (decomposition of multi-joint movements), and dysdiadochokinesis (impaired rhythmicity of rapid alternating movements; not applicable within the first year of life).

Athetosis (literally 'without fixed position')

Slow, writhing, continuous, involuntary movements. This is part of the spectrum of dyskinetic movement disorders (choreoathetotic vs dystonic). It also occurs in one subtype of cerebral palsy (see Chapter 27).

Chorea (literally 'dance-like')

An involuntary, continual, irregular hyperkinetic disorder in which movements or parts of movement occur with a variable rate, direction, and distribution (all body parts may be involved); typically unpredictable and random.

Ballismus

Involuntary, high amplitude flinging movements typically occurring proximally; they may be brief or continual. It may be an extreme form of chorea. If, as usually happens, one side of the body is affected, the term 'hemiballismus' is used.

Dystonia

Dystonia is an involuntary alteration in the pattern of muscle activation during voluntary movement or maintenance of posture. It is, thus, a syndrome of sustained muscle contractions, frequently causing twisting and repetitive movements, or abnormal posture. Typically, both agonists and antagonists cocontract. Dystonia can be action- or posture-induced. Dystonic spasms can resemble tonic seizures and can be extremely painful. Status dystonicus is a medical emergency.

Myoclonus

Quick, shock-like movements of one or more muscles. The term is usually applied to describe positive myoclonus: sudden, quick, involuntary muscle jerks caused by muscle contraction. Negative myoclonus refers to sudden, brief interruptions of contraction in active (postural) muscles.

Parkinsonism

Characterized by the presence of two or more of the cardinal features: tremor at rest, bradykinesia, rigidity, and postural instability.

Startles

Brief, generalized motor responses, similar to myoclonus. Startle syndrome is a disease entity.

Stereotypies

Involuntary, patterned, coordinated, repetitive, nonreflexive movements that occur in the same fashion with each repetition, often rhythmic.

Tics

Involuntary, sudden, rapid, abrupt, repetitive, nonrhythmic, simple, or complex movements or vocalizations. Tics are classified into two categories (motor and phonic) and do not usually occur in the first year of life.

Tremor

Oscillating rhythmic movements about a fixed point, axis, or plane that occur when antagonist muscles contract alternately. Usually this involves oscillation around a joint and produces a visible movement. Pathological tremor is also rare in the first year of life.

INTRODUCTION AND CLINICAL APPROACH

Many different paroxysmal and nonparoxysmal movement disorders can occur in neonates and older infants (see Table 28.1). In most, diagnosis relies on clinical recognition (for paroxysmal disorders videos, including those made on mobile phones, can be particularly useful) rather than investigations. The most important differential diagnoses are, for paroxysmal disorders (Chapter 21), from epilepsy (see Chapters 16 and 20), and for persistent disorders, from cerebral palsy (see Chapter 27).

Table 28.1 Movement disorders in the first 2 years of life

Movement disorders	Paroxysmal	Nonparoxysmal
Neonatal	Jitteriness Doggy paddle/bicycling Benign neonatal sleep myoclonus Transient dystonia of prematurity	Floppy infant (hypotonia) Dystonias Stiff-baby syndromes Chorea
Infancy	Shuddering attacks Paroxysmal torticollis Benign paroxysmal upgaze Sandifer syndrome Benign tonic upgaze of infancy Spasmus nutans Opsoclonus-myoclonus Head banging (jactatio capitis) Stereotypies Gratification phenomena (Tics) Benign spasms	Head tilt Dystonia — generalized Lower-limb hypertonia Ataxia Tremor

PAROXYSMAL MOVEMENT DISORDERS IN NEONATES: CLINICAL APPROACH

Paroxysmal movement disorders can easily be mistaken for neonatal seizures (see Chapters 16 and 21). In certain conditions, such as pyridoxine dependency, both seizures and nonepileptic movement disorders can occur in the same infant. The differential relies on clinical assessment and electroencephalographic (EEG) recording, both ictal and interictal.

Jitteriness is a common, nonspecific feature which can occur in hungry infants but can also be a sign of hypocalcaemia, hypoglycaemia, drug-withdrawal syndromes, or a range of acute neonatal encephalopathies. It can be distinguished from epileptic seizures by being interrupted by sleep, by a change of body posture, or by restraint of the affected limbs. An exaggerated startle response can be an associated feature. Infants born preterm in non-REM sleep can also show excess startles.

- *Age at onset:* first week of life.

- *Age at resolution:* typically before 6 months.

- *Treatment:* underlying cause if appropriate; otherwise information/reassurance.

Bicycling movements of the arms and doggy-paddling movements of the legs, with or without tonic axial hyperextension (back arching), are nonspecific signs of acute or chronic encephalopathies due to any cause.

- *Age at onset:* any age.

- *Treatment:* underlying cause; positioning.

Benign neonatal sleep myoclonus is frequently mistaken for epileptic seizures (see Chapters 16 and 20). The main distinguishing feature is that episodes only occur while asleep. Typically, they are not stereotyped, so on one occasion only one limb may be involved while on others, more than one limb shows the typical jerking movements. The infant is otherwise neurologically typical. In cases of clinical doubt, a normal EEG record during an episode can be helpful. The outcome is also normal.

- *Age at onset:* less than 1 month.

- *Age at resolution:* latest 6 months.

- *Treatment:* information/reassurance; no treatment is needed.

PERSISTENT MOVEMENT DISORDERS IN NEONATES: CLINICAL APPROACH

Hypotonia (floppy infant) is a feature of many central motor and other disorders (see Chapter 24 for more details).

Dystonia manifesting as back arching and head retroversion, associated with obligate asymmetric tonic neck reflex and at least transient relaxation with neck flexion, is most commonly associated with severe chronic neurological impairment due to prenatal or perinatal brain injury (e.g. asphyxia, hyperbilirubinaemia). Back arching and head retroversion can also be a symptom of raised intracranial pressure from any cause, including hydrocephalus.

Transient dystonia of prematurity can occur in infants born preterm and consists of increased leg extensor tone and asymmetric axial tone with head lag when pulled to sit, but not when held prone; sometimes associated with fisting and exaggerated tendon jerks.

- *Age at onset:* few weeks.

- *Age at resolution:* 12 months in most; a minority continue with more definite signs of a cerebral palsy.

- *Treatment:* reassurance.

Stiff-baby syndrome is a rare condition most commonly caused by hyperekplexia, due to a mutation in the glycine receptor gene or the glycine transporter gene. Clinically, the diagnosis of hyperekplexia (or startle disease) is suggested by a non-habituating exaggerated startle response to repetitive nose tapping. The condition is lifelong, but symptoms usually change with age, with hypertonia becoming less prominent by 1 year of age and the appearance of exaggerated sleep myoclonus, 'freezing' to fright, and sometimes epilepsy. In neonates and young infants severe life-threatening episodes with apnoea can be aborted promptly by neck flexion. Prophylaxis with benzodiazepines, valproate, or phenobarbital can prevent episodes (see Chapter 21). The differential diagnosis of stiff-baby syndrome includes congenital disorders of neurotransmitter metabolism (often associated with oculogyric crisis) and congenital absence of the pyramidal tracts.

In the past, infants born preterm with chronic lung disease could develop a movement disorder with choreiform movements of the limbs, face, and tongue and a general restlessness, which settled when asleep. The aetiology was unclear. It is now rarely seen.

- *Age at onset:* third postnatal month; can persist or slowly resolve over 12 to 18 months.

- *Treatment:* clonazepam can help, especially if tongue involvement affects feeding.

PAROXYSMAL DISORDERS IN INFANCY: CLINICAL APPROACH

(See also Chapter 21)

Benign infantile shuddering attacks are best diagnosed by video footage. The child is otherwise unaffected with typical development. There may be an association with essential tremor later in life.

- *Age at onset:* infancy, early childhood.

- *Treatment:* information/reassurance

Benign paroxysmal torticollis consists of episodes of head tilt lasting several hours or days, associated with vomiting, abnormal eye movements, and in older children, ataxia. The child is unaffected between episodes. Posterior fossa tumours can cause similar symptoms so neuroimaging is essential. Sandifer syndrome (see below) should be excluded. Some cases are linked to mutations in the *CACNA1A* gene. Some also develop migraine in later childhood.

- *Age at onset:* first year of life.

- *Age at resolution:* by 8 years.

- *Treatment:* information/reassurance.

Sandifer syndrome often consists of asymmetric dystonic posturing, usually involving the neck with turning and torticollis followed by distress, which lasts a few minutes. Occasionally more of the body is involved with back and limb extension. Some episodes occur after meals. These are due to gastro-oesophageal reflux and/or a hiatus hernia.

- *Age at onset:* early infancy.

- *Age at resolution:* early childhood or after treatment.

- *Treatment:* drug therapy for reflux; often surgical fundoplication is needed.

Action dystonia can occur in some chronic dystonias including dopa-responsive disorders, but usually in older children. Paroxysmal and exertional dystonia can be a feature of GLUT1 deficiency, diagnosed by low glucose levels in the cerebrospinal fluid and treated by a ketogenic diet. Paroxysmal chorea can occur in Allan–Herndon–Dudley disorder (MCT8 deficiency), an X-linked thyroid transporter disorder seen in males and suggested by raised blood T3 levels.

Episodes of benign paroxysmal tonic upgaze of infancy can be associated with unusual head postures and ataxia. The infant is usually otherwise typical, with typical neurodevelopmental findings between episodes, but a minority can show developmental impairment.

- *Age at onset:* first year of life.

- *Age at resolution:* 1 to 4 years.

- *Treatment:* some may respond to L-Dopa.

Spasmus nutans consists of the triad of abnormal head posture, repetitive head nodding (at around 3Hz), most apparent during visual fixation on near or distant objects, and a shimmering nystagmus (at around 11Hz). The nystagmus is asymmetrical and may be monocular. Rarely, this may be mimicked by tumours in the visual pathway or region of the third ventricle, but visual impairment is usually also present in such cases. Computed tomography (CT) or magnetic resonance imaging (MRI) may, therefore, be necessary. Head tilt (without the other components of the triad) may be a presentation of a posterior fossa tumour.

- *Age at onset:* 3 to 12 months.

- *Age at resolution:* within a few months, but subtle nystagmus may persist for years.

- *Treatment:* none.

Episodic or persistent chaotic but conjugate eye jerking is an important feature of the opsoclonus-myoclonus syndrome (also known as the opsoclonus-myoclonus-ataxia, Kinsbourne or dancing eye syndrome) typically together with severe distress/dysphoria/misery that may appear as 'rage attacks'. Most cases are associated with occult neuroblastoma, and so need specialist investigation.

- *Age at onset:* usually after the first year of life.

- *Treatment:* symptomatic: immunomodulatory agents (e.g. steroid pulses); of underlying cause: resection of neuroblastoma, as above.

Head banging while awake is seen in a number of typically developing infants when bored or frustrated. It is not usually severe enough to cause any injury or bruising. The equivalent while asleep, jactatio capitis, is a well-recognized parasomnia. Usually the child is otherwise well and wakes completely rested but their parents may not be, as the sound has kept them awake! It may persist for years.

- *Age at onset:* first year of life.

- *Age at resolution:* any, but jactatio capitis can persist.

- *Treatment:* reassurance; protective padding against surfaces, such as a mattress against the wall.

Gratification phenomena are voluntary events when a child will sit or lie, often with their legs crossed, and adopt repetitive postures or movements. Some authorities postulate a link to infantile masturbation. During episodes, the child remains aware and the activity can be interrupted but will start again afterwards. Frequently the feet can adopt an inturned supinated dystonic posture.

- *Age at onset:* 3 to 12 months.

- *Age at resolution:* any.

- *Treatment:* reassurance.

Infantile stereotypies can appear very similar and consist of repetitive semivoluntary movements. Some occur in specific situations, such as while watching a washing machine spin. There can be an association with autism.

Tic disorders rarely occur in this age group.

PERSISTENT MOVEMENT DISORDERS IN INFANTS: CLINICAL FEATURES

Chronic head tilt can be due to torticollis (e.g. benign sternomastoid tumour, hypothesis: residuum of haematoma within the sternocleidoid muscle), posterior fossa-abnormalities, including cerebellar or cervical tumours, and abnormalities of the atlanto-axial joint. If palpation of the contralateral sternomastoid reveals a tumour and there is restricted extension, treatment is by regular gentle stretching. Otherwise sonography of the muscles, neuroimaging focusing on posterior fossa structures, and X-ray, CT, or MRI of the cervical spine are required, with surgical referral for any abnormal findings.

Chronic dystonia involving the trunk and limbs can occur in Lesch—Nyhan syndrome, ataxia telangiectasia, glutaric aciduria, Aicardi—Goutières syndrome, and mitochondrial cytopathies. All of these can be mistaken for cerebral palsy.

- *Treatment:* mostly symptomatic; in Lesch—Nyhan syndrome: allopurinol, L-Dopa; in glutaric aciduria: diet, riboflavin, carnitine.

Rarely, comorbidities can help to identify a specific aetiology. For example, dyskinetic movement disorder and hearing loss are the essential features that, in combination with paresis of upgaze and/or enamel dysplasia of the deciduous teeth, constitute the triad/tetrad of classic kernicterus and should prompt enquiry into neonatal jaundice and other risk factors. Variants lacking one of the essential features (auditory kernicterus and motor kernicterus) also occur.

Hypertonia of the lower limbs raises the possibility of a spinal cord lesion due either to a neural tube defect or a congenital spinal tumour.

If brain MRI is normal it is important to assess the spine. Similar findings can be due to dopa-responsive dystonias; biotinidase deficiency; hereditary spastic paraparesis (Strumpell—Lorrain disease) due to a variety of genes; purine nucleoside phosphorylase (PNP) deficiency; arginase deficiency; and L1 syndrome.

- *Treatment:* dopa (dopa-responsive conditions); biotin (biotinidase deficiency); otherwise supportive; symptomatic (e.g. for hypertonia); genetic counselling.

Progressive spasticity, dystonia, and/or ataxia can all suggest a leukodystrophy, such as Pelizaeus—Merzbacher disease and its variants, or Krabbe disease (see Chapter 29).

Additional features include nystagmus, optic atrophy, stridor, and seizures. If this group of disorders is suspected, MRI is an essential first step. In Pelizaeus–Merzbacher leukodystrophy, symptoms begin in infancy with hypotonia, nystagmus, and sometimes chorea, followed by hypertonia and ataxia. The more severe connatal form causes early stridor and seizures. In infantile Krabbe leukodystrophy, symptoms begin at a few months of age with marked irritability, feeding difficulties, vomiting, and developmental slowing. Progressive hypertonia, epileptic seizures, deafness, and blindness follow, with death by 2 years.

- *Treatment:* supportive; symptomatic (e.g. for hypertonia); genetic counselling.

Ataxia is rarely diagnosed in early infancy, partly because young children are intrinsically ataxic when their coordination is compared to older children, and partly because early disorders of the cerebellum more usually present with hypotonia and early developmental impairment. However, acute ataxia can be caused by infectious or inflammatory cerebellitis, intoxication, cerebellar tumours, and other rarer causes. Chronic ataxia can be a feature of hexosaminidase A and B deficiency or mitochondrial disorders. GLUT1 deficiency can also present in this way.

- *Treatment:* usually symptomatic; for GLUT1 deficiency: ketogenic or Atkins diet.

Tremor can be difficult to distinguish from chorea. Prolonged chorea can follow encephalitis, especially when due to herpes simplex, usually associated with recurrence of the encephalopathy. The exact mechanism is uncertain. Previously it was believed to be due to persistence of the herpes virus infection leading to recommendations of very prolonged acyclovir treatment. However, it is now recognized that the disorder may have another explanation such as an autoimmune cause. Choreoathetosis is also associated with glutaric aciduria type 1 and Lesch–Nyhan syndrome. Benign hereditary chorea can present in infancy with delayed walking and falls. The chorea improves slowly with age but can be replaced by myoclonus. If due to mutations in the *NKX2-1* gene it can be associated with chronic lung and/or thyroid problems.

SUMMARY

With a wide range of possible disorders, it is difficult to propose a common diagnostic approach. However, always considering a differential diagnosis, even in 'known cases' of 'cerebral palsy' or 'epilepsy', will avoid misdiagnosis. In addition, if the motor condition does not follow an expected course but, for example, shows progression, re-evaluation of the diagnosis is essential.

REFERENCES

Sanger TD, Delgado MR, Gaebler-Spira D, Hallett M, Mink JW; Task Force on Childhood Motor Disorders (2003) Classification and definition of disorders causing hypertonia in childhood. *Pediatrics* 111: e89–e97.

Sanger TD, Chen D, Delgado MR, et al. (2006) Definition and classification of negative motor signs in childhood. *Pediatrics* 118: 2159—2167.

Resources

King MD, Stephenson JBP (2009) *A Handbook of Neurological Investigations in Children*. London: Mac Keith Press.

Singer HS, Mink JW, Gilbert DL, Jancovic J (2010) *Movement Disorders in Childhood*. Philadelphia: Saunders Elsevier.

CHAPTER 29

Progressive loss of skills

Meral Topcu, Dilek Yalnızoglu, and Richard W Newton

Key messages

- Progressive loss of skills in a child with typical or near typical development may be the initial sign of a progressive neurometabolic/neurogenetic disorder.
- Always consider treatable inherited metabolic disorders in a child with progressive neurological deterioration, e.g. biotinidase deficiency in an infant with seizures; spinal muscular atrophy or infantile Pompe disease in an infant with loss of motor function.
- A careful history is mandatory when other family members are affected; a pedigree showing at least three generations is helpful.

Common errors

- Children with progressive neurological diseases may be incorrectly diagnosed with cerebral palsy or epileptic encephalopathy.

When to worry

- Faltering developmental progress and loss of previously gained skills identified in the neurological evaluation of the young child should alert us to the possibility of neurodegeneration.
- Onset of seizures, progressive deceleration or acceleration of head growth, hearing loss, visual impairment, hypotonia, dystonia, or spasticity are considered red flags.

INTRODUCTION

Any child, whether developing typically or showing an early pattern suggesting developmental impairment, will follow a predictable developmental trajectory. When developmental progress slows from this expected trajectory, the question of a progressive disease arises. If the child develops typically and then loses the previously gained mental and/or motor skills, the clinical picture is likely to reflect a progressive disease process. Poorly controlled epilepsy may also cause this clinical picture and mimic a progressive disease.

CLINICAL APPROACH

The *history* should explore current symptoms and any exposure to infective and toxic agents, previous medical history including prenatal, perinatal, and postnatal risk factors, and a family history (including parental consanguinity or other affected family members). A personal or family history of febrile or afebrile seizures should be sought. A detailed developmental history and current level of functioning should be documented. If the family history is uninformative, acquired, or sporadic, genetic disorders should be considered.

Physical examination should be undertaken with awareness of the possible relevance not only of clinical neurological signs (see Chapter 6) but also of abnormalities of respiration, dysmorphic features, or signs of a storage disorder, including cranial or other skeletal abnormalities, organomegaly, retinopathy, or heart murmurs; hair (coarse in Menkes disease, sparse in biotinidase deficiency); and skin (rashes or signs of a neurocutaneous syndrome) should be examined. The occipitofrontal head circumference is always an important observation to record and plot on a centile chart. Disorders of eye movements may provide clues to a wide variety of disorders.

The clinical picture of neurometabolic disorders may, however, be nonspecific, and with early onset it can be particularly difficult to be sure that the disorder is truly progressive.

Laboratory evaluation (see Chapter 10) in any child with early developmental impairment, with or without suspected regression, should include a complete blood count with differential count, glucose, calcium, phosphate, urea and creatinine, thyroid function tests, lead, amino acids, organic acids, a mucopoly- and oligosaccharide screen, and chromosomal karyotype or microarray. Comparative genomic hybridization (CGH), which measures DNA copy number differences between a test and reference genome, is now adding to the diagnostic yield, but is not available in all settings.

Further investigation of regression should be tailored to fit the clinical picture, as summarized in later sections of this chapter (see also Chapters 8–10). Capillary pH, plasma, and cerebrospinal fluid (CSF) lactate and mitochondrial DNA deletions should be considered if mitochondrial cytopathies seem possible; transferrin iso-electric focusing (abnormal in congenital disorders of glycosylation) should be considered for the combination of early developmental impairment with either unusual subcutaneous fat distribution or cerebellar ataxia with hypoplasia on cranial imaging or persistent absence seizures; white-cell enzymes for the lysosomal storage disorders; dihydroxyacetone-phosphate acyltransferase (DHAP-AT), phytanic acid, and very-long-chain fatty acids (VLCFAs) for peroxisomal disorders; and copper for Menkes disease. If the picture includes acute encephalopathy, include glucose, ammonia, acid-base status, and organic acids (see Chapters 14 and 15). For intractable epilepsy include plasma urate concentration, and a sulphite dipstick test on a *fresh* urine sample to exclude molybdenum cofactor deficiency (Chapters 10 and 15).

Neuroimaging studies (see Chapter 8) have revolutionized our approach to neurological disorders with a progressive course and, in particular, the leukodystrophies including two disorders of infancy that present with a slowly progressive megalencephaly combined with irritability, spasticity (sometimes preceded by hypotonia), epileptic seizures, and bulbar problems, Alexander disease, and Canavan disease (or aspartocyclase deficiency).

Electroencephalography (EEG) (see Chapter 9) and, when available, visually evoked potentials, electroretinogram, nerve conduction studies, and electromyogram can greatly narrow the differential diagnosis or help to confirm clinical suspicion when their use is tailored to the clinical presentation. Gene testing is now superseding peripheral neurophysiology.

As children mature and you observe the clinical signs or developmental profile, the emergence of an epilepsy or dystonia may allow investigation to become more focused and specific. Targeted testing may then be performed based on individual patient evaluation and the results of previous tests, including CSF analysis and tissue samples, as appropriate. For a guide on clinical presentation and approach to specific investigations on neurodegenerative conditions presenting in infancy, see Table 29.1

EARLY REGRESSION WITH PROMINENT SEIZURES

Several conditions present with progressive myoclonic epilepsies in which multiple seizure types, including myoclonic seizures, occur alongside abnormal neurological signs and progressive, although sometimes slow, deterioration. Biotinidase deficiency, if severe (<10% biotinidase activity) presents with neurological and cutaneous symptoms between 2 months and 5 months of age. Refractory seizures and hypsarrhythmia commonly occur as the only early manifestations. Chronic presentations may be steadily progressive or intermittent with lethargy, ataxia, and floppiness. Blood concentrations of biotinidase (measurable in a dry blood spot) is reduced. Biotin therapy may be started while awaiting biochemical confirmation.

Other possible underlying diagnoses include *early infantile neuronal ceroid lipofuscinosis* (NCL) (Table 29.1), *Tay—Sachs disease* or (clinically similar) *Sandhoff disease* (Table 29.1), *tetrahydrobiopterin (BH4) deficiency, Menkes disease*, and *progressive neuronal degeneration of childhood* (PNDC). In tetrahydrobiopterin deficiency, the epileptic encephalopathy may be associated with extrapyramidal features including hypotonia, dystonia, and oculogyric crises. Diagnosis is by CSF biogenic amine and pterin profile, along with a phenylalanine challenge. Treatment is with L-Dopa, and biotin, possibly with phenylalanine dietary restriction. Menkes disease is a rare, X-linked disease which presents with failure to thrive from the neonatal period or after 2 to 3 months. Seizures may include infantile spasms and hypothermia may be a feature. Hair is brittle, sparse, and silver or grey, although not necessarily from birth. Microscopy of hair shows twisted hair strands (*pili torti*) and blood levels of copper and caeruloplasmin are reduced. PNDC, also known as Alpers disease or Huttenlocher syndrome, may have onset of clinical problems before 12 months of age, but may not declare itself until the second year. After weeks or months of refractory seizures, epilepsia partialis continua or other forms of status epilepticus, there is progressive loss of developmental skills. Deranged liver function is suggestive but may be apparent only late in the illness. In those children in whom a specific underlying defect has been confirmed, nearly all are mitochondrial cytopathies due to mutations in the catalytic subunit necessary for the replication of mitochondrial DNA, (called DNA polymerase gamma [*POLG1*]), located on chromosome 15.

Table 29.1 The clinical presentation and approach to specific investigations in neurodegenerative conditions presenting in infancy

Condition	Presentation	Clinical course	Neuro-physiology	Neurometabolic and genetic investigations
Early infantile neuronal ceroid lipofuscinosis (CLN1, Santavouri—Haltia)	Towards the end of the first year, developmental arrest; infrequent seizures; evolving blindness; movement disorder; microcephaly	Irritability, hypotonia, dystonic spasms	Attenuation then loss of ERG with abnormal VEPs; characteristic EEG response to slow flicker	Histopathology: skin biopsy shows neuronal granular inclusions on electron microscopy Biochemistry: palmitoyl- protein thioesterase (PPT) assay

Table 29.1 (continued)   The clinical presentation and approach to specific investigations in neurodegenerative conditions presenting in infancy

Condition	Presentation	Clinical course	Neuro-physiology	Neurometabolic and genetic investigations
Krabbe leu-kodystrophy (common infant-ile form)	In the first months of life: severe irritability, dystonia, spasti-city with excess of extensor tone; developmental impairment	Regression pro-gresses, espe-cially with febrile illnesses; dis-tressing dysto-nia, decerebra-tion by 1 year, loss of reflexes, decreased visual awareness	Slow peripheral nerve-conduction velocities	Histopathology: needle-like inclu-sion bodies in macrophages; demyelination on nerve biopsy; foamy histiocytes Biochemistry: raised CSF pro-tein; WCE ana-lysis: low levels of galactocerebrosi-dase, beta-galactosidase
Tay—Sachs disease (classic infantile GM2 gangliosidosis)	4—6 months, motor weakness, visual failure; excessive startle to sound; macu-lar degenera-tion and cherry red spot in some	Rapidly progres-sive hypotonia, seizures by 6 months (frequent myoclonus), blind by 1 year, death in 4 years, macro-cephaly from year 2	EEG initially unremarkable, becomes very abnormal; VEPs abolished by 18 months; ERG nor-mal	Neuroimaging: white-matter abnormalities Biochemistry: low levels of hexosa-minidase A
Pelizaeus—Merzbacher disease	Dysmyelinat-ing disorder of white matter Classic and conatal (more severe) forms are distinguished by rate of progres-sion, with consid-erable phenotypic overlap	Early infancy: pendular nys-tagmus, spas-tic paraparesis and movement disorder (usu-ally dystonia) Stridor in severe forms may be mistaken for cerebral palsy as clinical pro-gression is often slow or very slow		Neuroimaging: hypomyelin-ation of cere-bral white matter Genetics: (X-linked); mutation in the PLP gene (75%)

Table 29.1 (continued) The clinical presentation and approach to specific investigations in neurodegenerative conditions presenting in infancy

Condition	Presentation	Clinical course	Neuro-physiology	Neurometabolic and genetic investigations
Metachromatic leukodystrophy (late infantile; sulphatide lipidosis)	18 months; regression, flaccid limb paresis with depression or loss of reflexes (peripheral neuropathy)	Within 3—6 months hypertonia, optic atrophy, decerebration, and decorticate posturing; death by 8—10 years	Slow nerve conduction; abnormal VEPs and SSEPs	Neuroimaging: MRI shows symmetrical demyelination (typically frontal and occipital horns) Histopathology: metachromatic sulphatides in nerves WCE: low levels of arylsulphatase A; raised CSF protein
Infantile neuroaxonal dystrophy (INAD*; Seitelberger disease)	Hypotonic infant with decreased limb reflexes	Evolution of progressive spasticity and dystonia; opisthotonic posturing; optic atrophy; death by 5 years	EMG shows anterior horn cell disease and denervation (nerve conduction studies normal) BAEPs, SSEPs, and VEPs progressively worsen; normal ERG	Autosomal recessive: PLA2G6 molecular genetic testing Histopathology: axonal spheroids on axillary skin biopsy MRI shows diffuse cerebellar hyperintensity and atrophy ± iron deposition in basal ganglia

Table 29.1 (continued) The clinical presentation and approach to specific investigations in neurodegenerative conditions presenting in infancy

Condition	Presentation	Clinical course	Neuro-physiology	Neurometabolic and genetic investigations
HIV-associated progressive encephalopathy	A developmental plateau appears with later neurological and general cognitive regression	There is evolution of corticospinal tract signs, hypokinesis, and evolving dysphagia with feeding difficulties		Raised CSF protein (60%) and IgG (80%); usually no cells (mononuclear cells in 25%); HIV antibodies detected MRI: hyperintense lesions are noted in the periventricular white matter and centrum semiovale on T2-weighted images These lesions are often patchy in the early stages becoming more diffuse with disease progression

*INAD is now regarded as a form of neurodegeneration with brain iron accumulation (NBIA).
BAEP, brainstem, auditory evoked potential; CSF, cerebrospinal fluid; EEG, electroencephalography; EMG, electromyography; ERG, electroretinography; HIV, human immunodeficiency virus; MRI, magnetic resonance imaging; SSEP, somatosensory evoked potential; VEP, visual evoked potential; WCE, white cell enzymes.

Rapidly expanding discoveries in genetics have enabled clinicians to diagnose complex neurogenetic and neurometabolic disorders; in addition, rare and novel diseases can be recognized. The clinician should particularly be aware of treatable conditions regarding inherited metabolic disorders. Early diagnosis and treatment of inherited metabolic epilepsies which have a specific treatment are crucial as the prognosis is dependent both on the management of seizures and appropriate treatment of the underlying metabolic disorder, such as pyridoxine-dependent epilepsies, glucose transporter deficiency, developmental impairment and epilepsy neonatal diabetes (DEND), creatine synthesis and transporter deficiencies, biotinidase deficiency, cerebral folate deficiency, biopterin synthesis defect, and serine biosynthesis defect.

INHERITED DISORDERS OF METABOLISM PRESENTING AS PROGRESSIVE DISORDERS

Nonketotic hyperglycinaemia (see Chapters 15 and 16) classically presents in the neonatal period with seizures, hiccoughs, and burst suppression on EEG. Blood concentrations of glycine and/or the CSF:blood ratio of glycine are elevated while other amino acids levels are normal.

Glutaric aciduria type 1 typically presents between 6 months and 18 months with an acute encephalopathy and paroxysmal episodes, often interpreted as seizures, but which are actually involuntary movements. The bouts are often precipitated by a mild intercurrent illness. It can predispose to subdural effusions with associated macrocephaly. Urinary organic acid analysis reveals elevated levels of glutaric acid. The condition may be stabilized by a special diet.

Late-onset urea cycle disorders typically predominantly present with recurrent encephalopathy associated with hyperammonaemia (see Chapter 15). Take note of any family history of unexplained death in male siblings.

Multiple carboxylase deficiency typically has dermatological features (rash, which may be subtle, and/or alopecia appearing around 3 months of age) as well as seizures and severe developmental impairment. Biochemical abnormalities include specific organic acidurias and may include lactic acidosis. Defects in utilization of biotin, a cofactor in four carboxylases in humans, underlie the disorder which may respond to biotin.

Neurotransmitter metabolism defects, including disorders of biogenic amine metabolism in which there is failure of synthesis of dopamine, serotonin, norepinephrine, epinephrine, or the cofactor tetrahydrobiopterin. Biochemically, each has a characteristic CSF neurotransmitter profile. They may present with epileptic encephalopathy or myoclonic epilepsy, intestinal dysmotility or feeding difficulties, early developmental impairment, microcephaly, central hypotonia, and peripheral hypertonia. Principles of treatment include the replacement of neurotransmitters, in particular, a trial of L-Dopa or the administration of a cofactor or precursor such as biotin, pyridoxine, or folinic acid.

OTHER DISORDERS WHICH MAY PRESENT WITH LOSS OF SKILLS

The *cerebral palsies* are static conditions, but their course is not unchanging; they may mimic progressive disorders. Cerebral palsy (see Chapter 27) is also the most common misdiagnosis in the child with progressive loss of skills without epilepsy. Other possible mimics of degenerative disorders include conditions that may become evident after a period of apparently typical development. Their onset may lead to a slowing or even plateauing of motor, cognitive, or social development, often associated with the emergence of seizures, motor signs, and involuntary movements. Nonetheless, their course may be stabilized and become static, particularly if appropriate treatment is offered.

Around 20% of children infected with human immunodeficiency virus (HIV) become severely symptomatic or die in the first year of life and 10% of HIV-infected children have signs of encephalopathy, usually including motor and early developmental impairments (Table 29.1).

Mitochondrial disorders: Leigh syndrome is clinically heterogeneous, but the onset is often in infancy with brainstem involvement (clinically apparent as loss of saccadic eye movement and sighing or sobbing respiration) plus a motor disorder (pyramidal and/or extrapyramidal). Stepwise deterioration, sometimes precipitated by intercurrent illness, is characteristic; occasionally a long period of stability can lead to misdiagnosis of cerebral palsy that is corrected when the disease leads to further regression.

Neuroimaging shows involvement of the brainstem and basal ganglia. As specific laboratory confirmation of the diagnosis becomes available in a higher proportion of cases (e.g. in cases of mutations in *POLG1*; see section above covering progressive myoclonic epilepsies), it is clear that the range of mitochondrial disorders in infancy is wide and may not correspond to an obvious textbook disease category. The diagnosis should be considered in progressive unexplained neurological disorders, especially poliodystrophies (i.e. those affecting grey matter).

Acute necrotizing encephalopathy (ANE) is an even rarer, dominantly inherited condition (see Chapter 17). Like Leigh syndrome, ANE has acute deteriorations with intercurrent illness and radiology that is superficially similar to Leigh syndrome. Involvement of the external capsule and brainstem is seen in ANE, but atypical for Leigh syndrome. Either may be misdiagnosed as an acute acquired encephalopathy. The importance of ANE lies in identifying presymptomatic, first-degree relatives who can benefit from immunization and prophylactic antibiotics to reduce the risk of acute deterioration.

Rett syndrome affects female infants only (see Chapter 26). After appearing to be initially typically developing, there is regression of functional hand movement between 6 months and 18 months of age along with sleep disturbance, agitation, and acquired microcephaly. There follows the evolution of severe cognitive impairment, stereotyped hand movements, progressive deterioration of gait, scoliosis, seizures, and nonepileptic 'vacant spells'. Respiratory rhythm disturbances including hyperventilation and respiratory pauses usually evolve after infancy. Identified genetic mutations include the methyl-CpG-binding protein 2 (*MECP2*) gene (85%) and, less commonly, cyclin-dependent kinase-like 5 (*CDKL5*).

RARE STATIC DISORDERS WITH SEVERE EPILEPSY AND DEVELOPMENTAL IMPAIRMENT

3-Phosphoglycerate dehydrogenase deficiency presents with microcephaly, severe early developmental impairment, intractable epilepsy, and a severely abnormal EEG. Magnetic resonance imaging shows a reduction in white matter.

Guanidinoacetate methyltransferase (GAMT) *deficiency* presents with intractable epilepsy, early developmental impairment, and an extrapyramidal movement disorder. Suspect this condition where there is a low plasma creatinine, although this finding may sometimes be a non-pathological reflection of reduced muscle mass in a small infant. Additional laboratory evidence for this condition comes from the demonstration of low urine creatinine/calcium and creatinine/protein ratios. Brain magnetic resonance spectroscopy shows an absent creatine peak. The condition may improve with creatine administration.

Progressive encephalopathy, peripheral oedema, hypsarrythmia, and *optic atrophy* is a recessive condition with hypsarrhythmia and optic atrophy. Magnetic resonance imaging shows atrophy of the temporal lobes and atrophy of the cerebellar folia.

MANAGEMENT OF NEURODEGENERATIVE CONDITIONS

Palliation

There are some issues common to all; palliative interventions may be nonspecific or disease-specific. They should include an explanation to parents of the condition involved in terms they can understand (see Chapter 26).

Common attendant problems and treatment include the following:

- Feeding difficulties (often requiring nasogastric feeds as the condition progresses; gastrostomy may or may not be appropriate).

- Sleeplessness (use of melatonin or sedation).

- Distressing irritability; initial assessment should rule out intercurrent conditions which may lead to pain or enhance a feeling of illness (e.g. ear or urinary tract infection, toothache, bone or joint pain, subdural collection, etc.); if present they should be treated. At times the irritability will be pervasive, intrusive, and upsetting (Krabbe disease being one notable example) in which case a clonidine or morphine infusion should be considered. Either may be delivered subcutaneously in the home setting.

- Seizure control, which can be very difficult. Benzodiazepines are good for myoclonus and clonazepam may also help control distressing dystonia. When the standard approach does not help, consider using phenobarbitone in high doses.

- Spasticity and dystonia. Benzodiazepines can relieve and are a good choice when epilepsy is also a feature.

- More detailed guidance on strategies for management of pain in the presence of central nervous system (CNS) impairments is beyond the scope of this chapter and recommendations may not be applicable in all countries (WHO, 2019). However detailed guidance applicable in some countries is given, for example, by Hauer and Houtrow (2017).

Community support networks or a *hospice movement* can be called on to help support the family and the family should be encouraged to express their wishes on whether they would prefer the death of the child to take place at home, in hospital, or in a hospice. The emphasis should always be on a good palliative approach for the child, and easing distress which in turn will ease distress for the whole family.

Prenatal screening is possible for several disorders such as lysosomal storage diseases and peroxisomal disorder wherever there is a neurometabolic or neurogenetic marker. Where parents wish to pursue this the result offers important information and choices. Pretest counselling is an important part of this process.

Interventions that modify the underlying disease process

These again may be nonspecific or disease-specific (e.g. enzyme-replacement therapy for Pompe disease). Detailed consideration is beyond the scope of this book, but general principles include:

- **Reducing the metabolic load** on the affected pathway (e.g. dietary manipulation). Miglustat is a small iminosugar molecule that reversibly inhibits glycosphingolipid synthesis, and is approved for the treatment of progressive neurological manifestations of Niemann-Pick disease type C (NP-C) in both children and adults with the disease.

- **Correcting product deficiency** (e.g. biotin in biotinidase deficiency).

- **Decreasing metabolite toxicity** (e.g. sodium benzoate and sodium phenylbutyrate in hyperammonaemia; L-carnitine in organic acidaemias; substrate reduction therapy is used with some success in animal models of Tay−Sachs disease).

- **Stimulating residual enzymes** with cofactors.

- **Pharmacological enzyme replacement** (e.g. glucocerebrosidase for Gaucher type III). This and other enzymes are targeted for uptake by the mannose-6-phosphate receptor system present on the surface of nearly all cells, which facilitates their entry. The blood/brain barrier still offers the greatest hindrance to progress with many enzymes. Recombinant human tripeptidyl peptidase (cerliponase alfa) is an enzyme-replacement therapy that has been developed for treatment of neuronal NCL type 2 (CLN2) disease.

- **Gene therapy**, e.g. oligonucleotide gene-reading modification for spinal muscular atrophy (see Chapter 24).

- **Transplantation** cell-mediated therapy brings significant improvement in CNS pathology in the lysosomal storage diseases, largely through release of enzymes by transplanted cells for uptake by deficient cells. This can be enhanced through gene overexpression and the use of receptor-mediated uptake systems. Direct implantation of cells and the use of bone marrow transplant to deliver microglial/ brain macrophage precursors to the CNS have resulted in improvement in animal models. Neural progenitor cells coupled with enzyme overexpression show promise and but do not yet have any place in clinical practice.

REFERENCES

Hauer J, Houtrow AJ (2017) Pain assessment and treatment in children with significant impairment of the central nervous system. *Pediatrics* 139: e20171002.

WHO (2019) Web statement on pain management guidance. https://www.who.int/medicines/areas/quality_safety/guide_perspainchild/en/

Resources

Arzimanoglou A, ed (2018) *Aicardi's Diseases of the Nervous System in Childhood*, 4th edn. London: Mac Keith Press.

King MD, Stephenson JBP (2009) *A Handbook of Neurological Investigations in Children*. London: Mac Keith Press.

Pearl PL (2018) *Inherited Metabolic Epilepsies*. New York: Demos Medical Publishing.

APPENDIX 1

Growth charts

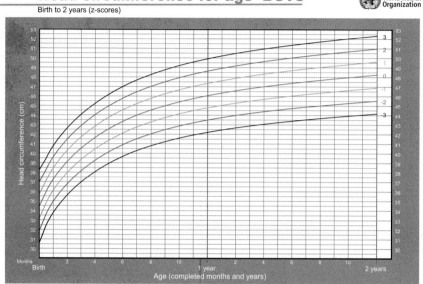

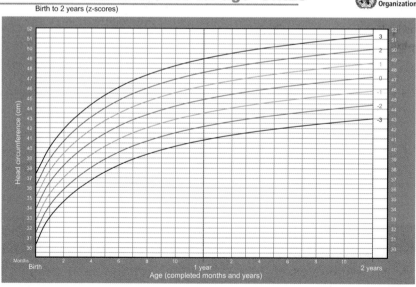

WHO Child Growth Standards

Length-for-age BOYS
Birth to 2 years (z-scores)

World Health
Organization

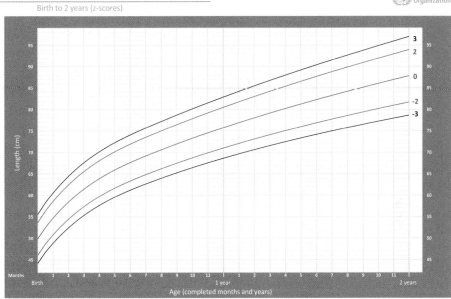

WHO Child Growth Standards

Length-for-age GIRLS
Birth to 2 years (z-scores)

World Health
Organization

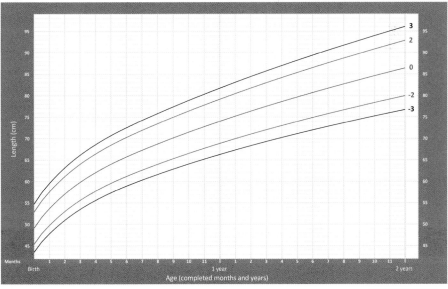

WHO Child Growth Standards

Weight-for-age BOYS
Birth to 2 years (z-scores)

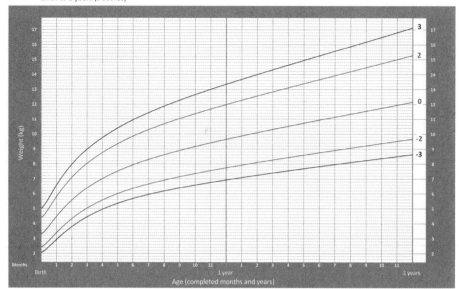

WHO Child Growth Standards

Weight-for-age GIRLS
Birth to 2 years (z-scores)

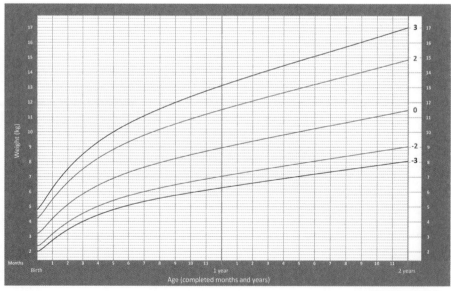

WHO Child Growth Standards

Index

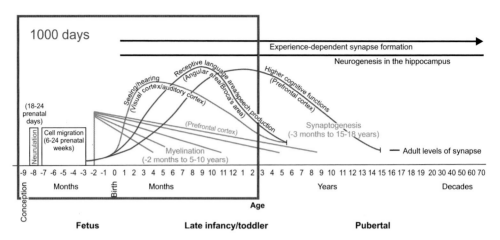

Plate 1 (Figure 4.1) The course of human brain development. (Adapted from Thompson and Nelson, 2001 with permission from the American Psychological Association.)

Plate 2 (Figure 27.1) Figure 27.1a plots motor performance on the y-axis against age in years on x-axis. The five curves correspond to the five levels (I—V) of the Gross Motor Function Classification System (GMFCS; Russell et al. 2003; Palisano et al. 2008). A careful history and repeated clinical assessments provide the basis for estimating the likely trajectory and brain imaging within the first two years will provide additional information. The graph provides parents, caregivers, and the multidisciplinary team with a vehicle for discussion of management options for the individual child and a means of visualizing the projected future course of the child's motor development. The basal green curve represents therapist input to which orthoses/aids (bright green), oral medication (yellow), botulinum toxin (orange), intrathecal baclofen (red), and orthopaedic surgery (blue) can be added as necessary. The thickness of the lines A to D indicates an approximation to the percentage (0—25%, 25—50%, 50—75%, 75—100% respectively) of patients having the need for each type of therapy with a broken line indicating an intermittent requirement. Bear in mind, however, that (1) the GMFCS level calculated before the age of 2 years may subsequently change, especially in milder cases, and (2) that the phenotype of cerebral palsies in infants born preterm became less severe between 1990 and 2005 (van Haastert et al. 2011) and may well be continuing to change. Figure 27.1b gives the indications, principles, and summary of limitations of the different treatment options indicated by the different coloured lines in Figure 27.1a, illustrated by examples. Indications for selective dorsal rhizotomy are not shown. For each treatment, the potential benefit has to be weighed against the limitations. These figures can be downloaded from Heinen et al. 2010, supplementary data. BSCP, bilateral spastic cerebral palsy. (Reprinted from Heinen et al. 2010 with permission from Elsevier.)

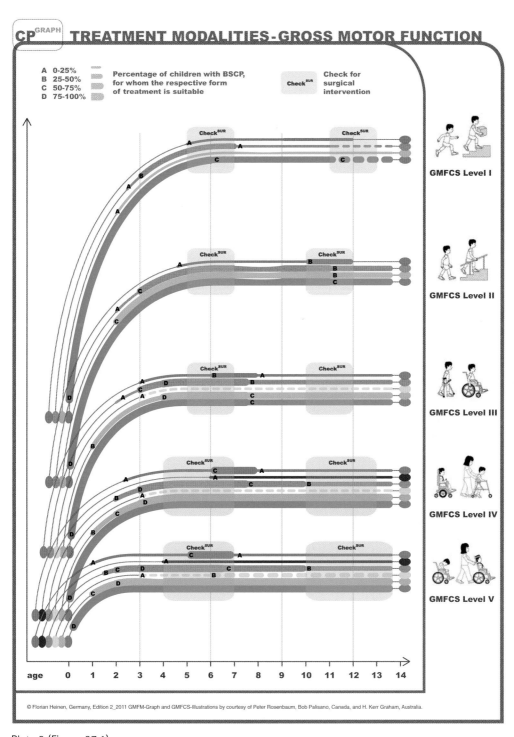

Plate 3 (Figure 27.1)

INDICATION, PRINCIPLE & LIMITATION

- Treatment indication: Established for each level of severity. Surgical intervention: The higher the GMFCS level, the earlier it should be considered.
- Aim: Correction of spasticity-induced structural misalignments involving one or more joints (multilevel) to prevent secondary bone deformities. In the case of irreversible bone deformities: Reconstruction for functional improvement or to facilitate care and ameliorate secondary injuries.
- Principle: The experienced paediatric orthopaedic surgeon is the key-member of the decision making team.
- Limitations/controversies: Irreversibility, morbidity, repeat surgery, lack of evidence.

Orthopaedic surgery

- Treatment indication: Starting with higher GMFCS-Levels (III) - IV, - V.
- Aim: Reduction of spasticity to enhance quality of life - extent of side effects and complications depend on the experience of the centre. Functional improvement: Improved ability to sit up, increased mobility, orthosis tolerance. Improved quality of life: Simplified care, pain relief, improved sleep, lower sedative doses, weight gain. Prophylaxis: Contractures, hip (sub-) luxations, scoliosis.
- Principle: Agonist of the inhibiting neurotransmitter GABA-B: Modulation at spinal circuits. Intrathecal administration with programmable drug pump via a spinal catheter enables effective treatment using 100 to 1000 times lower doses than with oral administration.
- Limitations/controversies: Technical complications, infection. Possible negative influence on scoliosis.

Intrathecal baclofen

- Treatment indication: Established for each level of severity.
- Aim: Correction of dynamic spastic misalignments over one or more joints (multilevel).
- Principle: Local inhibition of acetylcholine release as messenger for the motor end plates and muscle spindles, and hence reduction in tone of injected muscle (dose-dependent). Reduction in muscle strength of approx. 20%. Duration of effect approx. 3-6 months (or more). Adherence of 1/2 to 2/3 of patients, treatment will be renewed 1 (-3) times a year.
- Examples: GMFCS I-III: Functional indication: Reduction in muscular hypertonia, and hence prevention of imbalance between flexors and extensors given (still) passively correctable or repositionable deformities in the legs or arms. Structural indication: Delay in development of contractures, improved orthosis tolerance. GMFCS IV-V: Functional indication: Rarely, possibly improved operation of accessories. Structural indication: Reduced pain, simplified care, improved orthosis tolerance. Reduced salivation.
- Limitations/controversies: Focal treatment for non-focal disease, potential for distant action and systemic action of substance, only acts in active dynamic muscle. Action in muscle and its control circuits only partially understood. Ongoing discussion on labeling, please see[1] for update information.

Botulinum Toxin

- Treatment indication: Rare, time-constrained treatment option for higher levels of severity starting with GMFCS IV (rarely III), e.g., benzodiazepine, oral baclofen (if intrathecal baclofen treatment is contraindicated), etc.
- Aim: Tone reduction, e.g., to relieve pain, facilitate positioning and care, bridge treatment in acute situations.
- Principle: Reduction in spasticity/GABAergic action.
- Limitations/controversies: Cognitive side effects/sedation, development of tolerance.

Oral medication

- Treatment indication: depending on more national standards, interdisciplinary, continuous cooperation with experienced paediatric orthopaedic surgeons and (paediatric) orthotists.
- Aim: improvements in function and participation, prevention and/or reduction in muscle contraction (contracture formation and bone deformities) to minimize surgery.
- Principle: Extremities: Functional improvement and maintenance via maximum utilization of functional reserves. Trunk: Propping up through stabilization and trunk support.
- Limitations/controversies: Lack of evidence, Compliance and adherence, no international standards, variability of concepts even on national level between treatment centers.

Orthoses/aids

- Treatment indication: Concomitant treatment by a qualified therapist.
- Aim: Assist motor development, handling instruction, to avoid development of joint misalignments caused by spasticity.
- Principle: Problem-related focus of treatment depending on the severity of the disease: Define objective, repeat targeted, functional exercises, document changes. Muscle activation immediately after botulinum toxin treatment and subsequent strengthening of paretic, non-injected musculature. Conversion of change in muscular equilibrium (between agonists and antagonists) in everyday life toward functional objectives/participation. Treatment breaks (to avoid compliance loss) as reward for achievement of treatment objective.
- Limitations/controversies: lack of evidence, concept is only partly based on scientific foundation, bias to tradition and ideologies.

Functional therapies

1: European Medicines Agency (EMEA: www.wmwa.europe.eu), The German Federal Institute for Drugs and Medical Devices (BfArM: http://www.bfarm.de), Swiss Agency for Therapeutic Products (Swissmedic: www.swissmedic.ch), Food and Drug Administration (FDA: www.fda.gov).

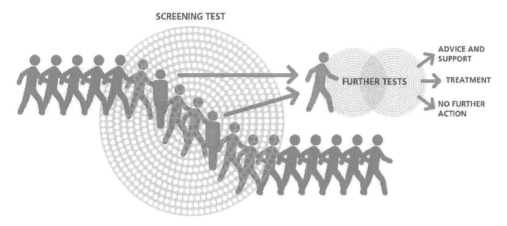

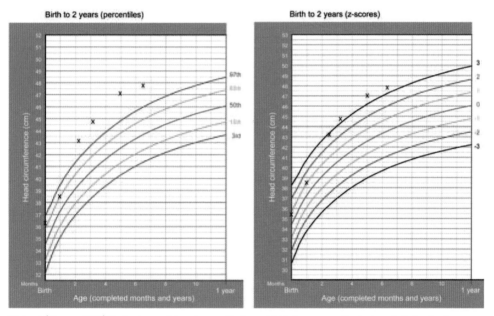

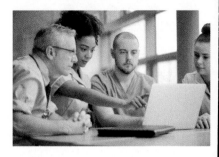
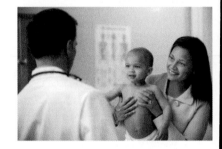
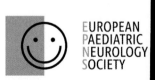

Other titles from Mac Keith Press www.mackeith.co.uk

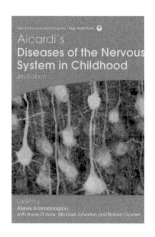

Aicardi's Diseases of the Nervous System in Childhood, 4th Edition
Alexis Arzimanoglou, Anne O'Hare, Michael V Johnston and Robert Ouvrier (Editors)

Clinics in Developmental Medicine
2018 ▪ 1524pp ▪ hardback ▪ 978-1-909962-80-4

This fourth edition retains the patient-focussed, clinical approach of its predecessors. The international team of editors and contributors has honoured the request of the late Jean Aicardi, that his book remain 'resolutely clinical', which distinguishes *Diseases of the Nervous System in Childhood* from other texts in the field. New edition completely updated and revised and now in full colour.

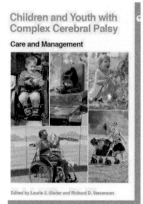

Children and Youth with Complex Cerebral Palsy: Care and Management
Laurie J. Glader and Richard D. Stevenson (Editors)

A Practical Guide from Mac Keith Press
2019 ▪ 404pp ▪ softback ▪ 978-1-909962-98-9

This is the first practical guide to explore management of the many medical comorbidities that children with complex CP face, including orthopaedics, mobility needs, cognition and sensory impairment, difficult behaviours, respiratory complications and nutrition, amongst others. Uniquely, contributors include children and parents, providing applied wisdom for family-centred care. Clinical Care Tools are provided to help guide clinicians and include a Medical Review Supplement, Equipment and Services Checklist and an ICF-Based Care: Goals and Management Form.

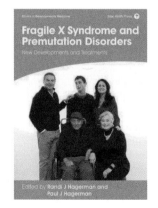

Fragile X Syndrome and Premutation Disorders: New Developments and Treatments
Randi J Hagerman and Paul J Hagerman (Editors)

Clinics in Developmental Medicine
2020 ▪ 192pp ▪ hardback ▪ 978-1-911612-37-7

Fragile X syndrome results from a gene mutation on the X-chromosome, which leads to various intellectual and developmental disabilities. *Fragile X Syndrome and Premutation Disorders* offers clinicians and families a multidisciplinary approach in order to provide the best possible care for patients with Fragile X. Unique features of the book include what to do when an infant or toddler is first diagnosed, the impact on the family and an international perspective on how different cultures perceive the syndrome.

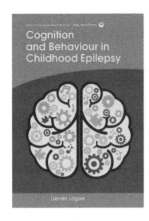

Cognition and Behaviour in Childhood Epilepsy
Lieven Lagae (Editor)

Clinics in Developmental Medicine
2017 ▪ 186pp ▪ hardback ▪ 978-1-909962-87-3

For many parents, cognitive and behavioral comorbidities, such as ADHD, autism and intellectual disability, are the real burden of childhood epilepsy. This title offers concrete guidance and treatment strategies for childhood epilepsy in general, and for the comorbidities associated with each epilepsy syndrome and their pathophysiology. The book is written by experts in the field with an important clinical experience, while chapters by clinical neuropsychologists provide a strong theoretical background.

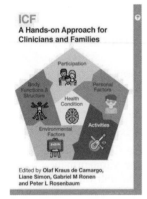

ICF: A Hands-on Approach for Clinicians and Families
Olaf Kraus de Camargo, Liane Simon, Gabriel M. Ronen and Peter L. Rosenbaum (Editors)

A Practical Guide from Mac Keith Press
2019 ▪ 192pp ▪ softback ▪ 978-1-911612-04-9

This accessible handbook introduces the World Health Organisation's International Classification of Functioning, Disability and Health (ICF) to professionals working with children with disabilities and their families. It contains an overview of the elements of the ICF but focusses on practical applications, including how the ICF framework can be used with children, families and carers to formulate health and management goals.

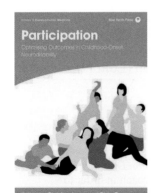

Participation: Optimising Outcomes in Childhood-Onset Neurodisability
Christine Imms and Dido Green (Editors)

Clinics in Developmental Medicine
2020 ▪ 288pp ▪ hardback ▪ 978-1-911612-17-9

This unique book focuses on enabling children and young people with neurodisability to participate in the varied life situations that form their personal, familial and cultural worlds. Chapters provide diverse examples of evidence-based practices and are enriched by scenarios and vignettes to engage and challenge the reader to consider how participation in meaningful activities might be optimised for individuals and their families. The book's practical examples aim to facilitate knowledge transfer, clinical application and service planning for the future.

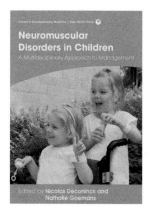

Neuromuscular Disorders in Children: A Multidisciplinary Approach to Management
Nicolas Deconinck and Nathalie Goemans (Editors)

Clinics in Developmental Medicine
2019 ▪ 468pp ▪ hardback ▪ 978-1-911612-09-4

Neuromuscular Disorders in Children: A Multidisciplinary Approach to Management critically reviews current evidence of management approaches in the field of neuromuscular disorders (NMDs) in children. Uniquely, the book focusses on assessment as the cornerstone of management and highlights the importance of a multidisciplinary approach.

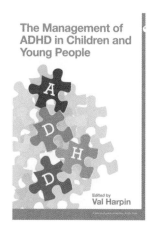

The Management of ADHD in Children and Young People
Val Harpin (Editor)

A Practical Guide from Mac Keith Press
2017 ▪ 292pp ▪ softback ▪ 978-1-909962-72-9

This book is an accessible and practical guide on all aspects of assessment of children and young people with Attention Deficit Hyperactivity Disorder (ADHD) and how they can be managed successfully. The multi-professional team of authors discusses referral, assessment and diagnosis, psychological management, pharmacological management, and co-existing conditions, as well as ADHD in the school setting. New research on girls with ADHD is also featured. Case scenarios are included that bring these topics to life.

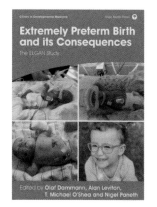

Extremely Preterm Birth and its Consequences: The ELGAN Study
Olaf Dammann, Alan Leviton, Thomas Michael O'Shea and Nigel Paneth (Editors)

Clinics in Developmental Medicine
2020 ▪ 256pp ▪ hardback ▪ 978-1-911488-96-5

The ELGAN (Extremely Low Gestational Age Newborns) Study was the largest and most comprehensive multicentre study ever completed for this population of babies born before 28 weeks' gestation. The authors' presentation and exploration of the results of the research will help clinicians to prevent adverse health outcomes and promote positive health for these children.

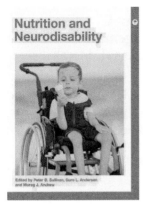

Nutrition and Neurodisability
Peter B. Sullivan, Guro L. Andersen and Morag J. Andrew (Editors)

A Practical Guide from Mac Keith Press
2020 ▪ 208pp ▪ softback ▪ 978-1-911612-26-1

Feeding difficulties are common in children with neurodisability and disorders of the central nervous system can affect the movements required for safe and efficient eating and drinking. This practical guide provides strategies for managing the range of nutritional problems faced by children with neurodevelopmental disability. The easily accessible information on aetiology, assessment and management is informed by a succinct review of current evidence and guidelines to inform best practice.

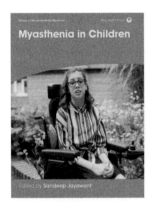

Myasthenia in Children
Sandeep Jayawant (Editor)

Clinics in Developmental Medicine
2019 ▪ 144pp ▪ hardback ▪ 978-1-911612-30-8

Myasthenia is a rare, but underdiagnosed and sometimes life-threatening disorder in children. There are no guidelines for diagnosing and managing these children, especially those with congenital myasthenia, a more recently recognised genetic condition, but there have been significant developments in identification and treatment of myasthenia in recent years. This book will help clinicians and families of children with this rare condition direct management effectively.

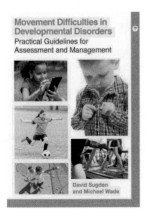

Movement Difficulties in Developmental Disorders
David Sugden and Michael Wade (Authors)

A Practical Guide from Mac Keith Press
2019 ▪ 240pp ▪ softback ▪ 978-1-909962-95-8

This book presents the latest evidence-based approaches to assessing and managing movement disorders in children. Uniquely, children with developmental coordination disorder (DCD) and children with movement difficulties as a co-occurring secondary characteristic of another development disorder, including ADHD, ASD, and Dyslexia, are discussed. It will prove a valuable guide for anybody working with children with movement difficulties, including clinicians, teachers and parents.